How To Conceive Healthy Babies – The Natural Way

Second Edition

Belinda ('Nim') Barnes

First published in 2009, Foresight as *Beautiful Babies, Fabulous Families Wonderful World*

All paper used in the printing of this book has been made from wood grown in managed, sustainable forests.

ISBN13: 978-1-78003-698-4

Printed and published in the UK
Author Essentials Ltd
4 The Courtyard
South Street
Falmer
BN1 9PQ

A catalogue record of this book is available from the British Library

Cover design by Jacqueline Abromeit

CONTENTS

Introduction	by Prof John Dickerson, PhD, Hon DSc., R.Nutr, Emeritus Professor of Human Nutrition	1
Foreword	by Dr Patrick Kingsley, MB, BS, MRCS, LRCP, FAAEM, DA, D.Obst. RCOG	3
A Personal Message	from Nim	7
Chapter 1	How it all began... and where we have got to!	11
Chapter 2	Nutrition	21
Chapter 3	Hair Mineral Analysis	71
Chapter 4	Voluntary Social Poisons	126
Chapter 5	Contraception, including the Pill	162
Chapter 6	Genito Urinary and other Infections	183
Chapter 7	Allergies and Intestinal Parasites	199
Chapter 8	Electromagnetic Pollution – or 'electrosmog' to you and me	221
Chapter 9	Chemical Hazards	242
Chapter 10	Talking to the 'powers-that-be' on what could be done to help	265
Chapter 11	Onwards!	277
Appendix 1	Useful addresses	293
Appendix 2	Recommended reading	300
Appendix 3	Specific Anomalies and relevant Research	358
Appendix 4	Article by Jean Philips from Powerwatch.org.uk	375
Appendix 5	A Survey of Foresight Results 1997–1999	385
Appendix 6	Foresight Research 2010	388
Appendix 7	Extract of University of Surrey Research Paper 1993 by Dr Neil Ward	392

INTRODUCTION

by Professor John Dickerson

One of my main scientific interests, throughout my academic career, has been in the effects of nutrition on growth and development. Studies in experimental animals, as well as observations and studies in children, have clearly shown that deficiencies or excesses of energy, protein and a variety of minerals and vitamins can have important effects on these processes. Human beings are very special 'animals', and a successful marriage can depend to a large extent on the partners being able to produce normal, healthy children. The 'National Health Service' cannot provide the support and detailed investigations of both partners which may be necessary to identify and deal with nutritional and other problems which may be the cause of family disappointments and distress.

I count it a great privilege to have known Belinda Barnes, and in a very small way to have been associated with the growth of 'Foresight', which came into being in 1978, to help childless couples. It was designed to help such couples to identify the causes of their problems and to provide the necessary advice and help to deal with them.

This book, written by Belinda Barnes, radiates the knowledge and enthusiasm for her subject which she has accumulated over the years. Her writing style is inimitable and an expression of her own commitment and personality. The book is illustrated throughout with real 'case histories'. It is more than an account or 'biography' of Foresight, and can be warmly recommended as a textbook for all those interested or concerned with helping hitherto disappointed couples to realise their ambitions, or longings, to have a family.

Professor John WT Dickerson Ph.D., Hon. D.Sc., R.Nutr.
Emeritus Professor of Human Nutrition
University of Surrey
Guildford, Surrey

FOREWORD

by Dr Patrick Kingsley, MB, BS, MRCS, LRCP, FAAEM, DA, D.Obst. RCOG

My father was in General Practice for about four decades in the middle of last century, and I remember discussing with him the subject of miscarriages at a time when I was studying for an Obstetrics and Gynaecology post-graduate examination. He had practised in a small town where the GP knew everything about his patients. He was so respected by everyone that he was often consulted about non-medical things such as whether to buy a house or not or whether such and such a job was right for a person. The church was packed to the rafters when we finally said goodbye to him.

He told me that a miscarriage was a rare event in his early practice years, but that it was becoming more common as he was getting closer to retirement. He had always found it hard to console a couple that had suffered a miscarriage, and he had found it so much harder when a woman had her second. He was always aware that the husband often suffered as much as his wife, something that is not always appreciated nowadays.

Not so long ago I heard that a woman is not referred for specialist investigation until she has had her third miscarriage. Just how desperate she would be by then is hard to imagine. The only way I was able to help at the time was to say that perhaps the physical body of the child was not ready for this world but its spirit was, and that it would find its way into the world in due course. Such a thought often helped a bit at a time of great mourning, but I would also say that perhaps her body was not quite in the perfect condition to receive the baby. After all, the onset of a period has been described as the 'weeping of the disappointed womb'. How much more might that be so with a miscarriage?

If miscarriages are becoming more frequent as the facts would suggest they are, and a full term pregnancy must surely be

3

considered to be the normal outcome expected of a pregnancy, what on earth is going on? Why is it happening, for there must be a reason? It would seem that many other medical conditions are becoming more common at the same time. I remember reading an article that was reprinted from a medical journal of sometime around 1900. It described a famous Consultant Physician with a group of medical students and young doctors round the bed of a patient in a hospital ward. The Consultant told them to study the case carefully because it was very rare and such a case was not likely to be seen again. He declared the patient had had a heart attack!

When I was a medical student I knew I had to learn anatomy and physiology but found it a bit boring. My student colleagues and I desperately wanted to be in the hospital wards dealing with sick people – patients. We were sure that was where our talents lay. When we did reach that stage, we were shown how to make a diagnosis and apply the correct treatment, usually a surgical operation or a prescription drug. Basically we were shown how to 'correct' the abnormality. What was rarely ever discussed was why the problem had developed. Nor were we shown how to try to return the abnormality back to the normal. That just wasn't anywhere in our teaching.

Most of my medical practice has been investigating the 'why', by taking a detailed history and asking questions not normally asked, certainly not in the five or seven minutes a GP may be allocated with each patient. Yes, it took a long time, but then it was worth it and my patients certainly appreciated my approach. So many of them kept saying that they wanted to know why their condition had developed and were not interested in merely taking a drug to suppress the symptoms, with all the risks of adverse effects that so many drugs have. I found it unnecessary to prescribe drugs although I was aware they were sometimes of value.

This approach of mine was why Nim Barnes asked me to become her first Medical Adviser all those years ago. I had always wanted to specialise in Obstetrics and Gynaecology, and to be involved in guiding prospective parents to achieve a successful pregnancy and a healthy beautiful child was a real honour. I felt that when I delivered a baby I was helping the fruits of other people's labours!

Nim Barnes' Foresight has undoubtedly helped very many parents. I don't think it is ethical to do double-blind studies on such an issue, but you can compare Foresight's results with the rest of the country, in which case they stand out as highly successful, especially when you consider that couples that try a Foresight programme have nearly always already had a sad outcome, so to begin with they are 'worse' than an average group with which a comparison is being made.

The Foresight programme looks at the whole body and tries to identify any problems the mother and the father may have, looking at their life styles in particular. When you read through this wonderful book you will see the approach Nim has worked on. Over the years she has identified what has prevented some women from getting pregnant in the first place or from holding on to their pregnancy or from producing a full-term healthy infant. We should all apply that approach in our daily lives to be more healthy.

Nature endowed all animals and man with the ability to reproduce their species. When habitats are destroyed by man's activities, species die out because their environment is no longer conducive to their survival. Television programmes remind us of this all the time. Why should man be any different?

Unfortunately people still go to their doctor and say, 'Doctor! I have a problem. Will you fix it for me please!' Anyone who follows the Foresight programme will have to take charge of their life, will have to think what they are doing, think what they are putting into their mouths and consider what they may be doing wrong. By writing this wonderful book, Nim has started this whole process by pointing out what someone can do. All her experience is here for everyone to read. It is a treasure trove of information. It is what I have practised for over thirty years. I know it works because my patients tell me it does.

A Personal Message from Nim

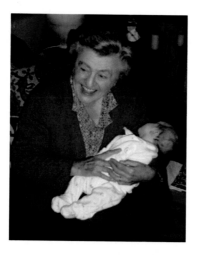

So you want to have a baby? You feel you have secretly loved and waited for your baby all your life and you can't wait to see him or her. Yet... your baby doesn't seem to be coming along? Well, hopefully we can help. We usually can. Foresight has helped hundreds of families for over 30 years.

I adore babies. This is why I founded Foresight in the first place. It was not originally to help with infertility; it was to try and ensure that **all** babies were born healthy and normal, able to realise their full potential, physically and mentally, and therefore able to have a wonderful, happy and productive life. However, along the way, we discovered that our programme also solved infertility in about 89% of cases.

In the course of this book, we will devote a chapter to each aspect of the environment that can be problematic, **why** it could be damaging, **why** it reduces fertility, and above all, **what to do about it.** I will introduce work by co-authors who are more authoritative in their writing than I am – I thank them, and everyone who helped me on the Foresight journey, for their generosity and help. I will also tell you my own take on everything – the point of view of the ordinary woman and mother.

All of the pieces of the health jigsaw that we have found important are in here including references to all the science that lies behind the Foresight programme. Not all the aspects apply to everybody as you are all individuals – you are all as different as your faces! This is what makes helping you all such a complex business – but so interesting. That is what makes having babies so fascinating too – they all arrive so different to each other!

I would read through the whole book and take from it what particularly applies to you. If you still need help, you can ring Foresight up and discuss with them exactly what your individual problems are and then they will help you find a solution!

We need to take stock. It would be magical to arrive at the dawn of an era where common sense breaks through and where people take control of their lives back into their own hands and realise they don't have to be ill, tired, dependent, nervous or 'below par' in any way.

Women need to find quiet times to be themselves again, and to tap into the Soul of Womanhood and into the love of your mother, grandmothers, and all the women who helped to create you down the centuries. They will be supporting you and spurring you on as you make the effort needed to turn things around. Mothers have always been the ones to carry evolution forward. They kept themselves well and fertile – or you would not be here!

Fertility is natural. Being healthy and happy is natural. Every little female mouse in the cornfield, every singing bird in the trees, every bison grazing on the prairie, every lioness striding the savannah, even the father penquin shuffling around on the ice, keeping the egg warm against all the odds, they all know how you feel. They feel with you. Tap into this enormous planetary emotion and let them all carry you forward. You are not alone. The world turns on the strength of this special love and universal effort

This knowledge will give you the patience and the strength to succeed. From the Big Bang until now, this is what has carried the world forward. Some of the book (my bits) are written from the soul and some of it (the science bits) are written with the help of more erudite beings. Go with the bits of the jigsaw which best suit

8

your style – but don't discard the rest of it. If you put all the bits in place, you have your Plan for your future family.

I feel the human race needs to get back to how we were meant to be. Let's get together, get well-fed, get rid of all the 'drugs, bugs, plugs and fugs', as I term all our bugbears, and make a start on it! If you are impatient to find out about a healthy diet go straight to the Chapter on Nutrition but read the rest later.

I wish you health and happiness – and of course healthy babies. Onwards!

With love to you all

Nim

CHAPTER 1

How it all began... and where we have got to!

Before my marriage, I had been a nursery nurse in a day nursery for some years, so babies were already a large part of my life. I became determined to spend the rest of my life finding out what parents needed to know to prevent disaster from afflicting their beloved babies and I wanted to give them this information in time. For this reason I founded Foresight. The journey has been a mental and logistical marathon, but here we are!

To give a little of the background, back in the late 1960s, when my youngest started school, I had some time and space to start on my mission which became a series of significant milestones. In 1973 I read an article by Roger McDougall, the playwright, in the Friday *Telegraph Magazine* in which he related how he had overcome his multiple sclerosis (MS) by going on a gluten-free, milk-free diet and taking supplements. My eldest son was a coeliac, but in those days the gluten-free diet was very little heard of, almost nothing was available ready-made, and the taking of supplements was regarded as strictly for 'cranks'.

Nevertheless, this sounded too significant to be ignored and I felt I could help. At the time, we were living next door to a Cheshire Home where there were 11 people suffering from MS. I knew the cook there quite well as I used to go round with superfluous vegetables from our garden (being an enthusiastic albeit disorganised gardener). I showed John, the cook, the Telegraph cutting and being a diabetic, the fact that modifying a diet could help an illness was not a mystery to him. 'I can help with gluten-free recipes – I am used to it.' I said. He replied, 'We could really help them, I would love to do that.'

We went to see the Warden. My first rude awakening to the frequently encountered opposition to health improvement was in his immediate reaction: 'It is all very fine, but what will happen to my wheelchair allowances if they can all get out and walk about?'

We assured him that, when inspectors were scented, they could all jump back into their wheelchairs!

For a while we were allowed to help them and all, bar one patient, made huge improvements. Three, who had homes to go to, went home. Then the policy was reversed (by the powers that were) as 'it was not scientifically proven', and patients relapsed.

Meanwhile, my friend Gilly Gibbons and I made copies of four pages of diet information and recipes and sent them round to all the other Cheshire Homes. One, to our knowledge, took it up and had great success. Eventually, the local neurologist took up the idea, as did several private physicians, and I believe now the regime is used with quite a lot of MS patients.

However, it took years of delay for 'research' to emerge – sadly too late for many. All this made us realise the tragedies that stemmed from the huge, financially involved and hierarchical nature of the health care machine. It was a structure not well suited to the sensitive, individual and immediate needs of people with health problems. It was inhibited by possessiveness and power structures, statutes and pecking orders which often produce total intellectual paralysis. This was over 40 years ago – slowly, things have advanced.

I am telling you all of this so you may better understand the complications of founding an organisation for achieving perfect health in preparation for a perfect pregnancy! Nowadays, a perfect pregnancy is almost always possible. There are wonderful people all over the country who have become involved in many different aspects of natural health care. This has brought forth colleges of nutrition, osteopathy, homeopathy, reflexology, acupuncture, naturopathy etc. From these, every year, there emerges a whole new army of people, mostly women, very well informed on all aspects of natural health enhancement. However, your babies still rely on **your** individual effort, willingness and free thinking.

Being lucky enough to have moved close to the sister and the wife of Professor Humphrey Osmond was my second milestone. Humphrey, at that time, was pioneering nutritional approaches to mental illness. Initially he worked in Canada with Dr Abe Hoffer and later in Alabama. At that time, he was **mainly** giving vitamins B6, B3 and C. His sister, Dorothy, who was one of my greatest friends, told me about this. She felt it would help my hyperactive, dyslexic, coeliac son and she was right. The difference it made to him was life-changing for the whole family. It opened all our eyes to the interdependence of nutrients and brain function.

I then met the irreplaceable Father Dunstan of Barrow Hills in Witley, a Roman Catholic priest who was trying to help priests suffering from alcoholism. A great character, highly intelligent, compassionate and with a great sense of humour, he was anxious to try anything new that would help. I was able to introduce him to Humphrey Osmond and Abe Hoffer, and to their work with nutritional support for mental illness and addictions. Dunstan started giving vitamins and minerals as well as emotional support to the priests and found it made the world of difference. Later, he went on to establish WACA, the Westminster Advisory Centre on Alcoholism, which flourishes today, although sadly Father Dunstan has passed on.

Jane, Humphrey's wife, and I went up to Surrey University to talk to Professor Parkes about Humphrey's work. In the course of the meeting he said to us, 'Never underestimate your own power. Never give up. If you write one letter a day for a year, if one person in 100 is interested, by the end of the year you will have three or even four people on your side. Take it from there.' He also introduced us to John Dickerson, Professor of Human Nutrition, who was a wonderful support and ally. He became our first advisor and encourager when the Foresight organisation was formed and, although now retired, is still a source of knowledge and encouragement. At this time he gave me access to the wonderful library of Surrey University. I remember the light pouring in down the stairs when I first walked up them, praying so hard I would find what I needed to help the babies. Down the years, what I read there has been endlessly useful.

The next significant development took place when Humphrey Osmond suggested I look at the Journal of Orthomolecular Psychiatry. From its pages I found another great friend and guiding light – Dr Elizabeth Lodge-Rees of California. She had

13

written an article on allergy, coeliac condition and hyperactivity which rang so many bells with me, I asked her over to stay with us for a holiday in England. To my joy, she said, 'Yes! Never been to England. Sounds like fun!' A few weeks later I was picking her up at Heathrow! She was pioneering nutrition and allergy work with hyperactive children and her luggage was heavy with books which provided further valuable contacts and information for my journey.

Some years prior to this in the UK, Vicky Colquhoun and Sally Bunday had formed the Hyperactive Children's Support Group. Gwyneth Hemmings had formed the Schizophrenia Association of Great Britain, and Marjorie Hall had founded the help group Sanity. Dr Jean Munro, later a household name for her work with allergic illness, was part of this scene, and all were pressing ahead with finding out more about the harmful effects of food additives, lead, chemical pollutants and allergenic foods on brain function. That most manifestations of mental aberration are biochemical in origin is now generally accepted in the 2010s, but this was rejected by the establishment in those days. It was a long search to find doctors who were interested. If these findings had been examined and accepted at that time by the establishment, millions of families could have been happier and years of acute personal suffering by the children and parents could have been avoided.

Those who were lucky enough to come across a doctor who understood nutrition and allergy pulled through.

I belonged to all these organisations and we had superb help from a small cohort of doctors who were pioneering the work and were sympathetic to our aims, and generous with their time and knowledge. We are forever in their debt. At the outset, as well as Dr Jean Munro, we knew particularly well Dr Patrick Kingsley, Dr Damien Downing, Dr Pam Tatham, Dr Stephen Davies, Dr Lambert Mount, Dr David Owen, and Dr Mark Payne. There was also the superb Latto family – four enormously enlightened doctors who were part of the core who created the resurgence of Sir Robert McCarrison's work in the 'McCarrison Society'.

Sir Robert was an army doctor in India at the beginning of the last century. He noticed how in certain areas of India there were diseases peculiar to that area. In other areas there were different diseases or much less disease. He was intelligent enough to link the bodily breakdowns to that which was lacking in the diets eaten in the different locations. This led him to study, with the analytical methods available to him at that time, what vitamins and minerals were present in which foods, and exactly what they did for the people who ate them. His book *Studies in Deficiency Disease* is a mine of glorious information (and often comes up for sale on eBay!). Alternatively, you can read much of his work on the society's website, www.mccarrisonsociety.org.uk. It is as relevant today as it was then and is well worth reading.

The first significant episode, in order to help repay Surrey University for their kindness to us, I volunteered to collect a huge parcel of placentas from St George's, Tooting, and bring them down to the university for study. Suffice to say that by the time I arrived at the university forecourt, the parcel had fallen apart (it was a hot day)! Don't even think about It... 'Security' found me freaking out in reception. Dr Neil Ward arrived to my rescue with a small army of quite saintly young students who produced gratitude, commiseration, disinfectant, soapy water and determined elbow grease in equal amounts, and in due course my car was driveable again. This resulted in a long and cheerful association with Surrey University which gave us the excellent study reproduced at the back of the book. And as you will see for yourselves, this research makes it quite clear how relevant mineral metabolism is to fertility, reproductive health and indeed health generally.

Key areas of concern:

Whilst every couple is different, you got this book because you care about conceiving a healthy baby. We all need to pioneer our own way through to fertility and the birth of healthy babies, by achieving the nutritional and mineral status within our own body that will build a healthy foetus. We need to give the sperm and the ova the nutrients they need, eliminate a load of unnecessary and potentially damaging toxins, get rid of any bugs, suss out any allergies or parasites that may be impairing either parent's absorption, and eliminate any electromagnetic pollution. (This pollution can impair fertility and also can cause malformations, leukaemia and other cancers. It has been implicated in chromosomal disorders like Down's Syndrome.) We also need to go over the home for any toxic chemicals and eliminate them.

Michelle's Story:

After suffering three miscarriages, Michelle read an article in the national press about the work of Foresight. However, it wasn't until she became pregnant again, which sadly ended in a stillbirth, that she decided she had to do something that would ensure the best for her own health as well as that of any future baby.

Michelle contacted Foresight and so began the Foresight Preconception Programme. Although there was no heavy metal toxicity reflected in her hair mineral analysis, both her calcium and magnesium levels showed up as being very low, but not as low as her selenium and zinc levels. Three lots of hair mineral analysis later, the levels of these minerals had improved enough for a pregnancy to occur.

This time the pregnancy held, and an 8 lb 1 oz baby boy was safely delivered after spontaneous labour. 'He is feeding well and is a really happy, smiley and very contented baby, and so strong!' says Mum.

'The changes to my diet were not difficult – the most difficult thing was to remember to take all the supplements,' said Michelle. 'I think that people should follow the Foresight programme to ensure optimum health for both the parents and ultimately their child. For me it was not a sacrifice to give up certain things from my diet and to take all those pills but an honour, so that I could give the best start in life to my baby.'

So what do we do to get it right?

- You need to be eating well. Good food that suits you. Good food that will nourish your baby. No harmful additives. No pesticides – so everything organic. No genetically modified food. No excess sugar. Clean water.

16

- You need to have a hair analysis, and supplements and cleansing programme, to ensure you have plenty of all the essential trace minerals the baby needs to make himself, and as little as possible of the toxic metals that could harm him.
- You need *not* to be taking in a lot of 'voluntary social poisons' that clobber you and will seriously harm the baby, like tobacco, alcohol, street drugs, caffeine, or over-the-counter medical drugs.
- You need to avoid use of the contraceptive pill and/or the copper coil. If they have been used in the past, you need to specifically address the deficiencies that this will have created. Whatever you do, learn natural family planning. That way, *you* are in control in the future, and your fertility and health are left intact. See www.fertilityet.org.uk
- You need to be free from bugs, such as genitourinary infections, candida and parasites.
- You need to recognise and eliminate any allergens.
- You need to be free from electromagnetic pollution from underground rivers, cracks in the substrata or from the many man-made sources (such as mobile phones etc.).
- You need to recognise the plethora of toxic substances in cosmetics and everyday household goods, and learn how to avoid them.

On many occasions we find the Foresight programme will sort out polycystic ovaries. They are often due to low zinc, B6 and essential oils. Low sperm counts may be due to nutritional factors, but also to genitourinary infections (GUI), allergies, electromagnetism (especially from mobile phones) etc.

Sometimes blocked fallopian tubes respond to the programme; i.e. you cure the GUI, look for cow's milk allergy (and eliminate the use of milk and milk products), plus get some reflexology or acupuncture. This will help to activate the tubes and clear the mucus.

Homeopathy will often manage to combat hidden infections. If the health problems in the parent generation are coped with, any health problems in future babies are pre-empted or at least minimised.

Julie's Story:

They had it planned nicely. Four years after the wedding they had a lovely daughter. It was straightforward with 'no problems'. Two years later, after conceiving again, Julie felt so sick, so nauseous and so very ill, she miscarried at 11 weeks due to 'blighted ovum'. Devastated, she took a long time to get over the miscarriage, both mentally and physically.

A year passed and Julie felt ready to try again. Once again, debilitating tiredness and that terrible nausea. An eight-week scan at the Early Pregnancy Unit showed that there was something very wrong. A week later everything was removed from the womb, and tests and treatments were performed until her hormone levels returned to normal.

Julie's mum got in touch with Foresight after seeing an advert, and shortly after this, the information pack arrived with 'loads of literature'. From then on, both Julie and her husband focused on health and diet, and had regular reflexology. They had their hair analysed, and both took all their supplements.

Once she was signed off from the Charing Cross Hospital in April, Julie conceived at the first attempt! Although there was some nausea and sickness, it was nothing like that which she endured prior to her miscarriages. The six-week scan showed a healthy heartbeat. 'We were so elated. Really elated seeing that little heartbeat!' In the fullness of time, a 9 lb 9 oz baby boy was safely delivered to overjoyed parents.

'He is totally different from my daughter; he is so calm, so much more content. Now we have one of each. I keep pinching myself, it's so wonderful, he's such a joy!'

The 2007 ONS (Office of National Statistics) discloses figures of 45,000 premature babies, 4,500 left with a lifelong disability -this is not a situation that should be allowed to continue. The ONS states that one baby in 84 is born malformed, but this is accompanied by a helpful letter pointing out that the Government has ordered a change in the categories, and doctors are told NOT to report a whole long list of sadnesses such as 'spina bifida occulta' and so on. The true figure for anomalies of any kind is nearer to one in 17. Where no action is taken preconceptually, approximately one family in nine is likely to have a little person starting life with a problem they will have to overcome. Mostly, they do so magnificently, but how much happier it would be if these agonies could be avoided in the first place.

With the full Foresight 'works', pregnancies can take place more naturally. Babies need *not* be so frequently miscarried (our statistic was 3.5% at our last count-up, as against 17%-19% nationally), nor born prematurely, brain-damaged, or with allergies or other ongoing problems.

The last 50 years has seen a regression in human intellectual ability, as well as in health. Dr Bernard Rimland, whose position was to test the intake to the American Army for their intelligence, found the average IQ dropped one point every year... Over 30 years this gets worrying. Quite simply, this has been because, if the unborn baby's body is badly affected by deficiencies, toxins, exogenous hormones, bugs and radiation, this will also affect his or her brain cells. At a national level, a general intellectual deterioration could lead to the inability of mankind to progress.

Children's bodies are often badly affected by crucial deficiencies which lead to allergic reactions. These cause them ongoing miseries such as asthma, eczema, epilepsy, irritable bowel syndrome and migraine. Later in life this general level of poor health can lead to more obesity, diabetes, heart disease, cancer, auto-immune diseases such as poor thyroid function, arthritis, MS and ME etc.

Children's brains are affected similarly by the same toxins and deficiencies (also by vaccinations). This can lead to hyperactivity, dyslexia, ADHD, Asperger's and autism. Later in life this can also lead to severe forms of mental illness and criminal behaviour.

My prayer is that if preconceptual care becomes the norm, reproductive tragedy, child ill-health and indeed ill-health generally can become largely a thing of the past. Let us all take this forward together.

Onwards !

Lisa's Story:

It only took three months for them to decide they wanted to start a family so when Lisa miscarried early on in the pregnancy they were devastated. Changes in lifestyle were made and they tried again six months later. Nothing. One year later, a laparoscopy revealed that Lisa had a blocked fallopian tube but she was assured that this was not a problem, so they carried on trying for a baby, unsuccessfully, for another year.

Thumbing through a magazine, Lisa read that nutrition can play a big part in fertility. She found a nutritional therapist who just happened to be a Foresight practitioner. Lisa also took reflexology sessions before trying to conceive and throughout the pregnancy.

Both partners went onto the Foresight programme. What little alcohol they drank was stopped, they ate organic foods, used a water filter and took all their supplements. It took a year to get his very high lead and copper levels down and Lisa's age was against her. As soon as their levels were optimised, it was decided that it was now or never, and 'bingo' – Lisa became pregnant at their first attempt.

Their Foresight baby daughter was born after a lengthy labour weighing 6lb 3oz. Six months later they decided that their daughter needed a sibling. They went straight back onto the Foresight programme in preparation for conception. Four months later, Lisa was ready once again and conceived straight away. Foresight baby daughter no.2, weighing 7lb 3oz, was safely delivered after a short labour.

'I had very healthy pregnancies. The girls are very bright, so aware of their surroundings and so astute! Having been told that there was "no reason" for infertility, we felt left in the dark and really crest-fallen. Foresight was fantastic in being proactive. They were a real boost, and we felt that we were once again doing something. Thumbs up to Foresight and we recommend Foresight to everybody. It's a fantastic thing to do; any child deserves such a good start.'

CHAPTER 2
Nutrition

What you need to eat – Why you need to eat it – What to avoid – How to avoid it – to achieve a healthy pregnancy

'If all prospective human mothers could be fed as expertly as prospective animal mothers in the laboratory, most sterility, spontaneous abortions, stillbirths, and premature births would disappear; the birth of deformed and mentally retarded babies would be largely a thing of the past.'

So said Roger Williams in the 1970s, pondering the very question I had posed to John Dickerson at about the same time: "why did we not take as much trouble with our human prospective mothers as we did with laboratory rats?" I remember shrieking with joy when I saw that paragraph in Roger Williams's book (he was professor of human nutrition at Texas University at the time.) My two favourite books of his are *Nutrition Against Disease* and *The Wonderful World Within You*. A pithy and witty writer, his books are still available on Amazon and are really rewarding reading – not just for achieving a healthier family, but also to achieve a healthier old age!

Good nutrition is the foundation of the Foresight approach to preconception care. It is vital for health, development and successful reproduction at all stages of life – from cells in the embryo to old age. It can help to clear the body of poisons, such as lead. It can help to protect against infection by building a healthy immune system. It is important for mental well-being.

Nutritional Research

It is not always easy to do nutritional research for ethical and scientific reasons. Animal studies can provide valuable data to help understand the human situation, but it is not always possible to extrapolate the findings to humans. However, it has been found that in all types of animal life, from insect to mammal, a diet which supports normal adult life is not necessarily sufficient to support reproduction. There is no evidence that human beings are different i.e. to be a mum, you need a bit more of everything as you are making another person as well as keeping yourself going. Examples of the truth of this philosophy are apparent in the work of three pioneers in nutrition.

Three pioneers in nutrition

Some of the most remarkable research into the effects of nutrition on health was done in the 1930s by Drs Weston Price, Francis Pottenger and Sir Robert McCarrison (see the bibliography – all their books are available on Amazon). Although they worked independently, their main conclusions were the same – good health depends on good nutrition. Their research findings have never been disproved, though they were for a long time ignored by the medical profession, the food industry, dieticians and governments. For many years, those who accepted them were labelled 'cranks'. Only for the last few decades or so has poor nutrition been recognised as a factor in ill health. The National Advisory Committee on Nutrition Education (NACNE), the British Medical Association (BMA) and the Health Education Council all issued reports in the 1980s and 1990s which advocated some changes in the national diet, though each fell well short of the recommendations of our three pioneers. However, thank God Jamie Oliver and some other TV chefs are waking the country up a little bit.

- **Dr Weston A Price** was an American dentist who was distressed by his profession's inability to find the *cause* of dental caries and periodontal disease. He discovered that people who did not live in industrialised parts of the world had good teeth, so he took time off from his practice and travelled for ten years collecting evidence from all the races of the world. His subsequent book covered many aspects of nutrition, including the vitamin and mineral content of food, soil fertility, nutrition and pregnancy, vegetarianism, the effects of processing food, and the inadequate foods which produced severe degeneration. His book is not just about nutrition – it is a history of various tribes, an anthropological study, a book on agriculture, covering work that has never been written about since. Not for nothing is he known as 'the Darwin of Nutrition'.

His findings are all the more significant considering they apply regardless of the native diet he was studying. No matter who the people were, he found that as soon as they started to eat white flour and white sugar and other processed products such as tinned foodstuffs, they began to suffer ill health and there were increasing dental and skeletal changes and other problems, including mental problems, in the children. The actual contents of the original diets varied considerably, from the fish and seal eaten by the Eskimos to the oatmeal porridge, oatcakes and seafood of the Gaelics, to the rye and milk products diet of the Loetschental Swiss. However, whatever the constituents of the original diet, when a modern diet was adopted the number of health and fertility problems increased dramatically. Why? Because our refined, packaged, processed 'dead' food does not have the vitamins, minerals and therefore enzymes that we need to 'run a body'. He wrote a wonderful book covering all of this in the 1940s – *Nutrition and Physical Degeneration.*

- **Dr Francis Pottenger** was an American physician whose work with cats confirmed Price's findings. He observed that cats fed on scraps of raw meat were healthier than those fed on cooked meat. This led him to some remarkable research over ten years, spanning many cat generations and involving hundreds of cats. Basically, he compared the effects of feeding one group on cooked meats, pasteurised milk and cod liver oil, and another group on raw meat, raw milk and cod liver oil. The latter group were healthier, had good skeletal structure, and produced healthy offspring. The former group had a high level of sickness, including allergies, birth defects and poor skeletal structure such as misshapen skull, narrow palate and jaw. They also exhibited serious behavioural problems, such as poor mothering and feeding. With each succeeding generation these problems increased. Even when placed on a raw meat diet, it took four generations of breeding before the inherited damage triggered by the cooked meat and pasteurised milk was corrected (so we had better buck up!)

23

Following these discoveries Pottenger turned to the study of human nutrition. He was particularly concerned with the effects of chemical fertilisers and processed foods, including cooked foods. He knew from his earlier work that a healthy soil was important and that this was dependent on good manure. The growth of weeds in the runs of the cats fed on raw meat, after the cats had vacated them, was luxuriant whilst little growth was seen in the runs of those fed on cooked meats. Clearly, the quality of excrement, reflecting that of the diet, was an important factor. Pottenger became renowned for his work with patients, advocating the benefits of raw food in the diet.

- **Sir Robert McCarrison** was a British doctor who served in the Indian Army, during which time he conducted many experiments in nutrition, showing how human health is dependent on the wholeness of food. Having noticed that most Sikhs, Pathans and Humzas were healthy and well-developed, while the Bengalis and Indians in the south were disease-ridden and underdeveloped, he investigated the possible reasons, using colonies of rats. Feeding them the equivalent diet of the various Indian groups, he found that each rat colony replicated the health status of the group whose diet it had been fed. He kept meticulous notes on diets, weights, health and condition at death. Those who were given a diet which deviated from the principle of eating healthy food grown on healthy soil, in as near its natural state as possible, suffered ill health. These were the rats that had numerous diseases, reproductive failures and behavioural problems, in one instance resorting to cannibalism. He concluded:

'I know of nothing so potent in maintaining good health in laboratory animals as perfectly constituted food; I know of nothing so potent in producing ill-health as improperly constituted food. This, too, is the experience of stockbreeders. Is man an exception to the rule so universally applicable to the higher animals?'

Thus we have three men whose research findings all concluded that the quality of food was vitally important in good health, and for whom quality meant wholeness. If the food was treated in such a way that it lost something, by refining, tinning or heating, health would be affected. They also understood the importance of a healthy soil in providing good food.

It is interesting to digress here for a moment, and ponder on the findings, until so recently studiously ignored by most of the establishment, that the quality of the food had a bearing on the quality of the **behaviour.**

The quality of the food eaten by many people in the western world has altered enormously over the last 40 to 50 years. More food is tinned, bottled, packeted, precooked and frozen than ever before. Much has travelled thousands of miles from where it was produced. On the way over, it will have lost valuable vitamins and enzymes. It will, in fact, be dead (which is why many people dislike vegetables as when stale they taste so bitter!). Fruit will be picked unripe, so it will travel better, but as a result it will taste sour, so children may refuse to eat it.

Let's just go back to the observation of Robert McCarrison,that rats who lacked essential nutrients resorted to violence and even cannibalism. This is not normal 'rat culture', however, no doubt there is a deep physical/mental/emotional instinct where the basic and primitive part of the brain says, 'We do not have enough food – fight for yourself – get out there and grab.' As our vitamin and mineral status is reduced, do we see more of this 'me first, out of my way' mentality emerging? Is there more 'elbowing in' and more 'passing by on the other side' than there used to be? I think so. We are hearing all the time about mayhem in some of the schools, gun battles and knife attacks in the streets with people in some areas afraid to leave their homes at night.

Where food does not provide well for basic mental and physical energy, do we crave alcohol, coffee, cigarettes, Mars bars, which give a brief boost of energy, followed by a precipitous fall as we run out of endorphins. Feelings of exhaustion lead to irritability, inefficiency, paranoia, or gross acts of cruelty. Relationships fail, jobs are lost and things take a turn for the worse. This will then be described as 'depression'. If this leads, via the GP, to Seroxat,

Prozac and the like, we are on the rocky road to mental illness and even, possibly, suicide.

However, how to prevent all of this was all there and demonstrated for our benefit in the rat world nearly 100 years ago. So let's take it all on board, once and for all, and create a well-nourished, strong and sane new generation without any of these problems. **It is all up to us!**

The concept of biochemical individuality

Dr Roger Williams, the American biochemist referred to at the start of this chapter, was also an important name in the history of nutrition. In his research he found that we are all biochemically different. This means that everyone has needs for levels of nutrients that are individual to them alone, especially in respect of vitamins and minerals and amino acids. It is an important principle often overlooked in medical studies and dietary advice. Research has shown, for example, that some individuals may need many times the Recommended Daily Allowance (RDA) of a vitamin or mineral if they are to remain healthy. Also, importantly, in certain conditions, such as pregnancy, requirements will alter.

The importance of food before pregnancy

It is essential to eat properly during pregnancy, but it is better to start, if possible, before conception. Good nutrition in the man helps to ensure healthy sperm and optimum sexual activity. Poor nutritional status in the woman can cause ovulation failure and other problems with fertility, as birth-rate studies during famines have shown. The woman will need to have her body packed with all the nutrients the embryo will require to develop into a healthy foetus. Ideally she should be neither very overweight, nor underweight, since both can have adverse effects on pregnancy outcome (NB: however, as some of us are greyhounds and some of us are St Bernards, we should not be too harassed about our weight by officious officialdom!)

The importance of food during pregnancy

The work of our three pioneers has shown how important the right food is in pregnancy. Subsequent studies have confirmed this. Women on good diets have better pregnancy outcomes than those on poor diets.

A success story:

We got married in 2001, and by early 2002 we started trying for a baby. Conception was swift but so was miscarriage. After the second miscarriage, my sister mentioned Foresight which we dismissed as nonsense.

After yet another miscarriage, we felt that there was a problem and perhaps IVF would diminish the chances of another lost pregnancy. Sadly, after both IVF and ICSI, I miscarried yet again. It was at this point that we were reminded of Foresight. However, undeterred, we attended a meeting at a fertility clinic to seek further advice and we were told that we would 'not have children naturally' and that we should consider other options like egg donation, adoption etc. We asked about Foresight. The advisor told us that it was a mad idea, but if we wanted to waste £300 on overpriced minerals then we could do!

We left the clinic with our world having fallen apart. Next day I called Foresight and spoke to both Nim and Tanya in floods of tears, but after two hours felt hope yet again.

That evening we sent off our hair samples and embarked with gusto and a 100% on the Foresight programme. We had a geo survey, turned organic, grew our own vegetables and really took it to the extreme.

The Foresight hair analysis results were shocking, showing very low levels of zinc, which Nim explained was probably the main problem. We set about correcting these. We also sought fertility advice from a fertility consultant.

Within a very short time I found that I was pregnant again. I wasn't excited; I just didn't believe anything could come of it. Throughout the pregnancy I was as sick as anything and loved every minute of it! It was an anxious time and I didn't truly believe I was having a baby until our son was delivered by caesarean section...

It only took 48 hours for me to start panicking that our son would be an only child! Just six weeks later I conceived again but sadly miscarried. Was it because I hadn't followed up with the Foresight programme and had let myself go so much? Calling Nim once again, I was put back on the Foresight programme with even more tablets than before, and a short time later became pregnant once again and in due course our daughter was safely delivered.

We know what we did worked. We feel better for the lifestyle changes that we made thanks to Foresight and we still follow a healthy organic diet – I have just extended our veggie patch!

- **Lawrence Study**

  174 women who had previously given birth to an infant with spina bifida were recruited and were followed up through their subsequent 186 pregnancies. They were divided up into those on a 'Good Diet', those on a 'Fair Diet' and those on a 'Poor Diet'. Outcomes were as follows:

	Good Diet (no. 53)	Fair Diet (no. 88)	Poor Diet (no. 45)
Miscarriages	0 (0%)	3 (3.5%)	15 (33%)
Spina Bifida (terminated)	0 (0%)	0 (0%)	8 (18%)
TOTAL:	0 (0%)	3 (3.5%)	23 (51%)

  Of those on a 'Good' or 'Fair' diet, only 3 babies were miscarried out of 141 – making 1 pregnancy in 47. This compares well with the UK average of 1 in 17 or 19. Of those on the 'Poor' diet, 23 out of 45, or just over half the babies, were lost. This work should be more widely known than it is. The message is that this tragic deformity is entirely preventable. Why is that which is basically good and important news so often buried or ignored?

- **Canadian Study**

   This is the birth record of a poor mother in Montreal. The birth outcomes were recorded before and after a nutritional programme provided by the Alice Higgins Foundation. This consisted of dietary advice, and the provision of a pint of milk, an egg and an orange per day.

   Before: Of the first eight children she gave birth to, before dietary advice and food allowances were given, six were below 2,500 gms, none were above 2,750 gms, two were below 1,750 gms and one of these died. All eight were neurologically damaged and the seven survivors had to be institutionalised.

   After: after the Alice Higgins programme, however, the next three births were much happier. The weights ranged between 3,500 gms and 3,750 gms, and all three children were mentally sound.

   The supplement programme cost $125 per child. Up to the 1980s, the institutionalising of the seven handicapped children had cost the State $300,000 – and counting.

The above is an extreme case, but it is not atypical of what is going on worldwide. So many children are being born subtly or overtly handicapped and the family grief is total, and the taxpayer's impoverishment is spread over lifetimes. This is likely to escalate unless we make a concerted effort to take things in hand.

Weight gain in pregnancy:

In this situation, small is NOT beautiful! Research has shown that the old idea that a woman should not put on much weight was wrong. In a London study, mothers in Hampstead who had higher calorie intakes than mothers in Hackney had babies who were in some cases 2 lb heavier. Dr Ebrahim, Institute of Child Health, London, found that mothers who gained more than 30 lb had the best birth outcomes. Other research which has given food supplements to women has found that those who took them had bigger babies.

Janet's story:

Janet married at 23 and didn't give the possibility of not being able to conceive a second thought. So when she and her husband decided to start trying for a family, and it didn't happen, she was devastated. She began to panic.

Two years later they began all the usual investigations which reveal 'unexplained infertility'. A 'satisfactory sperm count' did nothing to start bells ringing. The couple decided to go down the IVF route in 1997, but the first IVF failed due to hyper-stimulation and Janet was admitted as an emergency to hospital. She decided to never go down that route again.

They then decided to adopt, and adopted a little boy at six months old. Whilst going through the process, Janet fell pregnant but suffered a miscarriage at 12 weeks. A second conception took place 18 months later which was tragically terminated as the scan showed the baby had died.

A few months later Janet read about Foresight, and although her husband was concerned that Janet had been through so much already, they decided to do the Foresight programme. Although both were eating a very similar diet, their individual nutritional status was radically different. Foresight advised them to use natural family planning until both their mineral levels were improved. They both followed the programme meticulously and Janet soon found that she had conceived.

A beautiful baby girl, weighing 8 lb 6 oz, was born after ten years of trying for a family. Two years later, Foresight Baby no. 2 arrived; she weighed 8 lb 4 oz and was doing really well.

'I felt that I had Foresight on my side, so a big thank-you to you all for everything over the last few years.' Janet, Newcastle.

Women who are underweight at conception, and who gain less than 11 kg, or 24 lb, during pregnancy, often have babies who are small-for-date or growth-retarded. (NB: If you have been anorexic, when you come to Foresight, tell them this. They need to know to be able to give maximum help.)

Clearly, if you eat a great deal more, without exercising more, you will put on weight. But it is important to eat the right foods. Besides taking in extra calories for growth and energy, you need extra vitamins, minerals, essential fatty acids, and amino acids. Moreover, if you eat the right foods, you will have less of a problem in losing the weight after birth, while breastfeeding, without a special slimming programme. It is therefore a good idea to eat the most nutritious food you can.

A Healthy Diet

There are many misconceptions about a healthy diet, which have arisen mainly because we have strayed from the teachings of our three pioneers. In reviewing the importance of nutrition pre-conception, Foresight originally drew from their work and that of Roger Williams, Carl Pfeiffer, Adelle Davis, Isobel Jennings, Eric Underwood, Lucille Hurley, Donald Caldwell and Donald Oberleas.

It is really quite simple to eat properly, as any wholefood cookery book shows (we recommend *The Foresight Wholefood Cookbook*, which gives good basic guidance on diet and an excellent selection of recipes, and is obtainable from Foresight). A good diet comprises carbohydrates, fats, proteins and clean water. Within these groups are found the various vitamins and minerals that are essential for well-being.

Carbohydrates:

Carbohydrates should be unrefined, 'with nothing added and nothing taken away' – i.e. brown! They include starches, sugars and fibres. They provide energy, B-complex vitamins and many of the essential minerals. Contrary to popular belief, they are not fattening if they are eaten in the form of complex carbohydrates. This is good news, as they are also cheap!

However there is a horrible substance called phytate, which lurks in raw grains and, unless dealt with in a pre-emptive way, can prevent the uptake of the zinc, calcium etc. by the gut. The way to deal with phytate is firstly by soaking muesli overnight in the fridge. Just put your portion into a bowl and add as much water as it can soak up by the morning. This has the added advantage that it is a bit quicker to eat in the morning – not quite such a laborious

31

chew! Secondly, when flour is used to make bread, phytate will respond to 'proving' with the yeast. This is probably why bread has been traditionally made with yeast for hundreds of years – or maybe it was just a happy accident! Either way, if you make your own bread, make it with yeast rather than sourdough, as yeast is more effective against phytate.

Good sources: Complex carbohydrates, including whole grains (wholemeal flour, millet, wholemeal bread, oatmeal, buckwheat, brown rice, maize meal), fresh vegetables and fresh fruit.

Poor sources: Simple carbohydrates, including sugars, white flour, white bread, white pasta, sweets. These are all poor in fibre, vitamins and minerals.

Proteins:

Proteins are sometimes called 'building blocks', as they are used to build or repair enzymes, muscles, organs, tissues and hair. Proteins are made of amino acids which are broken down in the body to form other amino acids. We are only just beginning to realise the potential of amino acids in health. Two amino acids, spermidine and spermine, play a major role in the synthesis of semen. Their levels have been found to be low in men who have low sperm counts. Fortunately, with the right foods and supplements, it is usually possible to raise the levels and help improve sperm count quite quickly (many other factors are also involved in the production of healthy sperm which will be discussed in following chapters).

Amino acids are especially important in digestion as they form the enzymes necessary for the digestive processes. Thus if they are in short supply, digestion may be affected and this may result in malabsorption, causing shortages of other nutrients in the body. Such shortages can interfere with various processes including fertility and pregnancy. Animal products and fish contain all the amino acids. However, to get the full range from vegetable sources you need to combine nuts with pulses, or nuts with seeds, or pulses with seeds. Combining is an excellent way to improve the quality of protein eaten.

32

Good sources: Fresh meat, poultry, offal, fish, shellfish, milk, eggs, cheese, nuts, pulses and seeds (including whole grains).

Poor sources: Bought pies, TV meals, sausages and hamburgers, salamis, pâtés and other processed meats. Twice-cooked meat, as this is not fresh.

Fats:

Fats provide energy and build the cell walls. Although animal fats are sometimes linked with illnesses such as arteriosclerosis, heart disease and some cancers, we need both animal and vegetable fats as part of a healthy diet. Eaten in the correct proportion and as part of a wholefood diet, there is no need to eliminate animal fats, such as butter, unless there is a specific reason, e.g. cow's milk allergy. Polyunsaturated fats occur in vegetables, nuts, unheated vegetable oils and fish oils, all of which should be included in the diet (see essential fatty acids, below). Olive oil is best for heating. You do not, therefore, generally need to eat margarines high in polyunsaturates and often highly processed! (For those who do need alternatives to butter and cream, *The Foresight Wholefood Cookbook* is a useful resource).

Water:

Water if it is clean, contains useful trace elements. Sadly, much of our water is less than ideal, sometimes containing high levels of nitrates, nitrites, chemicals, copper, lead, aluminium, pesticides, fluoride and other toxins.

When we have done hair analysis, we usually have some clues about what your tap water contains. Over-high copper, usually with some lead, is the most common bugbear. High copper and lead, found together, can almost always be traced back to a corroding pipe. We can also see high levels of aluminium in some cases, which can be aluminium flocculants used to clear peaty particles from the water, although in other cases it may be from a deodorant.

It is now possible to obtain ABS plastic pipes, said to be safe for potable water. It is possible to get fibreglass and stainless steel tanks. Hopefully things are advancing. A lot more attention needs to be paid to the plumbing. The relevance of water quality to people's health appears to be much underestimated. There are many types of water filter now available – see the web.

Vitamins

We make no apology for what may seem to some readers a disproportionate coverage of vitamins.

As long ago as 1916, a doctor wrote in the *Lancet*, '*Whatever the nature and whatever the mode of action of these puzzling substances, it is beyond question that their absence from the food does profoundly affect not only the physical health, but the mental health also.*' How much attention has been paid, in nearly 100 years of escalating levels of illness and insanity, and of declining fertility, to this profoundly important finding?

In experiments with various species, if a specific vitamin or mineral was totally omitted from the diet during the first three months of pregnancy it was found that a particular defect appeared in most of the litters, regardless of the species. Deficiencies can also affect fertility.

I believe Nature is a lot brighter than we are. If a woman's body is not replete in the nutrients the future foetus is going to need, the ovaries say, 'No, not this month' and just switch off. The sperm beds evidently do likewise. Thirty years of Foresight work has shown us that, more often than not, they will 'switch on' again when nutrients are introduced. It is humbling to realise that something as small as a sperm can be a whole lot brighter than we are and know when the going is too tough, and be able to save us from the tragic outcome of a damaged or non-viable baby.

There is abundant evidence on the value of vitamin and mineral supplements before and during pregnancy and during lactation. The stores of trace elements built up by the foetus have a strong influence on the infant's copper, iron and zinc status. However, the liver does not accumulate manganese so the infant may be at risk of deficiency. The nutritional requirements of the newborn are strongly influenced by the foetal stores. Any level of deficiency can be serious for the infant, since the brain continues to grow and develop very rapidly for at least two years after birth. Under-nourishment, especially under four years of age, alters the brain development and activity and, if prolonged, can cause irreversible damage. Many research papers in the literature demonstrate the above. So voluminous is the research done on this that we can only concentrate below on a small proportion.

So many of you ask me every day on the telephone: 'What do they all **do**?' 'Are they really necessary?' 'Do they really make a difference to fertility?' and so on. So, I am printing for you here everything in the way of research that Gail Bradley and I put together, which answers all the questions. Happy reading!

Foresight recommends that all prospective parents and lactating mothers have a hair analysis and supplement with the Foresight vitamins and minerals, which have been specially formulated by the Foresight medical advisers and are made by G & G to provide a balance of essential nutrients. The only 'packers' used are organic vegetable powders. With the 'key' ingredient, e.g. zinc, we always provide the 'companion nutrients' that are used in its metabolism, e.g. manganese, B6, folate and vitamin A. In this way the absorption/utilisation of the key ingredient is enhanced, and it does not deplete the body of other nutrients as it is utilised. Foresight does not recommend exceeding the doses suggested, or taking any mega-doses, especially of individual substances, unless advised to do so by a person who is experienced in nutritional medicine, after appropriate tests. All the ingredients in the Foresight capsules are given on the label.

Fat-soluble vitamins:

These include vitamins A, D, E, K and the essential fatty acids, sometimes called vitamin F. Because they are fat-soluble, the body can accumulate stores of them against shortages. However, in pregnancy especially, these stores may need supplementing.

- **Vitamin A:** can be obtained directly from animal products in the form of retinol, or from vegetables in the form of carotene. Carotene is then changed in the body, with the help of zinc, to proplasma vitamin A, the form the body can use when it is needed. If sufficient zinc to complete this step is not available, it is possible to become vitamin A deficient.

Vitamin A is essential for healthy eyes, hair, skin, teeth, the mucous membranes, such as the lining of the mouth, and good bone structure. It plays a part in good appetite, normal digestion and the making of red and white blood cells, and helps to make the male hormones concerned with reproduction.

Deficiency problems in animals include increased susceptibility to infections, kidney stones and reproductive system problems in both males and females. In humans, the eyes and also the hearing are most affected, though there are numerous reports of other conditions being helped by vitamin A supplementation, e.g. mental illness, skin problems and sexual problems. In the animal foetus, **too little** vitamin A can result in eye defects, hydrocephalus, diaphragmatic hernia, cleft palate and cleft lip, undescended testicles, and heart defects. It is associated with neural tube defects and stillbirths.

Women with diabetes mellitus tend to have more malformed babies. Problems include microcephaly, hydrocephalus, cardiac defects, and cleft palate. Vitamin A deficiency may be involved. Vitamin A deficiency has been associated with nutritional anaemia. One study reported that 'Improvement in Vitamin A status may contribute to the control of anaemia in pregnant women.' Another study has advocated supplementing staple foods with vitamin A.

The measurement of vitamin A has been changed from the old 'iu' (international units) to the new 'European Correctness' of 'mcg' or micrograms, sometimes written as μg.

These two measurements do not reflect exactly the same thing. The international units were used to give the potency of the source (which can vary with the oil-soluble vitamins). The mcg only gives the weight. However, the powers-that-be have ruled that to convert iu of vitamin A to mcg, we divide by 3.33, and so, for all practical purposes, this will now have to serve us. To avoid confusion we will give both measurements, as you may find either in papers, or on tubs of supplements.

For pregnancy, Foresight advises 2,500–5,000 iu (833–1,501 mcg).

36

Vitamin A excess can be dangerous in pregnancy, but so can **vitamin A deficiency**. The dangers of vitamin A deficiency have been too little understood or published over the last few decades.

Scientific advice on what constitutes excess vitamin A in pregnancy is very variable. The Denner Report quoted 10,000 iu (3,003 mcg). Professor Merlyn Werbach of the University of California (arguably the world authority on foetal nutrition) says 40,000 iu (12,012 mcg). An Australian source gives 25,000 iu (7,507 mcg).

Foresight programmes are always very conservative, as the obvious approach is to give enough to avoid any danger of deficiency, while giving very little more than this, to be sure of staying within the safe limit.

Even our most generous programmes give less than half the most conservative upper limit, which was the Denner Report's 10,000 iu (3,003 mcg). France and Canada give 5,000 iu (1,501 mcg) as supplementation to all pregnant women.

It is interesting to note in this context that during the war (when, despite rationing, the diet of most people was more nutritious than that of today), the Government decreed all pregnant women should have 'a teaspoonful of cod liver oil' daily. It is hard to assess the amount of vitamin A, as a lot would have depended on the size of the teaspoon, but it is likely to have been in the region of 5,000 iu (1,501 mcg).

At the present time, in the USA, pregnant women are given 5,000 iu (1,501 mcg) vitamin A daily.

In some areas of Australia, they are given 10,000 iu (3,003 mcg). UNESCO campaigns for funding to give vitamin A to pregnant mothers in the Third World to stop babies from being born blind.

Both vitamin A excess and deficiency can cause deformities in experimental animals.

Both have been recorded by Dr Isobel Jennings, MRCVS of Cambridge, and by Dr Weston Price of California.

Isobel Jennings, Cambridge – Fetal animal studies by a veterinary pathologist.

Vitamin A – Excess and Deficiency

Excess	Deficiency
Cranial anomalies	No eyes
Cleft palate	Micropthalmias
Hare lip	Blindness
Eye defects	Hydrocephalus
Hydrocephalus	Cardiovascular anomalies
Spina bifida	Urogenital anomalies
Exencephaly	Diaphragmatic hernia
	Hydrospadias
	Cryptorchidism

Dr Weston Price, of California, lists vitamin A deficiency as causing problems with the development of the eyes, ranging from impaired sight, to blindness, to being born with no eyes (anophthalmia). Dr Price also reported damage to the nerves leading to the ears, and therefore impaired hearing, ranging to total deafness. Prolongation of the gestation period and long and difficult labour were reported in rats. Calves were reported as being born small and less likely to survive. Farm animals generally were reported to have had less successful reproduction and lactation, and less resistance to infection, where vitamin A levels were less than optimum.

Lack of vitamin A in the diet of pigs resulted in 'extreme incoordination and spasms', and a tendency to abortion and farrowing dead piglets. Another researcher quoted by Price showed that lack of vitamin A produced disturbances in 'oestrus and ovulation', leading to sterility.

Professor Hale of the Texas Agricultural Experimental Station found that as well as piglets being born blind, 'depriving pigs of Vitamin A for a sufficient period produced severe nerve involvements, including paralysis and spasms so the animals could not rise to their feet.' (Would this be relevant to cerebral palsy in the human infant?)

Professor Hale also found that if the sire of any species were deprived of vitamin A, he would become sterile.

Disturbances of the development of the upper and lower jaw and tooth decay were also reported in humans whose diets lacked vitamin A.

In 30 years of running Foresight we have not seen any of the deformities listed above in 'our' babies. I would not therefore be tempted to supplement above 5,000 iu (1,501 mcg), although you could probably take up to 10,000 iu (3,003 mcg) without harm. However, I think there could be a case made for a little more with the multiple births, especially triplets.

I would also not be confused or bullied into taking less than 2,500 iu (750 mcg), as this could lead to the risk of serious malformations. 22,000 babies (1 baby in 32) are now born in Britain with malformations annually. The largest groups include those with the malformations found in Isobel Jennings' research, which are proven by scientific research to be due to vitamin A deficiency. This is a tragedy probably greater than the thalidomide debacle, and it should be more easily preventable, as all the research is out there, and has been for many years.

At the present time, the Department of Health (DoH) say they *have no position on Vitamin A in pregnancy'*. They passed me on to the Food Standards Agency, who passed me back to the DoH. In the Summer of 2008 the FSA were advising not more than 2,100 iu daily, but in this they are at odds with every other country in Europe, the USA, Canada and Australia. Our level of premature birth and disability is also higher than that of these other countries.

We continue to advise you to take between 2,500 iu (750 mcg) and 5,000 iu (1,501 mcg) daily, before and throughout pregnancy.

You are welcome to take this information to your GP, midwife or health visitor if this would be helpful. If they have any scientific papers that contradict what I am saying, or support it, I would be particularly grateful to be sent a copy, as I would be very interested to study them.

Do note that both Australia and the USA advocate 8,000 iu (2,402 mcg) per day for pregnant women. Most European countries advocate at least 5,000 iu (1,501 mcg) per day. This safeguards the sight and hearing, prevents undescended testicles and other anomalies of the genitalia in little boys and makes other problems, as listed previously, less likely.

We do not want any Foresight baby ever to be less than perfect! We suggest sticking with supplementation between 2,500 iu and 5,000 iu. This way, you are safe from both deficiency and overdose.

Good sources: Vitamin A – fish oils, especially cod liver, fatty fish, egg yolk, organ meat, whole milk, butter, cream, cheese, yoghurt. Carotene – spinach, carrots, red pepper, broccoli, kale, chard, tomato, apricot, marrow, butter, cream.

It is best taken with full B-complex, vitamins C, D, E, essential fatty acids, calcium, magnesium, selenium and zinc.

Liquid paraffin prevents the absorption of vitamin A, **so should never be used**. Long, slow cooking of vegetables can destroy carotene.

- **Vitamin D:** is necessary for the growth and maintenance of bones and teeth. It also aids calcium and phosphorus absorption.

Lack of vitamin D in adults may lead to hot flushes, high sweats, leg cramps, irritability, nervousness and depression. Other signs include osteoporosis, osteomalacia, pains in the hips and joints, and dental caries. In children, rickets and tooth decay may be present. There may be other signs of bone deformities. Poor skull development can lead to impairment of brain development. (See Dr June Sharpe's study of high raised palates on page 42.) Poor jaw development may give buck or snaggle teeth. It may also inhibit the function of the Eustachian tubes, leading to constant middle ear infection. There may be receding chins or foreheads, or large bossing foreheads with deep-set eyes. The middle face may be cramped or narrowed, pushing the palate upwards and/or forwards. Price found that most retarded children and those with learning difficulties had high raised palates. Asymmetrical development of the skull may distort the membrane carrying the blood supply to the brain cells, and inlets for the blood supply may be occluded by deformed platelets. This can affect the supply of nutrients, oxygen and glucose to the brain.

Girls with insufficient vitamin D during childhood may have narrow pelvic development which may later in life make childbirth difficult.

Good sources: Vitamin D can be obtained in the food or through the action of the sun on oils in the skin. This latter method is important, since food sources tend to be poor. Hence, it is wise to build up stores during the summer months, by allowing the action of the sun on the skin. However, since the destruction of the ozone layer, we have to be more careful, but perhaps work is now underway to help to reduce this hazard.

Food sources include fish oil and fatty fish. There are small quantities in whole milk, free-range eggs and butter.

It is best taken with vitamins A and C, choline, essential fatty acids, calcium and phosphorus.

Liquid paraffin can prevent its absorption so should not be used.

Excess vitamin D can lead to a range of unpleasant symptoms.

- **Vitamin E:** prevents the oxidation (destruction by oxygen) of vitamin A and is needed for the utilisation of essential fatty acids and selenium. It can protect from scarring after burns, surgery and injury and is important in wound healing, such as the healing of abrasions after birth. Davies claims that some congenital heart defects will disappear if it is given from early babyhood. It has also been suggested that it has a protective effect against some haemorrhage in premature babies. Researchers at the University of Edinburgh have suggested it may be another factor that can be useful in the treatment of infertility in the male, since it is necessary for flexibility in the cell walls of the sperm; abnormal sperm are less flexible.

Without vitamin E, people can develop anaemia, and enlarged prostate glands. Premature aging can take place with liver and kidney damage, varicose veins and heart attacks. Phlebitis, strokes, protruding eyes, muscle degeneration and muscular dystrophy can occur.

Deficiencies in animals have caused muscular dystrophy, central nervous system disorders such as encephalopathy, vascular system defects, and foetal resorption. In rats, deficiencies lead to abnormalities including exencephaly, hydrocephalus, joined fingers and toes and oedema. In human babies, they lead to anaemia, jaundice, weak muscles, retarded heart development and squint.

A Small Study of Palate Height:
conducted for Foresight by Dr June Sharpe of Godalming, Surrey, UK, in the 1970s.

Palate Height – Normal Primary School – 95 Children Seen

Palate Height	Percentage
Normal	73%
Marginal	9%
High	18%

Palate Height – School for Children with Learning Difficulties- 95 Children Seen

Palate Height	Percentage
Normal	31%
Marginal	5%
High	64%

Palate Height- Home for Mentally Subnormal Children – 13 Children Seen

Palate Height	Percentage
Normal	15%
Marginal	15%
High	70%

NB: I think this breaks down to only two mentally subnormal children seen having a normally developed palate.

Vitamin E may prevent miscarriage and help to ease labour by strengthening the abdominal muscles. Labour prolonged because of weak muscles can lead to problems for the baby as it becomes starved of oxygen during the birth process.

Good sources: Unrefined (cold pressed) oils, whole grains, wheat germ, nuts, whole milk, egg yolk, green leafy vegetables, avocado. It is best taken with vitamins A, full B-complex, C, essential fatty acids, manganese, selenium.

- **Essential fatty acids (vitamin F):** cannot be made by, or in, the body and include, among others, linoleic, linolenic and arachidonic. They are important because they form a large part of the membranes of all cells, and they give rise to substances called prostaglandins. These are used to make sex and adrenal hormones and affect all systems in the body. They help in the absorption of nutrients and activate many enzymes.

Because of the wide role of these substances in the cells, deficiencies can give rise to a large number of disorders, including allergies, gallstones, diarrhoea, varicose veins, skin problems, and heart and circulatory conditions.

In reproduction, EFA deficiency may be a factor in pre-eclampsia. There may be infertility, especially in the male. In rats with deficiency, the pups were of lower birth weight than was expected.

Deficiencies have also been reported in hyperactive children, alcoholics and drug addicts.

Recently (in the 2000s), work on the omega-3 fatty acid has been centred on behaviour and intelligence in schoolchildren, and in juvenile delinquents. After supplementation huge improvements have been seen in youngsters who previously were failing in learning situations and behaving badly. If only they could all be given everything they need from the moment that the sperm and the ova start to form – could we perhaps have a problem-free world?

Good sources: Nuts, unrefined oils, nut butters, cold pressed oils, green leafy vegetables, seeds and fatty fish. They are best taken with vitamins A, C, D, E and phosphorus.

- **Vitamin K**: is generally made in the healthy intestine. It is essential for blood clotting, which explains why it has sometimes been given to mothers in injection form at the time of birth. It was felt that if the baby was short of this vitamin at birth, there could be a risk of bleeding. Later it was given to the newly born baby, since even small haemorrhages of the brain could be serious. More recently, however, there has been some controversy over this. Some studies have linked vitamin K injections to later development of leukaemia in the child (see recommended reading). Be sure to make your own decisions over this. If you have been short of vitamins A and E during the pregnancy (which could reduce the strength of the blood vessel walls) or have been taking aspirin or heparin (given to thin the blood and therefore to reduce the clotting) the risk of haemorrhage may be increased (be sure to read the Foresight leaflet on aspirin in pregnancy). If you have not been given aspirin the risk will be commensurately less. However, if a woman is healthy and eats plenty of green leafy vegetables, she should have a good store of the vitamin and will have a baby who has adequate stores. Also, vitamin K is included in the Foresight Vitamin Supplement.

Water-soluble Vitamins

Water-soluble vitamins include the B-complex and C. Since these are readily absorbed in water, they are easily lost to the body through urine (except B12). However, the body does have limited stores.

- **B-complex**: B vitamins should never be taken on their own, but always in conjunction with other B vitamins because they are linked in function. Dosing with one alone may lead to a greater need for usage of others, thereby creating a deficiency. In nature, no B vitamin is found on its own. However, it is possible for any person to have a greater than usual need of any one, since we are all biochemically different.

During stress, infection, pregnancy, lactation and childhood, there is an increased need. Lack of almost any B vitamin can lead to blood sugar problems causing reactive hypoglycaemia.

Some of the B vitamins can be made in a healthy intestine or liver, though it is not certain how much of that synthesised can be used in the body. This does not happen where the gut is not healthy. For example where there is undiagnosed coeliac condition, candidiasis or the use of alcohol or certain drugs (antibiotics and sulphonamides). These circumstances can exacerbate any shortfall in the diet.

B-complex is best taken with vitamins C, E, calcium and phosphorus.

- **Vitamin B1 (thiamine)**: is needed to break down carbohydrate into glucose. Deficiencies lead to mental symptoms such as depression, irritability, temper tantrums, failure to concentrate and poor memory. There may be fatigue, feeling listless, muscle weakness, aches and pains, anorexia, neuritis, digestive problems, heart problems and shortage of breath.

Deficiency in animals has been linked with sterility, relative infertility, low birth weight and stillbirth. In pregnancy, a shortage can lead indirectly to loss of appetite and vomiting in the mother, which may cause the baby to be born with a low birth weight.

Good sources: Wheat germ, rice polish, whole grains, brewer's yeast, nuts, dry beans, peas, lentils, seeds, rice, heart, kidneys.

It is best taken with full B-complex, vitamins C, E, manganese and sulphur.

- **Vitamin B2 (riboflavin)**: assists in the breakdown and utilisation of carbohydrates, fats and proteins. It is essential for healthy eyes, mouth, skin, nails and hair. It works with enzymes in cell respiration.

Signs of deficiency are sensitivity to light, sore and bloodshot eyes, broken capillaries in cheeks and nose, wrinkled or peeling lips and dry upper lips. There may be cracks at the corners of the mouth and dermatitis. Experimental animals have developed cataracts, possibly because without vitamin B2 they could not use their vitamin A. Since it works in conjunction with other nutrients and enzymes, deficiency symptoms may not disappear on straight supplementation. It should be given in conjunction with B-complex.

In animal reproduction, deficiency has been found to cause sterility, stillbirths, small misshapen foetuses, reduced oxygen consumption in the liver and reduced enzyme activity. Rats have been born with blood disorders, misshapen jaws, cleft palates, joined claws, oedema, anaemia and degeneration of the kidneys. In humans, vitamin B2 deficiency is considered to be one of the worst in pregnancy, with cleft palate and shortening of limbs as risks. These are both seen in smokers' children, especially the shortening of limbs. (NB: If you are a smoker's child like me, you can't purchase a garment without having to take up the sleeves. Maddening!)

Good sources: Brewer's yeast, kidney, tongue, leafy green vegetables, whole milk, fish, butter, egg yolks, nuts.

It is best taken with full B-complex and vitamin C.

Vitamin B2 is sensitive to light, so it is destroyed if exposed to light in glass bottles. This is no longer such a problem as most milk is now sold in containers.

- **Niacin or nicotinamide (sometimes known as B3):** – aids in the utilisation of energy. It is important for a healthy skin and digestive system, and the normal functioning of the gastrointestinal tract. It is also needed for proper nerve function, as a co-enzyme and for the synthesis of sex hormones.

Deficiencies have often been linked with the three 'D's – dermatitis, diarrhoea and dementia. There can also be a coated tongue, mouth ulcers, anorexia, dyspepsia or intermittent constipation. Mental symptoms include depression, confusion, hostility, suspicion and irrational fears. Sufferers become tense, nervous, miserable, subject to dizziness, insomnia, recurring headaches and impaired memory.

Nicotinamide deficiency in rats has been found to produce young with cleft palate and/or hare lip and hind limb defects.

I have always been puzzled by cleft palate being more commonly seen among agricultural workers' and market gardeners' children. Why should this be? Then I read a paper by MK Johnson, of the Medical Research Council (no less), which told us that nicotinamide was the only nutrient that would take the organophosphate pesticides out through the liver. Then I realised that people using organophosphate regularly would be using up their nicotinamide on liver function, and this could be starving the sperm of this essential nutrient.

How meticulous is Nature, that when a man produces 100 million sperm, each one will be perfect, if the environment is uncontaminated. Yet still how primitive are we that we splash pesticide and industrial chemicals around, we swallow drugs, additives, alcohol and inhale smoke, inhalants etc and we never even pause to wonder what it all does?

What a work of art a sperm must be and so full of spirit. It is awe-inspiring to realise that someone so tiny should be suffering a deficiency. We should be much more thoughtful on their behalf than we are.

Good sources: Brewer's yeast, lean meats (not pork), liver, poultry, fish, wheat germ, whole grains, nuts, especially peanuts, whole milk and whole milk products.

Nicotinamide is best taken with full B-complex and vitamin C.

- **Pantothenic acid or B5**: is needed for every cell in the body as, without it, sugar and fat cannot be changed into energy. It is important for a healthy digestive tract, and essential for the synthesis of cholesterol, steroids and fatty acids and the utilisation of choline and PABA. It can help the body to withstand stress.

Deficiency causes a wide variety of complaints. The adrenal glands do not function, leading to a paucity of adrenal hormones which regulate balances in the body. This may cause low blood sugar and low blood pressure. There will be a shortage of digestive enzymes, slow peristaltic action (movement along the digestive tract), indigestion and constipation following as a result. Too little pantothenic acid is also linked with food allergies.

As with all the B vitamins, the mental symptoms of deficiency are many, including depression and causing the sufferer to be upset, discontented and quarrelsome. There may be headaches and dizziness. These symptoms are common with low blood sugar.

In animals, deficiencies have given rise to a variety of foetal abnormalities, which mainly affect the nervous system. Also, cleft palate, heart defects, club foot, lack of myelination, and miscarriage have been noted. Sterility is also mentioned. Similar problems in humans are suspected.

Damage to the myelin sheath, which protects the nerves, is present in multiple sclerosis (MS). Maybe making sure people have enough B5 before birth and throughout their lives could give some protection against this terrible condition?

Good sources: Organ meats, brewer's yeast, egg yolks, legumes, whole grains, wheat germ, salmon, human milk, green vegetables.

It is best taken with full B-complex, vitamin C and sulphur.

- **Vitamin B6 (pyridoxine):** is needed to make use of the essential fatty acids and many of the amino acids. It is essential for growth and the synthesis of RNA and DNA. It helps maintain the balance of sodium and potassium in the body and is necessary for nerve and muscle function. It helps to prevent tooth decay, kidney stones, atherosclerosis and heart disease, if it is present in abundance.

Lack of B6 can mean less use is made of minerals such as zinc, magnesium and manganese (see below). There may be headaches, halitosis, lethargy, pain and cramps in the abdomen, rash around the genitals, anaemia, anorexia, nausea, vomiting, diarrhoea, haemorrhoids, dandruff, dermatitis of the head, eyebrows and behind the ears, sore lips/tongue, and a rash round the base of the nose. Hands can become cracked and sore. Night-time problems include insomnia, twitching, tremors, leg and foot cramps, nervous lethargy and inability to concentrate. Premenstrual tension syndrome (PMT) often responds to B6 supplementation, as do nausea, vomiting, oedema and the convulsions of eclampsia in pregnancy.

Foetal abnormalities, including cleft palate, have been linked to B6 deficiency. Babies born with B6 deficiency have low scores on general condition ratings. There may be seizures in the newborn.

Good sources: meats, whole grains, organ meats, brewer's yeast, blackstrap molasses, wheat germ, legumes, peanuts.

It is best taken with full B-complex, vitamin C, magnesium, potassium, linoleic acid and sodium.

Unfortunately, once again (as with vitamin A), inaccurate information has meant a panic in official circles about the safety of B6.

In huge doses, such as 250 mg, given over some weeks, too much B6 can induce 'neuresthesia' or lack of feeling in the fingers and toes. This problem disappears in a few days if the high doses are discontinued.

In any case, in practice, B6 is not used in this way. Women who suffer very bad PMT have sometimes taken doses of 250 mg or more for a couple of days before their period was due and for the first day of their period. I am not aware of this ever causing any side-effects, and the PMT relief was found helpful. Researchers then tried giving these very high doses, 250–500 mg, for weeks on end. This did prove problematic and based on the evidence of these studies, vitamin B6 preparations may be forbidden over 10 mg. This now appears to be the case.

Motivation for these types of studies has to be considered. Possibly removing this simple solution will increase the sales of HRT, which fell due to research revealing links with cancer, thrombosis, migraine and osteoporosis.

When faced with an unaccountable situation, the French used to say, 'cherchez la femme' – 'look for the woman involved'… Now people say, 'follow the money'. Yes, lots of scares regarding natural therapies and nutrients are much publicised because the natural therapies work and lots of little illnesses disappear. This is hugely frustrating for those who make vast fortunes out of selling medicaments for these lucrative little illnesses!

Good Sources: meats, wholegrains, organ meats, Brewer's yeast, blackstrap molasses, wheat germ, legumes, peanuts

It is best taken with full B complex, Vitamin C, magnesium, potassium, linoleic acid and sodium

- **Para-amino benzoic acid (PABA)**: is unique in being a 'vitamin within a vitamin', occurring in combination with folic acid. It stimulates the intestinal bacteria, so they make folic acid, which is then used in the production of pantothenic acid. It helps with protein breakdown and use, and the formation of red blood cells. It is important in skin and hair colouring. It can soothe burning, especially sunburn.

Lack of PABA can cause 'patchy'-looking skin, as it is needed for smooth skin pigmentation. As it is also needed for hair colouring, shall we see if it can help us to avoid grey hairs naturally? Because we're worth it!

Good sources: brewer's yeast, wheat germ, whole grains, liver and yoghurt, organ meats, green leafy vegetables.

It is best taken with full B-complex and vitamin C.

- **Biotin:** is necessary for the body's fatty acids and carbohydrates. It also helps in the utilisation of protein, folic acid, pantothenic acid and vitamin B12. It is useful in the treatment of candidiasis.

Deficiency is linked with depression, panic attacks, extreme fatigue, muscle pain, nausea, pain around the heart, dry peeling skin, hair loss, conjunctivitis, loss of appetite, pallor of skin and mucous membranes and lower haemoglobin. In children there may be stunted growth, and adults may become thin to the point of emaciation. In rats, biotin deficiency is linked with reabsorption of the foetus and death in the first few days after birth, due to damage to the liver, heart and blood vessels.

Some autopsies were done on very young American soldiers who were tragically victims of the war in Vietnam. Many were found to have degeneration of the heart and blood vessels typical of biotin deficiency. This research was available then. A daily B vitamin tablet is all that it would have taken to prevent so much tragedy. Why ignore all the superb research, done at great expense, coming out of universities all over the world? Why do governments pay for it to be done (with our money!) if they are not going to act upon the enormously useful results?

Good sources: Egg yolks, liver, unpolished rice, brewer's yeast, whole grains, sardines, legumes.

Raw egg white destroys biotin.

It is best taken with full B-complex, vitamin C and linoleic acid.

- **Inositol**: is needed by human liver cells and bone marrow cells. It is necessary for fat metabolism and transport, as well as healthy skin and hair. It combines with methionine and choline to make lecithin, a substance needed for the myelin sheath – the protective covering for the nerves. Lecithin also carries vitamins A, D, E and K around in the blood.

Lack of inositol may cause falling hair, eczema, abnormalities of the eyes, constipation, irregular heart action and a slowing down of the digestive system. Again, could we pre-empt ME and MS?

Good sources: Whole grains, citrus fruits, brewer's yeast, molasses, meat, milk, nuts, vegetables and eggs.

It is best taken with full B-complex and linoleic acid.

- **Choline**: is needed for the formation of DNA and RNA and for making nucleic acid in the centre of the cell. It is used in normal muscle contraction. It is used to make lecithin (see above) and is involved in nerve functioning.

Lack of choline can lead to headaches, dizziness, strokes, haemorrhage in the eye, noises in the ear, high blood pressure, awareness of heartbeat, oedema, insomnia, constipation and visual disturbances.

Because of its role in acetylcholine, a neurotransmitter, deficiency is linked with mental disorders. Animal experiments have shown a lack can cause fatty liver and haemorrhages in the heart muscle and adrenal gland. It is linked with the development of stomach ulcers, liver cancer and kidney damage in young animals.

Organophosphate (OP) insecticides, which are in common use, deactivate choline-containing enzymes, which are necessary for manganese absorption. This prevents the uptake of manganese by the plants. This can lead to manganese deficiency in the food and thus in the human who eats it! 'Rust' on lettuce stalks is a sign of a lack of manganese.

Eating organic food, and thus avoiding much contact with/consumption of OP pesticides, will make the absorption of inositol and choline easier. Lecithin granules available from health stores are a good way of boosting your intake, if you have been exposed to too much 'pesticide drift' from neighbouring fields or gardens. At the same time, I would use nicotinamide with magnesium to help cleanse the liver of organophosphates.

Although, I am told, the use of pesticides has fallen to about half what it was 20 years ago, the problems of drift remain with us. Hopefully, lots of us buying organic food and/or growing our own will contribute to a further decline in pesticide use. This will help everybody.

Good sources: Egg yolks, organ meats, brewer's yeast, wheat germ, soya beans, fish, legumes, green vegetables.

It is best taken with vitamins A, full B-complex and linoleic acid.

- **Vitamin B12 (cyanocobalamin)** is needed for the production and regeneration of red blood cells, and carbohydrate, protein and fat metabolism. It helps with iron function and is used with folic acid in the synthesis of choline. It is involved in the synthesis of RNA and DNA.

Although it is often said to occur almost exclusively in animal products, this is not true. It also occurs in well-water which has been exposed to the soil. Dr John Douglass reports that, *'People who consume peanuts and sunflower seeds have adequate levels of B12. This indicates that the B12 is synthesised in the gut when the diet includes these foods. Eating seeds and sprouted seeds apparently provides the necessary nutrients to promote B12 synthesis.'*

Unfortunately, however, there has been 'genetic modification' of peanuts, and for some people this appears to have made them into a very allergenic substance. Tales of anaphylactic shock, a potentially lethal allergic reaction involving the heart, have become all too common. There has been a huge decline in the population of little song-birds such as blue tits. Has putting out peanuts for them contributed to this, by making them ill or sterile? Sadly, I think it may have.

We gather it was proposed in 2008 that GM foods could come over from the States and be sold in this country **without being labelled** as such — eg soya, peanuts and maize. This was presumably planned because the UK public had **not** been buying the GM stuff – with very good reason!

More recently, we have been told that maize is being made into biofuel in the USA. So have there been some adverse reports on using it as a food? We are not going to be told, I guess. I would avoid peanuts, or try to track the origin. We may have to do the same with sweetcorn and soya. We have been told that adverse effects have been noted in experiments with animals so **we need to be very alert about all of this.**

 The Soil Association certified organic foods are NOT GM. Look for their little 'knickers in a twist' logo on produce. This may prove to be very important.

Deficiency of B12 causes pernicious anaemia, deterioration of nervous tissue, sore mouth and tongue, neuritis, strong body odour, back stiffness, pain, menstrual disturbances and a type of brain damage. A very severe deficiency leads to deterioration of the spinal cord, with paralysis finally appearing.

In pregnancy the foetus does not seem to be affected by variations in the mother's level. However, it has been noted that if *several generations* of rats are kept deficient, the death rate in young animals rises sharply and their weight at four weeks old is reduced. The young of deficient mothers are often hydrocephalic and have eye problems. NB: We do not know how many generations of our relatives have been deficient SO FAR! Let's stop the rot, before the situation gets worse!

Good sources: Organ meats, fish and pork, eggs, milk, cheese, yoghurt. For vegetarians, useful quantities can be found in soy sauce, tempeh, miso, dulse, kelp, spirulina, seeds, sprouted seeds. Some types of brewer's yeast also contain small amounts.

It is best taken with full B-complex, vitamin C, potassium and sodium.

- **Folic acid**: is needed for the formation of red blood cells in the bone marrow, the making of antibodies and the utilisation of sugars and amino acids. It is also important for the formation of nucleic acid, a substance essential for the growth and reproduction of all body cells, so it plays a crucial role in pregnancy. It helps the digestive process. It works with B12 in making haemoglobin in the blood. It is essential for zinc metabolism.

Deficiency in the adult can lead to pernicious and other types of anaemia, depression, dizziness, fatigue, pallor and susceptibility to infections. Anaemia in pregnancy can be a factor in smaller placentas, urinary tract infections and premature birth.

Folic acid deficiency is common, and pregnancy exacerbates it. Foetal abnormalities in the young of deficient animals include spina bifida, cleft palate and hare lip, deformed limbs, malformations of the heart, diaphragm, urogenital system, blood vessels and adrenals, malformations of the eye, skeletal deformities, underdevelopment of the lung and kidney, cataracts, brain deformities, oedema and anaemia. Foetal death and miscarriage or rebsorption may occur.

In litter animals, if folic acid is given at the time of rebsorption of some of the foetuses, others may survive to term but may have hydrocephalus.

If deficiency occurs during pregnancy, microcephaly can be seen in the newborn rats.

In humans, folic acid has been the subject of much attention in pregnancy, especially in relation to neural tube defects, such as spina bifida. A number of studies have been done which suggest that women who are given supplements of folic acid in the month before conception and for the first 8–10 weeks afterwards are less likely to have a malformed baby.

Many of the research methods of these older studies were criticised as not proving the value of folic acid supplements. However, research has led the Government to recommend folic acid supplements for pregnant women.

Taking all the research into account, there can be little doubt that folate deficiency in the mother, especially in the early stages of pregnancy, can be a major contributory factor in neural tube defects. But Foresight recommends that folic acid supplementation needs to be considered as part of a balanced supplementation programme. Eating wholefoods that contain a balance of vitamins is preferable with balanced supplementation as required. (See also manganese and zinc.) 400 mcg of folic acid daily has been part of the Foresight programme since 1979. However, it is always given in conjunction with other B-complex vitamins, as they all help each other.

Good sources: Green leafy vegetables, brewer's yeast, organ meats, whole grains, wheat germ, milk, salmon, root vegetables, nuts.

It is best taken with full B-complex and linoleic acid.

NB: I am sure we have all seen the appeals in the newspapers for the poor little scraps with their hare lips and (probably) cleft palates. We are told these can be reversed for £150. Maybe, but they could have been **prevented** with a good multivitamin for about £14. No anguish, no pain or shock. It's a no-brainer, really, isn't it?

Tracy's story:

'He is lovely!' says Tracy, referring to her three-month-old son. 'He was 8 lb 13 oz at birth, long and big and strong, and has been gaining weight steadily since birth. He is feeding well and I feel so blessed.'

Before coming to Foresight, Tracy became pregnant naturally. Unfortunately pressure from a fibroid caused her waters to break, which led to a termination at 23 weeks. During the next six years no further conception took place, so Tracy and her husband went to seek medical advice. The IUI specialist informed them that Tracy was fertile and that she was producing many eggs, but unfortunately the IUI failed.

A homeopath by profession, Tracy attended a Foresight Practitioners Training Day which she found very interesting. So much so that she decided that both she and her husband would go onto the Foresight programme themselves. The first hair mineral analysis results showed that her husband had high levels of lead and even higher levels of copper in his system, which could account for the specialist saying that her husband's sperm, although high in quantity, had very low motility.

Their supplement programme began just after Christmas and by the following April, Tracy knew she was pregnant!

'It's so simple when you compare it to IUI and IVF,' says Tracy, who is still on the programme. 'I am also healthier and have more energy, and I would recommend it to anybody; far better than bombarding the body with drugs and compromising the body systems. If more people knew about it, it would be fantastic. I am 40 years old, and if I decided to have another baby, I would certainly do the Foresight programme again.'

- **Vitamin C**: keeps the collagen (connective tissue) healthy and resistant to penetration by viruses, poisons, toxins such as lead, dangerous drugs, allergens, and/or foreign materials. It promotes healing after surgery, infection or injury, including broken bones. It keeps the capillary walls intact. It helps the absorption of iron, preventing anaemia. It is important for mental health.

Deficiency symptoms include scurvy, dandruff, haemorrhages on the thighs, buttocks and abdomen, swollen and bleeding gums, leading to infection, ulceration and loss of teeth. There may be spontaneous bleeding. Children who are short of vitamin C are prone to infections and have poor teeth and gums. Their bones break easily, they bruise easily and quickly tire and become irritable. It has been linked with miscarriage.

Good sources: Citrus fruit, rose hips, sprouted alfalfa seeds, tomatoes, green peppers, broccoli and other green vegetables, blackcurrants, strawberries and other soft fruits, bananas, apples, pears, carrot, cauliflower, new potatoes eaten with their skins and parsley.

Vitamin C is lost in storage. It is best taken with all vitamins and minerals, bioflavonoids, calcium and magnesium.

So what can we do? Luckily there is plenty we can do. (For information on MINERALS see Chapter 3)

Food and Beyond

Food purchase and preparation:

Knowing the contents of a healthy diet, you want to ensure that you do not spoil them with the wrong sort of preparation. Again a good wholefood cookery book will help, but here are some very basic guidelines:

1. Buy everything you can 'organic'. It has more nutrients in it, it is less toxic i.e. it has less chemicals such as pesticides in it and if it has the Soil Association logo it will not be GM contaminated. These are three major benefits.

2. Avoid packet, tinned, precooked and generally stale food.

3. Buy everything you can fresh, keeping 'sat on the shelf stuff' to a minimum. When you do have to buy manufactured stuff, use the Foresight booklet *FIND OUT* to check out the additives.

4. Buy carbohydrates whole where possible: whole-wheat flour bread, cakes and biscuits, brown rice etc. Sweeten with brown sugar, maple syrup, honey or molasses.

5. Eat as much food as you can in its raw state – most vegetables and fruit are delicious raw. If you cook it:

   - Steam rather than boil.
   - Stir fry rather than deep fry.
   - Grill, roast or stew rather than fry.
   - Prepare food as near to eating it as possible
   - *The Foresight Wholefood Cookbook* gives you lots of really good recipes.

Conclusion:

It is often said that 'We are what we eat', and, like most clichés, there is an element of truth in it. If we want to be healthy, we must eat healthy food. If we want to have healthy children, we must recognise that this means providing the best ingredients – that is, the best food. This means food which is grown on good soil, or reared in healthy conditions, and eaten as near its natural state as possible. Fortunately, there is a rapidly increasing awareness that organic produce is superior and it is becoming much more available. Enjoy it, knowing that this was the type of food our three pioneers found to promote well-being and productive success! But also recognise that with modern lifestyles, it is unlikely to give you all you need to prepare for pregnancy and lactation; you will need to supplement it.

THE FOUR GOLDEN RULES

1. **Eat Organic. Whenever you can.**   *Think Green!*
2. **No refined carbohydrates.**   *Think Brown!*
3. **No hazardous additives.**   *Think Colour-free!*
4. **Filter the water.**   **Think Transparent!**

Here are some interesting bits of relevant research:

Henry Schroeder, Battleborough, Vermont
Refined Flour Contains:
(as a percentage of amounts found in whole-wheat flour)

Thiamine	23%
Riboflavin	20%
Nicotinamide	19%
Pyridoxine	29%
Pantothenate	50%
Folic acid	33%
Vitamin E	14%
Magnesium	17%
Chromium	13%
Manganese	9%
Iron	19%
Cobalt	13%
Copper	10–30%
Zinc	17%
Molybdenum	50%

Avoid, as far as possible:

- **processed, tinned and packet foods**
- **microwaved foods**
- **excess tea and coffee**
- **ersatz drinks with sugar substitutes**
- **artificial colouring and flavourings**
- **confectionery and white flour products**

Basis of Balanced Diet (take into account individual allergies)

5 helpings per day of:

Fruits and vegetables – organic, raw, cooked, dried and juiced.
Seeds, nuts and nut butters. (Soil Association label)

2 helpings per day of:

Meat, poultry, fish, game, shellfish, molluscs.

4 helpings per day of:

Grains – whole or crushed, raw or cooked. Cereals, bread, flour products, Rice Dream, Provamel. (If allergic to gluten, avoid wheat, oats, barley and rye.)

3 helpings per day of:

Dairy products – cow, goat and sheep; milk, yoghurt, cheese, butter, crème fraiche, cream.

Eggs – hen, duck, goose and quail.

(If allergic to dairy, avoid as necessary. Substitute with 'Rice Dream with Calcium'. Some people who are allergic to cow's milk can manage goat's or sheep's milk and products.)

Avoid white flour and sugar

Avoid excess tea, coffee, chocolate

Avoid excess canned and packet foods

FILTER DRINKING WATER (to avoid lead, pesticides, nitrates, oestrogens and excess chlorine and copper)

If you are not allergic to gluten, there are wonderful brown breads, pitta breads and even whole-wheat organic pizzas! There is so much organic and wholegrain stuff out there!

With meat and poultry, remember to stick to organic. They have had a better life, and they will be much better for you too, not being laced with antibiotics, growth enhancers, extra hormones and so on, which can be a cause of feminisation of men, and infertility in women – quite apart from the cancer risk.

Get a few cookbooks, old and new. The Foresight one is good (I can say this as I did not write it myself!). It was written by Norman and Ruth Jervis who were, respectively, head chef and his wife, the latter being the daughter of the founder of Enton Hall, the first of the 'health hydros' – they had a lifetime of relevant experience!

**For more information and ideas,
see *The Foresight Wholefood Cookbook*.**

Daily menu suggestions – just some ideas from which to pick and choose:

BREAKFAST			
Whole carbohydrates Bread crisp-breads or cereals	fruit fruit juice yoghurts Bananas dates or prunes	Black molasses honey maple syrup	If allergic to milk, use milk alternatives: Oatly Rice Dream Provamel Almond milk Hazelnut milk.
Cooked (beneficial if lunch is not a major meal): fried whole-wheat bread or potatoes mushrooms tomatoes bacon, egg or fish – cooked as preferred.	**On bread or toast:** butter olive oil spread nut butters	low-sugar marmalade jams jelly honey	Fry in a small amount of oil or grill
LUNCH – Main meal			
Meat poultry fish offal shellfish etc.	Potatoes rice polenta pasta	Two vegetables. one bulb (leek or onion) one root (beetroot, parsnip, carrot, swede), one legume (runner or dwarf beans, peas, butter beans), one leaf or flower (cabbage, spinach, greens, kohlrabi, broccoli, cauliflower).	Green salad tomatoes peppers celery and apple sultanas other dried or fresh fruit.

Dessert			
Dairy and fruit: yoghurt custard junket milk jelly rice /semolina /sago/tapioca cornflour blancmange etc	Sponge, crumble or pastry puddings or pancakes can be made with whole-grain flours. Fruit raw, stewed, cooked or fruit fool	Cheese and fruit	Fruit raw, stewed, cooked or fruit fool

LUNCH – Secondary meal

Whole-wheat bread protein sandwich with salad :
    ham
    egg
    sardine
    salmon
    prawn
    pilchard mackerel
    trout
    nut butter
    cheese
    tongue
    corned beef, chicken etc
	raw fruit and yoghurt cheese & wholegrain biscuits simple fruit juice smoothie.	Keep in a fridge if taken to work.
		Meat can 'go off' if kept in a warm office.

TEA

Major meal			
hot soup cold meats fish or poultry and salad fish & chips grilled tomatoes baked beans Peas broccoli	wholegrain flour: cakes biscuits bread pancakes pastry puddings: sponge, crumble dairy pudding fruit nuts dried fruits whole-wheat biscuits & cheese.	Herb tea juice milk or milk substitute Marmite / Bovril or other beefy hot drink	Use Marmite and similar yeast spreads if yeast is not a problem.

Snack meal			
Whole-wheat: bread cakes scones biscuits.	dried or fresh fruits nuts salad dollop of Greek yoghurt in hot soup	Juice herb tea milk Rice Dream or as above soup yoghurt	Alternate butter with oil-based spreads. Use nut butters, cream cheese, goat's cheese, honey, sugar-free jams and jellies.
SUPPER			
Main meal See above			
Snack meal See abpve			

Ruth Jervis's Invaluable Practical Tips for the Kitchen

1. Eat food fresh. Avoid storing fruit and vegetables wherever possible. Where inevitable, store in a cool place.

2. Avoid preparing in advance.

3. Use mineral water for boiling and for soups or gravy.

4. Do not overcook. Heat destroys B-complex vitamins and vitamin C.

5. Do not cook at all if it can be eaten raw! (You can *graze* mustard and cress!)

6. Make bread with yeast. Shop-bought bread made with bicarbonate of soda contains phytates which interfere with the absorption of zinc and calcium.

7. Soak muesli in the fridge overnight to destroy phytates.

8. Boil the water first and add vegetables to minimise oxidation and loss of vitamin C, or preferably steam them. (Yes, they taste better steamed, too.)

9. Serve foods promptly after cooking.

10. Use stainless steel, enamelled or glass cookware. Aluminium is a toxic substance which accumulates in the body.

11. Grill rather than fry food; if frying, use oil rather than hard fats. (Discard oil after use.) Stir frying in a minimum of oil is the frying method of choice.

12. Many vegetables can be braised in the oven in a closed dish, moistened with stock.
13. Avoid microwaved foods, as microwaving can destroy vitamins and enzymes in the food.
14. Filter all drinking water and cooking water, or use bottled water.
15. Avoid hazardous colourings and other food chemicals.
16. Use eggs from free-range hens, preferably organically fed.
17. Peas, beans and lentils and the pectin from apples are natural ways of increasing the elimination of toxic metals.

Having bought all this Very Good Food, are you going to like it? Is the family going to like it? Will they eat it? Or will they complain?

- You have to **explain why** to everybody. Explain that it will make them better-looking, nicer, and much more clever – because it will!
- If you have to make big changes, **make the changes gradually** over a few weeks. Do not be too sudden! If you are changing over from white to brown flour, for example, change a quarter of the recipe at a time.
- **Get them all to join in**! If you are making bread, for example, involve them in it. They will be keener on the loaf they kneaded for themselves!

Growing Your Own

Producing 'own produce' can be hard work, but it can also give a great sense of achievement!

If you are going to try growing your own, try adding rock dust for minerals and liquid organic seaweed manure and compost and horse manure to your soil. Every positive move you make enhances your garden's basic fertility, and this will enhance your own as you eat the produce! You can buy organic rock dust, organic manure, organic compost and organic water-on seaweed liquid manures. If you have stables near you, find out about horse dung. If horses ride near you in a rural situation, take a plastic bag and a trowel with you for a walk! This way you get it for free! If you have even a small amount of garden that is doing nothing, have a go! Why not?

I have found the easiest things to grow are runner beans; they are so prolific and go on and on for ages. You can buy little plants about 3 inches high in February or March. They need some sticks or netting to grow up. If they are in a prominent part of the garden, you can push in some climbing nasturtium pods here and there amongst them for visual effect! Or you could plant some sweet peas, and they will all look quite jolly and decorative together. Tomatoes can be put in a tub or growbags along a sunny wall or fence. The growers are becoming quite innovative and you can now get climbing ones that have tiny little tomatoes, and keep on producing them, while growing up a rambler rose or similar.

If you can get four to six sweetcorn plants they can all stand together and will produce several cobs each. You can then pick them and sit in the garden and eat them raw, which is lovely and much nicer than cooked. They even have their own little handle, so you don't have to bother with skewers!

The same goes for lettuce – the leaves taste so much better when really fresh and the same applies to baby spinach and beetroot leaves which you can eat with chicory, nuts and pine kernels. Home-grown lettuce is not bitter. If you need to pull it a while before you eat it bring it in roots and all and put the roots in water in a vase. Like a flower, it will go on living for a bit, and you can pull leaves off as you need them. If the garden is just outside the door, you can pull leaves off as you need them, as with spinach, baby beetroot plants and so on. I saw a TV programme about a girl who had a balcony to her town flat where she grew salad in large pots and sat amongst it all, eating freshly picked leaves! .

The bottom line is to make it all interesting and delicious and fun. Am I the only person who finds leaves dull without dressing them up a bit? But there are all the old sauces and garnishes: redcurrant jelly on cabbage; mint jelly on lots of things; red onion garnish and apple sauce. Put sultanas in salads and use nut butter with chopped apple too. Put marmalade on coleslaw (yes it is lovely!). Watch MasterChef etc and pinch all their lovely ideas. Chop up celery, lettuce, apple and plum and mix them with nuts and/or pine kernels or make a 'dip' out of cream cheese and onion. Eat your own grown coleslaw with redcurrant jelly, sultanas, soaked prunes or apricots, a scoop of nut butter or a dollop of Greek yoghurt. Cut up celery and lettuce with grapes or pears and add nuts and pine kernels. Mix with cream cheese, or yoghurt, mayonnaise or honey, balsamic vinegar and oil. If you are more conventional, add herbs such as chervil. Have a go!

Bland ingredients can be mixed with tasty sultanas, chopped apples, orange segments, grapefruit, cherries, plums. Raw plums with avocado and lettuce are lovely, mixed with mayonnaise, yoghurt or cream cheese. Raw cabbage could be shredded up and mixed with redcurrant jelly – or sultanas and apple, or orange and grated carrot. If green leaves are a bit dull, mix them with something you do like. Grated cheese, if you are not milk-allergic, tomato puree, chopped-up apple, apricots, orange segments – bits of any fruit you like! Mix it all together; use a bit of honey, and imagination! For savoury salads, prawns, sardines, crab, salmon and fried scallops are delicious (and full of zinc!).

I find leeks and beetroots are very easy to grow. You buy little things about an inch high and put them in with a teaspoon. I like teaspoon gardening; it is not too onerous. Peas, however, I find, tend to be eaten by mice, but perhaps if you have a cat you will be luckier! We have tried brassicas, but if you are organic you have to try and cover them up with lots of muslin-like stuff, as otherwise you find you are running a white butterfly farm which non-organic neighbours might find irritating – a bit like a college of burglary.

Gooseberry bushes don't take up too much space; neither do a few raspberry canes and you can get terracotta tenements for strawberries. Just do what you can in the space you have. If you have space for a tree anywhere, even a little one, this is wonderful. The blossom is so pretty and picking your own fruit is one of the most cheerful occupations I know. I am sure many of you will be much more enterprising and innovative than I have been. Foresight would love to share your ideas with others.

Useful organisations:

- Garden Organic   www.gardenorganic.org.uk
- The Soil Association   www.soilassociation.org
- Good Gardeners Association   www.goodgardeners.org.uk

Food Preparation

Cooked or raw food

Many famous doctors and naturopaths have advocated the benefits of raw foods, including Max Bircher-Benner, Max Gerson, Kristine Nolfi, John Douglas and more recently Gabriel Cousins. Most of them recommend a vegetarian diet comprising 75% raw food and 25% cooked, though some are not averse to between 75% and 100% raw, depending on the individual. Why do so many of them advise that 'cooking may damage your health'? There are many reasons quoted, some of which we can list:

- Cooking destroys vitamins: eg if you cook fresh peas for five minutes, you destroy 20–40% of vitamin B1 and 30–40% of vitamin C. (peas are delicious raw!)

- Cooking destroys enzymes: these are essential for the efficient metabolism of food. eg the phosphatases in milk, which break down the phosphorus-containing compounds as in lysine, are destroyed when milk is pasteurised. The result is that most of the calcium that milk contains becomes insoluble, making milk constipating.

- Other proteins are deformed, with some of the amino acids being destroyed, while others may be altered so they are useless.

- Fats heated to high temperatures change their structure from the 'cis' type, which the body needs and uses, to the 'trans' type, which the body cannot use, and which causes harm to health.

However, not all foods *can* be eaten raw. So cooking does have some advantages:

- It destroys harmful organisms, especially in meat, poultry and some shellfish. It breaks down toxins in red and black beans. It changes the tough connective tissue in meat to gelatine, making eating easier.

Balance is the key, with plenty of raw food in a varied diet.

Microwave ovens

Microwave ovens 'cook' food not by the application of heat to it, but by generating heat from within it. There is no reliable work on how cooking in microwave ovens affects the nutritional value of the food. However, we do know some of the effects of microwave energy.

Regulations about leakages are strict. You may buy a detector to check for leakages but there are no standards for such devices. Some work well, others do not. It is advisable to have a qualified repairman service your oven annually. If you must use one, do not stand near it when it is on; do not cover food with plastic to cook. We know that microwaves affect cells inside the body but we do not know the 'safe' limit of microwave exposure. However, we do know that the officially pronounced 'safe' level has been dropping steadily over the last 20 years.

Personally, I would get rid of it. A Danish study on mice showed that after eating microwaved food they got stomach cancer. Do we need this? Other studies have said microwaving destroys all vitamins and enzymes in the food. If this is true, it does us no good at all, and what is wrong with good old-fashioned cooking – especially if we are eating a lot of our food raw anyway?

To conclude:

Now we know which deficiencies cause which malformations and health problems in the babies; now we know why Nature will switch off the ovaries when you are not sufficiently nourished. The ovaries are just saying, 'You can't get pregnant this month – you haven't enough zinc/selenium/manganese. It could mean disaster for the baby!' They then turn off – an age-old instinct I suspect. It happens in the wild, in times of famine, when another mouth to feed would be unwelcome.

Once you get well, if the delay has not been too long, the ovaries will turn on again. In a few cases, they need to be reminded by a little reflexology or acupuncture, which can stimulate them by sending extra energy in their direction.

Helen's story:

Two miscarriages and two ectopic pregnancies made a natural conception impossible when both severely damaged fallopian tubes were removed.

Helen knew that natural conception could never take place, so her only course of action was to take up the offer of three IVF attempts on the NHS. The first IVF attempt failed. The second embryo transfer was also rejected. After four years of infertility and with one more IVF attempt to go, Helen decided to seek help.

Following a car crash, Helen was trying acupuncture for her back and at the same time seeking a remedy for infertility. Her acupuncturist suggested Foresight. After surfing through the Foresight website both Helen and her partner joined the Foresight programme. Helen by now had stopped working full-time.

It took six hair mineral analyses and supplement adjustments before both partners were nutritionally and mentally ready, and attempted their third and final free IVF. Behold, the pregnancy held! An 8 lb 8 oz baby girl was delivered by caesarean section.

Helen said: 'We burst into tears and just couldn't take it all in. We had a wonderful baby. Today she is a very alert little girl, taking everything in around her, very content, thriving really well and sleeping through from 7 pm to 7 am from 16 weeks old! She is the first grandchild on my mother's side. She is cherished.'

The same applies with the sperm. Zinc and selenium are particularly important. Once the sperm are all well fed, they become strong and purposeful.

As your nutrition improves so do your looks. Your hair will become like that of the girls in the adverts for hair products! People have come to Foresight with hair problems, like big bald patches or receding hairlines and in a few months it has all grown back again. One lady was completely bald and came to us wearing a wig but after a few months on the Foresight programme, it came back so fast, it was reported to us as being: 'so thick, but so short, it looks like rabbit's fur!' It had to go through the growth stage, of course, but she was absolutely delighted!

Nature is brilliant. Lovely hair, smooth skin, bright eyes – and what happens? Men will fall in love with you and you can take your pick – just as Nature intended!

The same with the chaps! A lot of Foresight fathers get promotions or do really well at what they are doing – as well as fatherhood! Strong and healthy means efficient, as well as virile!

It is a shame, and a huge waste of money, all the girls having Botox for shrivelled lips (lack of B2), having 'breast implants' for sagging bosoms (too little food generally), and paying huge sums of money to get facelifts (wrinkles due to a lack of vitamins E, A and zinc). Beauty glows through from the inside out; just get the diet into gear and watch it happen.

The soil has been overworked, and for this reason the food has been poor quality and low in nutrients – even what we assume to be the 'good' stuff. **But we can all make a brilliant recovery!** It is important that we do ASAP! As a country, we cannot cope with any more years of depression, excess drinking and drug taking being the norm!

We are flagging in energy and breeding sick children. We are running the NHS ragged and it is running out of all of its (our) funds, and we are doing ghastly things to the wildlife. Billions of pounds' worth of toxic substances are being urinated and flushed into the drains and it is all going out to sea or being absorbed by the soil, causing ecological mayhem.

We must get back to natural food, clean water, brighter, better-looking productive people, happier children... there is a lot to be done.

What a marathon of a chapter this has been! Hopefully, however, it will have given you solutions to many of your ills, as well as those of friends and family. I also hope it has inspired you to find the vital spark to go a bit wild in the kitchen with the right ingredients!

Onwards!

CHAPTER 3
Hair Mineral Analysis

Essential Minerals and Toxic Metals

Hair analysis provides an accurate assessment of the concentration of minerals in the body – those that are toxic in any amount, those that are essential, and those that are necessary in small amounts, or toxic in larger amounts. This non-invasive technique readily determines exposure to toxic substances such as mercury, lead and cadmium. The correlation between mineral concentrations in the internal organs of the body and levels in the hair is much more reliable than the correlation between intracellular mineral concentration and the levels found in serum and urine specimens. Normal trace element concentrations, as detected in the serum or the urine, may be quite variable; however, hair analysis gives accurate readings of the intracellular concentrations of these substances.

From the book *Prescription for Nutritional Healing*, by James Balch, MD
(Member of the American Medical Association and Fellow of the American College of Surgeons)

Hair mineral analysis is arguably the most important part of the Foresight programme. It is one of the main reasons why I founded Foresight.

In the 1970s, my friend Gilly Gibbons and I had taken the outstanding American paediatrician Dr Beth Lodge-Rees to see Winchester Cathedral and on our way home we were discussing the formidable strengths of the men who had built it. Without the machinery to help them, we reckoned the strength they needed must have been phenomenal and ended up surmising about their diet...

'We are linking the quality of muscle meat now to the trace mineral content of the diet,' said Beth. 'They are taking samples of hair from the animals in the slaughterhouses. They are finding the levels of the essential elements in the hair relate to the quality of the meat. It seems to me that this could be a good way of looking inside people without the complication of cutting them open. I am thinking about this. I am wondering if there is some way I could do this for my kids.'

'YES!' we all said together. 'There will be!' We were so excited we nearly drove off the road!

Beth went back to the States, and within the year she and Dr Gary Gordon had started 'Mineralab', the first of the hair analysis laboratories. They were both in agreement that hair was the ideal sample material. Hair takes in the nutrients, that are present in the blood, at a steady pace. Those that enter the hair follicle grow out in the hair, where they are bound into the structure. Thus a one-inch sample of hair will give a good rough history of what has been going on in the body for approximately the previous 7–8 weeks. In most cases this is the most stable and useful record for examination. With the body fluids such as blood, saliva and urine, they are all in a constant state of flux. The blood is transporting minerals to an organ, or to storage in fat or bone. Thus a sample will show what was in the last meal. Urine will show what is being thrown out of the body. Saliva is somewhat akin to blood. About a quarter of all American doctors, apparently, now use hair analysis routinely.

The human body is quite volatile, and the levels of trace minerals are in a constant state of flux. Each meal, and with some minerals each breath, brings a fresh influx, and minerals are lost in outward breath, perspiration, urination and bowel movements. Minerals are carried round the body by the blood and lymph, and all the body fluids vary during the day, which is why hair is the most stable sample for information on mineral status.

Once we heard that the American lab had opened, we sent hair from hyperactive and allergic children and found that when we gave them the minerals they needed to correct their deficiencies we could help them a great deal.

A number of pioneering doctors, who were into diet, allergies and natural therapies generally, became interested, and a few years later two of them, Dr Stephen Davies and Dr Alan Stewart, set up 'Biolab' with Dr John McLaren Howard in London.

Some years after this, Foresight contributed to obtaining an analytical instrument and started working with it at the University of Surrey with Dr (now Professor) Neil Ward. We then did the study published in the back of this book. In this particular study we had 367 couples who participated, and we achieved 327 babies (89% success rate), all in good health, with no miscarriages or other mishaps. As you will also see, the data gave us a whole lot of other information regarding the parents' mineral status when they came to us, and how this related to their previous medical and reproductive history.

We have used this information ever since, and built upon it. It was a great shame it could not be published in the medical journals, but they rejected it on the grounds that there was **no control population**. A 'control population' would have had to be duped with fake pills called 'placebos', and this would have meant they would have been denied the supplements they needed – putting their babies at risk. The researchers would then have counted the index population's babies, and the placebo babies (or lack of babies, or miscarriages or whatever disaster occurred). This would have given them a 'scientific study'. Also a lot of very sad parents and possibly dead or damaged babies. **This is something Foresight will never do.**

Unfortunately, current medical training imposes these Draconian strictures, and a world of useful knowledge and healing gets blocked from the medics, which would otherwise be very helpful to them – and to us all. This serves the interests of the pharmaceutical industry, who fund the medical schools, as the more people are 'below par', with deficiencies, toxic metals, undiagnosed allergic illnesses etc, the more drugs get taken and the more money the pharmaceutical companies make!

Background information

There are things it is useful to know if you are doing analysis. Some minerals will 'override' or drive down others in the body if they become too dominant. Others act synergistically and help the absorption/use of another.

Some of them use the same 'binding sites' in the intestines. I feel this may act as a type of rough homeostatic mechanism for keeping them in balance; if too much of something has been taken in, maybe they shut down for that mineral and open up for another? (Empirical observation seems to point to this.)

However, if, due to environmental factors, the body gets swamped with a rogue element (such as lead, mercury, aluminium or cadmium), then much-needed elements can be denied absorption and then the body is in trouble. Needless to say, most of the sources of unfortunate environmental factors are man-made, albeit often inadvertently. Fortunately almost all of the excess levels are reversible, although it takes a little time.

The most obvious of these is lead. When we were first doing hair analysis in the late 1970s it was quite usual to see 5–7 ppm (parts per million) in the hair, even of children. Due to the tireless campaigning of Professor Derek Bryce-Smith for lead-free petrol, (which was successful after 29 years !) the average lead level in hair has fallen to approximately 2–3 ppm, and now only approximately 17% of people who come to us have a level that is of concern, even for reproduction. Lead damage to the foetus can include malformations such as spina bifida and mental retardation, hyperactivity, ADHD and autism.

In an ideal situation the needed trace minerals should be at or above the recommended values, and the toxic ones below the threshold values. We get people's levels as near to this ideal as we can.

Selenium protects the lungs, so smoking always reduces levels of selenium. Selenium is also necessary for sperm production, and is a mineral that guards against cancer and chromosome damage. This could be one of the reasons – perhaps the main reason – why children of fathers who smoke are more prone to cancer and also why parents who smoke are more likely to have Down's syndrome children.

These are just a few of the problems confronting the modern sperm and ova! They may be short of the minerals that they require to form properly, and they may be damaged or destroyed by toxic metals.

However, we all need to be aware of some aspects of hair analysis:

a) If the supplements significantly enhance the health of the person taking them, this may increase the rate of growth of the hair. Faster-growing hair may contain somewhat lower levels of some of the minerals we are looking at. This is, in fact, likely to be a more valid reading of the body status than the more optimistic levels shown in the reduced growth of the first sample! Further supplementation can achieve good levels even in the normally growing hair. These are then the optimum levels for healthy pregnancy.

b) If a person's hair analysis shows a high level of a toxic metal – lead, cadmium, mercury or aluminium – or an over-high level of the essential mineral copper, they will be given 2–6 'Vitamin C with Garlic' to reduce it. This can reduce other mineral levels also. This will be partly due to enhanced bowel actions, which may hasten the transit time of food. It will also owe something to the ability of the body to coat (chelate) the toxic substances with a non-toxic substance such as zinc or selenium to carry them safely through the liver and kidneys and out of the body. This will mean that, even though we have given some zinc and selenium, these may also go down along with the toxins. As the programme continues, they will return to normal.

c) It is the policy of the body to store any toxic metal to which it is exposed in large quantities, until such time as circumstances are more favourable to cope with the overload. When B-complex vitamins and minerals such as zinc, selenium, manganese, calcium etc. enter the body, sometimes the tissues start to evacuate larger stores of lead, cadmium, mercury etc. into the blood. This will take some months, rather than weeks, to clear, so the second hair chart may show some dumping of toxins. The more that is released, the better, as the quicker we can get it to leave the body, the better. However, one must be very careful not to become pregnant until this has been fully achieved. All of the toxic metals, if present in large amounts, can cause health problems with the baby. Do not be tempted to try to leave the metals 'in storage', however, as in response to pregnancy hormones they would be released into the body, and would be impossible to keep away from the developing embryo.

Sadly, we often see high levels of toxic metal in people who have come to us after the birth of a malformed baby. If only this work was done with one and all routinely, prior to every pregnancy, so much suffering could be avoided.

d) The body has ways of balancing the levels of the minerals so that no single one will predominate in the body. Zinc, selenium and manganese all share binding sites in the intestine. You therefore need to take a little of one when you take any other of these; for example, if you are taking zinc, you need to balance it with a little selenium, even if it does not show a low level in this reading, or the selenium will go down. Magnesium will enhance the utilisation of calcium, so giving either, without enough of the other, can result in the levels of the neglected element going down. It is not an easy matter to get the balance exactly right, and, with zinc in particular, one can sometimes struggle for several programmes. A lot may depend on the levels of lead, copper etc. in the drinking water and even the house dust, and nutrients in the diet. *Levels are often slow to rise in people who do not give up alcohol.* If water and/or dust need testing it is worth doing this at an early stage.

As you may have gathered, it is not always easy to achieve perfection in a short space of time. This is why it is unwise to take a hair analysis to an inexperienced person for interpretation. One can understand why they may be nonplussed or dismissive!

However, the babies who are ultimately born free from a toxic load of dangerous substances, and able to use any vitamin or mineral they require for their mental and physical integrity, are, unsurprisingly, perfectly formed and mentally and emotionally exceedingly bright.

I devoted my life to making it possible for all parents to achieve this, because I know it is worth it. Be patient – you will get there.

People have to use up their precious stores of essential minerals to chelate the toxins. As a toxin is released from storage, it will be wrapped around with zinc or similar to go safely through the liver or kidney. This stops the toxic metal from causing damage as it makes its way out of the body. However, it also may deplete an already parlous zinc level! So as you detoxify, you also have to back up with the essential minerals, to hang on to them as best you can!

Yet another problem is that organophosphate pesticides inhibit the uptake of manganese. Therefore low manganese can indicate there is some organophosphate contamination. Organophosphates are a nerve poison, so it is best to clear them from the body before pregnancy (or at any time, as they can cause epilepsy and have been linked to illnesses such as MS, ME, Parkinson's and Alzheimer's disease). We give nicotinamide as it is the only substance known to take organophosphates out through the liver (according to MK Johnson of the Medical Research Council, who has made a study of this).

It is best to be doing all the other components of the full Foresight programme as you are taking the supplements. If you improve your diet this backs up the supplements and makes success likely to happen more quickly. This helps us all, as you are understandably impatient for your precious baby to appear!

Tobacco and alcohol both increase the load of toxic metals, and cannabis is the worst of all! The weed appears to be full of both lead and cadmium, among other toxins. Alcohol removes zinc, and slows down liver and kidney function, making it more difficult to get rid of toxic metals. Cannabis can deposit aluminium, lead and cadmium.

The pill causes women to retain copper and lose zinc, and sometimes also magnesium and manganese. (Pfeiffer and Grant)

Mercury from dental amalgams or from eating tuna etc can lower positive minerals, especially selenium. Genitourinary infections, allergies and candida (which overuse zinc and cause malabsorption), and, of course, intestinal parasites, all lower the essential minerals.

Electromagnetic pollution which is increasing all the time is now believed to lower levels of zinc.

Many environmental chemical 'nasties' do the same – including aluminium from deodorants and fluoride from toothpastes, food additives, pesticides, toxins from cosmetics etc and medical drugs.

So there is every good reason for taking all the information on board and doing everything you can. If we work together we can get there sooner! When you see your programme of vitamins and minerals you may find it a bit daunting. If so, just start with one or two every day, and work up gradually. You will find you soon get used to it, and as you get into the full lifestyle, you will feel so much more energetic and on top of things, and it will all swing into place.

If you find it hard to swallow the capsules, they can be opened and their contents mixed with food. Many people seem to find capsules easier to swallow than the old-fashioned tablets.

Apart from the Vitamin C and Garlic, which contains two herbs, the ingredients in the Foresight range are just simple nutrients, given in quantities well below 'mega' doses and packed with organic vegetable powder. There are no artificial colourings, flavourings, preservatives or fillers.

The only large doses sometimes given are 2–6 of the Vitamin C and Garlic, as a cleanser of toxic metals and/or excess copper. This capsule contains garlic and milk thistle, which are excellent liver-supporting herbs. The level of vitamin C is well within the range advised by Linus Pauling, and also by Carl Pfeiffer, both of whom were world-renowned for their work with nutrient therapies.

Some people find that large doses of vitamin C can cause loose stools, especially if it is given to clean out lead, cadmium and/or copper. This is partly due to the metal that is coming out in the stool. If this becomes tiresome, drop the vitamin C for three days, and then start again, using one tablet for the first few days, and then working up gradually to using just as much as you can tolerate comfortably. This will make the process a little slower, so allow a few more weeks before retesting.

Some people find the zinc can be a little nauseating. If this is a problem, I would drop it for three days and then take one with meals, and work up over a few days, to find how many you can tolerate. Most people find they can get used to them. Foresight has added ginger to the zinc to help to counteract any nausea with the bigger doses, and given a mixture of zinc citrate (absorbed in the stomach), and zinc picolinate. Foresight believes that this has made it easier to handle but it depends on the individual.

It is extremely important that zinc levels in the hair are up to at least 175 ppm – preferably 185 ppm – to ensure both a healthy conception and a smooth pregnancy. Copper excess, coupled to zinc deficiency, can cause miscarriage or premature birth. If you feel you need to spread the programme out over a longer time-span, by all means do, but this may mean a longer time before conception would be advisable.

Whatever you do, let Foresight know exactly what you have taken and for how long when you retest so that the results can be examined in light of this information. It makes it easier to help you.

Energy levels soar on the Foresight programme with many saying they were promoted at work whilst on it and others saying: 'The house and garden have never been tidier!' They often share with me the ways in which they are preparing their 'nests', and I feel we are all part of one enormous explosion of love and life, and it is all enormously hopeful!

Interesting to think the little birds in the trees are also making their nests when they get to this bit! (Little male birds bring their partners lots of titbits as part of the courting ritual. Instinct is a wonderful thing. Presumably this tenderness gives her tiny ovaries the boost they need to spring into action!)

As the season arrives when they are foraging around gathering up little bits of moss and feathers to line their nests, people often tell me they are making a quilt, or re-covering a lampshade, or washing the curtains, and I feel we are all part of one enormous explosion of love and life, and it is all enormously hopeful and jolly!

Just as fertility can be repaired, so can many general health problems. I know that we can turn the general health around in so many families where the children are hyperactive or 'awkward' most of the time, due to the lack of preconceptual care.

In the same way, unwillingness to work, the 'sick-note culture', would respond to deficiencies, allergies, addictions and so on being addressed with hair testing and nutrients. Much chronic illness is likely to be due to lack of nutrients coupled to an overload of toxins, compounded by a significant intake of voluntary social poisons!

Thirty years of reading hair analyses and hearing about the outcomes of the Foresight programme at first hand has convinced me that balancing the minerals is the key to excellent reproductive health.

Getting rid of the toxic metals prior to pregnancy means the babies are guarded against deformity and brain damage. Getting the necessary minerals up to speed means they develop optimum physical and mental abilities.

As you become more familiar with the charts, the patterns will become more obvious. Low levels right across the board can show an inadequate diet – whether because of poor food choices. Many times I hear: 'I have to admit that I love Mars Bars – yes, I eat one for my lunch every day. No, I don't eat breakfast, I don't have the time...'; or because of anorexia: 'I don't want to look fat like my sister...'; or because of undiagnosed gluten or milk allergy: 'I have an upset tummy two or three times a week – some days I have diarrhoea up to six times, my doctor says it is nerves, he's given me some tranquillisers and told me not to think about my bowels but I can't really stop it – it just seems to happen anyway...'

These people will all have very low mineral levels – particularly zinc. Other charts will show up with high copper and lead, so they will need to test the tap water (see the internet for a reasonable lab). Sometimes there is a high level of aluminium – their deodorant may need to be changed. The very high mercury levels are usually seen in the dentists and dental nurses. High lead and cadmium are in the smokers – low zinc, again, will be linked to alcohol consumption or chronic illness. Low manganese indicates organophosphate pesticide contamination. Low chromium relates to high sugar concentration.

The high toxic metals send all the needed nutrient levels down. As you supplement your diet with helpful vitamins your body will perk up and repair itself – or just give you more energy!

I often hear: 'I've been getting a lot of praise at work – goodness, my supervisor said I was really getting down to it!'

'My husband has just been promoted – he was quite surprised really, but he's done so well lately. I said to him that it was the vitamins, but he's not going to admit it, because he was so against taking them...!'

'We've started running together in the evenings, and our little dog is so pleased. He thinks he persuaded us...'

...and as for the stories about the babies don't start me! But isn't this how it is meant to be?

A lot of you say to me, 'When the kids grow up, I'm going to start helping people with this myself. How do we learn about it?' Well, I think we're going to have to organise this because I think there could be a whole army of you out there, and you could be quite unstoppable! Join Foresight and get the Newsletters, and then take it from there. There are many satellite courses for hard-pressed mums who want to start from scratch, and there are courses on organic gardening and cooking on the television – and if time is an issue, there are some wonderful books available

To all of you who are practitioners (or would like to be), I would suggest you meet Colleen Norman if possible. I would also look at Alf Riggs's video (contact his son Roy Riggs) and contact Foresight about Foresight Information Days. Nutritionists, homeopaths, naturopaths, reflexologists, acupuncturists, herbalists – anyone can expand their area of expertise or find out who they can cooperate with to enhance their service. If you are a nutritionist or a naturopath, you could team up with a homeopath and a reflexologist, and all areas of the work can be covered.

What we have all got to do is find ways of helping people remove the road-blocks between where they are now and their perfect fertility and perfect health. We need to spread the word! You remove one road-block when you get the tap water right. You remove another when you stop smoking. You remove another when you change your deodorant. You remove another when you realise not to use copper algaecide at the swimming pool. You remove another when you bathe the dog and get rid of at least some of the anti-flea drops, and so on. Then you build the bridges you need to cross with nutrients, organic food and clean water – and the genuine goodwill that goes with it all!

On another tack, but still relevant, we are told that thousands of people are 'malingering' and living off benefits because they pretend to be ill, so as not to have to work. **I don't believe it.** Most would probably get better in a few months if (a) we cleared their toxic metals, and (b) we supplemented the minerals they needed, and (c) we did the rest of the Foresight programme with them!

They start off feeling below par, and because of poor brain development leading to lack of success at school, they see themselves as stupid. They are depressed and embarrassed about this, and either take to alcohol and street drugs, or 'go to the doctor' and get put on tranquillisers. Either way, their lives and their brains are bombarded with toxins, which makes them feel worse, and perform worse. With women, this may all be further compounded by the contraceptive pill.

As the cycle continues, they feel worse and worse. Some may have allergies due to early weaning. Some may have parasites. Some may have 'foetal tobacco syndrome' or 'foetal alcohol syndrome'. Others may be bombarded by electrosmog from nearby pylons, mobile phone masts, TETRA masts. This may keep them awake at night, and then they may be given sleeping pills which then join the other medicaments in plaguing their already harassed liver.

We need an army of New Health Pioneers to get them back on their feet, and having the courage to live real lives. Exhortation won't do it. Nutrients would. Can we get the powers-that-be to see this? The challenge is to get the next generation born road-worthy!

Those of you who are young, energetic and intelligent – help them! Just telling people about the Foresight programme is a step forward. Do what you can, however you can!

Toxic Metals (also known as heavy metals)
What they do, and how we stop them doing it.

Gail Bradley and I produced this research in the 1980s and it is as significant today as it was then. The modern environment is like a minefield for the foetus, but, by testing the hair and seeing what toxic substances, if any, are present in the prospective parents' samples, we can see what needs to be done.

All trace elements can be toxic if consumed in sufficient quantities. However, the term 'toxic metal' generally denotes *'those elements not recognised as having an essential function and known to have well documented deleterious effects.'* (Lodge Rees, 1983)

Man has been utilising these metals for building and industrial purposes for hundreds of years, but in the twentieth century new processes and products have meant a huge escalation in use. The result is widespread pollution with sometimes serious effects on health. The injurious effects of lead were recognised by the Victorians and lead was widely taken to procure abortion. In the 1980s, largely due to the unremitting effort of Professor Derek Bryce-Smith, the environmental effect was acknowledged with the introduction of lead-free petrol.

Although the dangers of cadmium are highlighted in discussions on soil levels, there was little apparent concern until very recently over its major source, cigarette smoking.

Dentists have been aware of the risks of mercury for decades now, yet some still continue to use amalgam fillings. Those at greatest risk are dentists and their assistants, and dentists' spouses. An association has been formed to campaign for compensation for dental nurses affected by mercury (www.mercurymadness.org).

The possible toxicity of aluminium has been highlighted in respect of Alzheimer's disease, but UK hospitals, especially those dealing with the mentally ill and geriatrics, serve large amounts of tea, a high source of aluminium. Aluminium serving pans are also still used in some institutions. The use of deodorants and antiperspirants grows, and these are sometimes high in aluminium salts, although it is possible to find them without. Once again, we need to read the labels. Also tell the shop managers about it!

There is the continual interaction between the elements in the body – and it is the beneficial relationship between the individual elements that is important in health. There are only a small number of studies which review these interactional effects as the work is difficult and expensive, but Bryce-Smith and his colleagues pursued it. (Ward, 1987) There is also the problem common to government health departments and the medical industry: the assumption that something is safe until it is proved otherwise. What is needed is a major shift to assume the opposite, namely that something with toxic potential is dangerous until proved safe! (Twenty-two years on from when this was originally written, we are still waiting for this shift!)

The major toxic metals which are known to adversely influence pregnancy outcome include lead, cadmium, aluminium and mercury. Also over-high levels of copper can be problematic.

- **Aluminium**

Sources: The major sources of aluminium include antacids (they are a stomach irritant – these are some of the many self-perpetuating medicaments), antiperspirants, food additives, and anti-caking agents found in milk substitutes and baking powder. Pearly, glittery cosmetics, especially eye cosmetics. Some toothpastes use it as an abrasive. In some places aluminium flocculants are added to the water to collect up the peaty particles; sometimes the 'comb' that is meant to catch it all as it leaves the reservoirs is damaged, and becomes ineffective, and there is some leakage of the gel into the mains water. If a patient's hair level is high, the water from their taps should be tested. Aluminium saucepans and other cooking utensils impart some metal if they are in contact with food, especially leaf vegetables, rhubarb, apple and other acid fruits. The pans seem polished when you have cooked them! Aluminium pressure cookers, although now relatively rare, are worse than ordinary pans. Kettles and aluminium teapots were potent sources, but happily in the last 17 years, there has been a shift away from aluminium kitchenware, though some people may still have old family possessions! Work at the University of Wales at Cardiff suggests that the major UK food source of aluminium is tea, since the tea plant thrives on alum soils, so the soil is fed with alum. Foil-wrapped foods can be sources. Foil-wrapped fats and acid foods are the worst. (Pfeiffer 1978, Millstone 1988) Food microwaved in aluminium foil containers is very bad news. Modern antiperspirants contain aluminium. Look at the labels.

Effects on health: Aluminium is easily absorbed, accumulating in the arteries. A study has shown that people living in areas with a high level of aluminium in the drinking water face a 50% greater risk of developing Alzheimer's disease. (Many who develop Alzheimer's in other areas may be suffering from pollution from any of the above sources.) How many people with chronic indigestion, likely to be due to an undiagnosed milk or gluten intolerance, habitually take antacids, for example? The aluminium they contain is a stomach irritant, leading to the sufferer needing another tablet a short time later. (The only one that does not contain aluminium, 'Nulacin', contains gluten!) Also, check vaccines, most contain it.

The following food additives are allowed in this country: E173 Aluminium (cl 77000), known to cause kidney stress and said to be 'not safe' for the brain. It is forbidden in Australia. E554 Aluminium Sodium Silicate is implicated with Alzheimer's disease, as is E556 Aluminium Calcium Silicate, E541 Sodium Aluminium Phosphate and Acidic Aluminium Phosphate. It is all unsafe for babies or people suffering from kidney or heart problems. There can also be skin reactions. It is also known to be a neurotoxin. As this is not suitable for babies under six months, it is advisable for pregnant and lactating mothers to avoid it also. E559 Aluminium Silicate has been implicated in Alzheimer's disease, which is hugely on the increase. *We should all be reading labels while we can!* Take *FIND OUT* and *WATCH IT* with you when you go shopping (obtainable from Foresight).

It is known that aluminium can destroy vitamins as it readily combines with other substances. It irritates and weakens the lining of the gut. Excessive amounts can lead to constipation, colic, excessive perspiration, loss of appetite, nausea, skin problems and fatigue. Adverse effects associated with the body's attempts to clear itself, in which aluminium salts are found in small quantities in the blood, include paralysis and areas of numbness, with fatty degeneration of the liver and kidney, as well as symptoms of gastrointestinal inflammation. Thus it seriously compromises nutritional status. It has been linked with kidney problems in babies, with researchers concluding that formula feeds should be aluminium-free for neonates and infants with reduced kidney function, in fact for any infants! Soya milk has been withdrawn for infants due to high aluminium levels. It has been associated with behavioural problems and autism. For the same reason it is vital that pregnant/breastfeeding mothers do not use antiperspirants. Mice fed large doses had no symptoms, *but* the next three generations of offspring had growth defects. (Cowdry 1989, Nutrition Search Inc. 1975, Freundlich 1985, Lodge Rees 1979, Ward 1992)

We recommend that the hair mineral analysis level should not exceed two parts per million.

- **Cadmium**

Sources: The main sources of cadmium are cigarette smoking – your own or even passive smoking. (NB: The law regarding no smoking in pubs is Very Good News!)

Cadmium is in processed foods, since in the refining of flour the zinc in the germ and bran layers is mainly removed, leaving a higher cadmium to zinc ratio.

It is widely used in manufacturing industries, including particularly those concerned with paints, dyes, batteries, television sets and fertilisers. Artists or housepainters should be aware that it is in yellow and red paints. Artists should not lick their brushes, as this can lead to tongue and throat cancer, also depression. Housepainters or those scraping down old paint need to wear protective gear, including masks and rubber gloves. It is found in shellfish from polluted waters and galvanised containers and can be released by coal-burning. It can come from burning rubber. This can occur where old rubber tyres are burnt to dispose of them, and on race-tracks, as the rubber can burn off the tyres as the pressure is on!

Effects on health: It is highly dangerous as it accumulates in the kidneys and liver slowly, unless nutritional measures are taken to remove it or reduce absorption. It particularly builds up in people who are deficient in vitamins C, D, B6, zinc, manganese, copper, selenium and/or calcium. (Pfeiffer 1978, McKie 1983, Colgan 1982, Pfeiffer 1975)

Cadmium is known to damage the unborn in animal studies. Elizabeth Lodge Rees reported cleft palate and/or lip, other facial malformations and limb defects in a number of species, testicular and ovarian necrosis, and renal disorders. This will explain why cleft lip and palate is more common in the children of smokers. In research studies, she noted pregnant animals developed toxemia, an observation which led her to wonder if 'one might suspect that toxemia in humans may be due to excess cadmium and/or a lack of nutrients that counteract the effect of cadmium'. She also mentioned that in humans it was associated with proteinuria, as well as low birth weight and small head circumference in the baby. Cadmium accumulates in the placenta, causing placental necrosis if large amounts are absorbed. (Lodge Rees 1983b) It also crosses the placenta. It has been found to impair reproduction in mice. (Bryce-Smith 1981, Schroeder 1971)

The importance of zinc in counteracting the effects of cadmium has been demonstrated in animal research on the effects of cadmium on the testes. Pre-treatment with zinc can abolish some of the adverse effects, though it does not reverse others. When cadmium is injected subcutaneously into female rats it produces marked changes in the ovaries, the adverse effects initially increasing over time, though the ovaries do return to normal eventually, when the cadmium leaves the body. (Samarawickrama 1983)

It seems likely from these observations that smokers' semen will contain excess cadmium, and that this could adversely affect their partners' ovaries. One more good reason to stop smoking!

Foresight recommends that the hair mineral analysis level should not exceed 0.14 parts per million (and when it does, we take steps to do something about it!).

NB: Cadmium is known to accumulate in the kidneys, and we frequently see high levels in people suffering from high blood pressure. If people were always given a hair analysis before being given medical drugs, so often the solution would be obvious. Cadmium can be removed from the body with vitamin C, garlic, milk thistle and B-complex vitamins, especially nicotinamide.

• Mercury

Sources: The main sources of mercury are dental fillings and vaccines, pesticide and fungicides, fish and industrial processes. The larger the fish, the greater the concentration of mercury with tuna and swordfish being the most common sources in the UK. People who consume tuna fish on a regular basis tend to have quite high levels of mercury in their hair. 'Freshwater' fish can also be contaminated if the river has been polluted by factory effluent, or water run-off from fields which have been treated with mercury-containing agrochemicals.

It is found in slimicides used in paper manufacturing to stop the growth of slime moulds.

It is in some cosmetics and other toiletries, antiseptic sprays, make-up removers, eye moisturiser and mascara. The worst dangers of all have come from the vaccines where mercury was used as a preservative. The recent work of Dr Viera Scheibner of Australia, who has followed research all over the world, makes clear that the damage done to the human brain, and therefore the human mind, by vaccines has been incalculable. Some of this was due to the mercury preservative thiomersal (although in part there may also have been problems with the viruses themselves, and with the animal lymph in which they were 'floated').

Dr Viera Scheibner also has evidence of how the most severe reactions occur approximately 16 days after the vaccination/immunisation. She has investigated thousands of cot deaths, and believes that apnoea attacks and cot deaths cluster around this inauspicious date. This needs much further – urgent – research.

A well-known London dentist, Dr Victoria Lee, has long been concerned about the mercury saga, and has made a huge study of the whole subject. She said to me: 'The phials which contain the vaccine have enough for five shots. Mercury is a heavy substance. It will fall to the bottom of the phial. The fifth baby is likely to be the unlucky one. He will get a big wallop of mercury. Is this why one child in five now has learning difficulties? I think so.' Although it may not be the full answer, it may be a big piece in some children's biochemical jigsaw.

The major controversy around the dangers of mercury concerns mercury-containing amalgams used in dentistry. (Ziff 1985, Kupsinel 1984) Dentists have been aware of mercury poisoning for many years. We have found that the people with the highest mercury in their hair are dentists, dental nurses, and dentists' spouses or partners. Unfortunately, the seminal fluid is an excretory route for toxic metals. This means that a wife often suffers from toxic effluent coming from her husband's occupation. The American Society of Dental Surgeons was opposed to mercury amalgams 150 years ago! Norway, Sweden and Denmark now ban mercury in dental work. It is time Britain followed suit.

Effects on health: There are three basic forms of mercury: elemental, non-organic and organic. The elemental and non-organic forms tend to be slowly absorbed and readily excreted, unlike the organic form which is easily absorbed and slow to be eliminated. Thus the main dangers lie in the organic, especially methyl mercury, although there are some conditions linked to elemental mercury. These include psychological disturbances, oral cavity disorders, gastro-intestinal, cardiovascular, neurologic, respiratory, immunological and endocrine effects. In severe cases there are hallucinations and manic-depression. Organic mercury exposure is linked with psychological symptoms which can develop into paralysis, vision, speech and hearing problems, loss of memory, lack of coordination, renal damage and general central nervous system dysfunctions. Eventually death can occur. Not exactly what you need put into your mouth on a permanent basis. Nevertheless, the British Dental Association refuses to admit it is harmful. However, there is a splendid Association for Mercury Free Dentists who have a website: www.mercuryfreedentistry.org.uk (The British Society for Mercury Free Dentistry, The Weathervane, 22a Moorend Park Road, Cheltenham, GL53 0JY / Tel: 01242 226918). I would contact them for help with finding a dentist who does not use mercury.

Metallic mercury vapour has been reported to affect men exposed to it in a serious way. In one study of nine men, exposed after an accident, all complained of loss of libido, lasting in some cases up to eight years. One reported temporary impotence for 18 months. (NB: Should we regard this as a failsafe mechanism of nature as toxic sperm can produce damaged children? Nature can be far more aware than we are.)

The damage mercury can cause to the foetus was highlighted in the Japanese tragedy of Minamata, in which 23 children were born with cerebral palsy-like symptoms, varying from mild spasticity to severe mental retardation, blindness, chronic seizures, and death. Their mothers, free from symptoms themselves, had been exposed to mercury while pregnant. Mercury is readily passed through the placenta and foetal blood often contains concentrations 20 per cent greater than the maternal blood. Foetal brain tissue concentrations may be four times higher than those in the mother's brain tissues. In the Minamata incident, adults and older children were also affected with a total of 46 dying.

Animal work by Dr Joan Spyker suggests that the adverse effects may be long-term. Mice exposed in utero did not appear outwardly different from controls until they were about 18 months old (middle-aged). The experimental mice then contracted severe infections, implying an immune system impaired prenatally. They lost all semblance of normality, ageing quickly and prematurely.

Only extensive investigation, magnifying the brain tissues 48,000 times, showed slight damage to the individual cells – yet this slight damage was responsible for their problems. Dr Spyker has pointed out that the Minamata victims are deteriorating just as the animal model predicted. (Elkington 1985, Kupsinel 1984, Norwood 1980)

• Lead

Lead has been known to be toxic to animals and humans for centuries and its use has been so great, it has been impossible to escape ingesting or inhaling it.

Sources: It is found in foods and in water which has coursed through old lead piping, or through lead-glazed earthenware mains. Sometimes it is found in copper piping where the joins of the pipes have been formed with lead-containing alloys.

Where high lead does arise now, it is often in conjunction with high copper, and is coming from the tap water. Joining copper piping to a lead connecting pipe from the mains, and joining copper pipes with a lead-containing solder, are now both illegal. However, this simply means that builders/plumbers cannot do this anymore. *It does not mean* that these problems have been rectified in the properties already built. I think from what we see on a daily basis that in the region of 10–20% of homes still have these problems. It should be part of the remit of the surveyors to look for this when the properties change hands. Better still, all houses should have a water survey as a starting point for the government's new drive forward on health! Expensive, maybe, but *what* it could save the NHS!

Cigarette smoking can increase lead uptake significantly, from the lead arsenate used as an insecticide in the production of tobacco. Occupational exposure can be a hazard, as lead is used in a number of industries. (Davis 1981, Pfeiffer 1978, Clausen 1977, El-Dakhakhny 1972) Builders can be high in lead from scraping down old paint, from roofing felt and from cement. Artists can get it from certain paints. Particular occupations such as making windows with 'leaded lights' and stained glass windows, glazing pottery can put workers at risk.

Some black hair dyes and black hair extensions, used when making hair into little plaits all over the head, can contain lead and/or cadmium. Always check, and reject those that do. Some popular hair products contain a lot of lead – on no account use them. Lead may also be in some powdered inks.

It is illegal to put lead into cosmetics in this country, but some people import a type of mascara made in India or Pakistan that contains it. Although it is illegal over here, people have too little understanding of why this is so. The danger to babies needs to be fully explained – ideally on television.

Animal research suggests that nutritional status may be a factor in lead absorption. Diets low in calcium, iron, zinc, selenium and manganese may actually enhance lead uptake. However, one study also suggests that cow's milk may increase absorption, since, although it is high in calcium, it is low in other trace minerals such as iron. (Kostial, 1979) The fact that lead can be removed from the body by nutrients further supports the idea that nutritional status is important.

Safety levels: There is no agreement on safety levels of lead in the body. Some researchers (who I find easy to believe) say that no level can be assumed to be safe. The Government sets limits for industry and the environment which are lowered from time to time as more is revealed about its toxicity. (Bryce-Smith, 1979) One problem in deciding toxicity levels is that for a long time there were no officially agreed ways to measure levels. Blood levels are not reliable as the lead is passed quickly into other tissues. Hair analysis is now accepted as a reliable guide, and is available through Foresight. Foresight recommends that the hair reading should be no more than 1.4 ppm (parts per million). None at all would obviously be the ultimate goal, but this is unlikely to be achievable in the present environment.

Further information on the effects of lead toxicity on health: It is now accepted that levels of lead in the body which do not manifest symptoms of 'classical lead poisoning' may still have significant effects on the body. Chronic 'low' lead exposure is implicated as a significant causative or contributory factor in a wide range of conditions, including cardiovascular disease, renal and metabolic disease, immune dysfunction, and a multiplicity of vague symptoms, such as lethargy, depression, muscle aches and pains, and frequent infections. Cancer can occur in the babies born to mothers with significant amounts of lead in their systems. Developmental abnormalities and learning, behavioural and central nervous system dysfunction in schoolchildren later in life are also linked to raised lead levels during the pregnancy. Lead interferes with the normal functioning of many trace elements, especially by inhibiting zinc-dependent enzymes, making its effects widespread. Other enzyme systems are also vulnerable. High childhood blood lead levels and smaller stature have been shown to be highly correlated.

Lead can affect both male and female reproductive abilities. Men exposed to high levels in their work have been found to be at risk of low sperm count, with more sperm likely to be misshapen and less mobile. High rates of infertility, miscarriage and stillbirth, congenital abnormalities including microcephaly, convulsions, early deaths and chromosomal aberrations have been reported in their children.

In women, lead's capacity for inducing abortions has long been known – *it was used for this purpose* about the turn of the century with, sometimes, blindness and brain damage in surviving babies as unwanted results. It was also this danger that eventually ensured women were not employed to work with lead.

In 1977, a study of placental lead levels by Wibberley at the University of Aston in Birmingham showed that there were greater amounts in the placentas of malformed stillbirths and neonatal deaths compared with normal babies surviving longer than a week. In the same year, two other researchers reported higher levels of lead (and cadmium) in stillbirths, using rib and pre-ossified cartilage for the analyses.

Needleman and his colleagues found lead exposure in utero and congenital abnormalities to be associated 'in a dose-related fashion with an increased risk for minor abnormalities.' (Needleman, 1984)

Prenatal exposure can result in lead intoxication in the newborn. In a study which measured the level of lead in umbilical cord blood at birth, subsequent mental developmental testing at the ages of 6 months and 12 months showed that the higher the level of lead, the lower the test scores. At neither age were scores related to *current* blood levels. The researchers concluded: 'Prenatal exposure to lead levels *relatively common among urban populations* appear[s] to be associated with less favourable development through the first year of life.' (Bellinger, 1986)

Another longitudinal study by the same researcher, which concerned lead exposure and early cognitive development, concluded, 'It appears that the fetus may be adversely affected at blood lead concentrations well below 25 ug/dl, the level currently defined by the Centre for Disease Control as the highest acceptable level for young children.' (Bellinger 1987)

Research by Doctors McConnell and Berry suggests why this should happen. They found that in rats lead tends to derange the development of the brain in a unique way, interrupting the process of forming neural connections. Other studies have shown that other parts of the brain closely involved with learning processes are also susceptible to damage by lead. Animal research with monkeys has confirmed that learning abilities are affected. In one study, monkeys in their first year of life showed no physical signs of toxicity, but all the lead-exposed ones showed performance deficits on reversal learning tasks. The researchers report that the effects are not the result of delayed maturation:

Data currently being collected in this laboratory indicate that the deficit can be observed at least three years beyond the final dosing. It therefore appears likely that this deficit represents a relatively permanent characteristic of the chronically lead poisoned monkey. (Bushell, 1977)

The most widely quoted study on the effects of lead on children is that done by Needleman and his colleagues. They showed that at levels below those which were considered to produce symptoms of toxicity, the performance of children in the classroom was adversely affected. A wide range of behaviours was examined, including distractibility, persistence, dependence, organisational ability, hyperactivity, impulsiveness, frustration, day dreaming, ability to follow and overall functioning, and it was found that the higher the lead level, the poorer the performance in every measure. Other studies have also indicated the negative effects of lead on learning abilities and classroom behaviour.

94

Alison's story:

They always enjoyed the weekend papers. On such an occasion, an article relating to age spots, mineral deficiency analysis and Foresight caught Alison's attention. Life went on as usual and she thought no more about it.

After trying for six months for a baby, conception occurred but unfortunately at six weeks the baby was miscarried. Although they tried, no further conception took place. Several months later, tests revealed that all was normal. With these findings, they were referred to a hospital for further investigation. They were informed that there would be blood tests as well as investigations of the fallopian tubes, antibiotics, painkillers, X-rays and dyes injected into the body – all in the name of searching for reasons for infertility. Both Alison and her husband had a science background, yet this did not feel right as it seemed too uncomfortable and too invasive. Both knew that there must be an alternative. Alison remembered the article she had read a few months earlier, searched for the article and luckily found it. Foresight was contacted.

'After speaking to Nim, who was so calm and supportive, we both started on the Foresight programme – after all, we had nothing to lose.'

Their first hair mineral analysis revealed that both had high lead levels and low zinc levels. The analysis was scientific and they became 'very dedicated' to the programme. The second analysis revealed that mineral levels had improved sufficiently for conception in about three months. Three months later, prompted by 'a feeling', out came the pregnancy test. All Alison heard from upstairs was 'Oh!' shortly followed by 'OH! Yes, you are pregnant. It works!' At the appointed time, a 6 lb 14 oz baby boy was born to them.

In a follow-up study, Needleman and his colleagues checked 132 students over an 11-year period (ending in 1989), concluding that the harmful effects of lead persist beyond childhood and the mental impairment from lead poisoning may be permanent. Decreased hand-eye coordination and shortened attention times, as well as physical effects, were seen in 45 adolescents and young adults with hair levels considered to be normal, with problems starting at levels as low as 10 ppm. Most laboratories class up to 15 ppm as 'normal'. His work was published in the New England Journal of Medicine.

A number of other studies have also suggested a link between hyperactivity and raised lead levels. In one, 13 children with no apparent cause for their hyperactivity were examined. Their behaviour improved when their lead levels were reduced using lead-chelating medication. A Danish study linked high levels with minimal cerebral dysfunction (MCD) – learning disabilities are often linked with hyperactivity or MCD.

(Davis 1981, Blamer 1980, Lacranjan 1975, Elkington 1985, Needleman 1984, Ward 1987, Wibberley 1977, Singh 1978, Bellinger 1986, Bryce-Smith 1979, Needleman 1979, Pihl 1977, Garnys 1979, Thatcher 1982, Yale 1985, Moore 1975, Gittelman 1983, Lin-Fu 1973, David 1976, Hansen 1980, Needleman 1990, Schwartz 1986)

Multi element studies

As far back as 1969 it was reported that *'Cadmium teratogenicity is dramatically augmented by lead when they are administered concurrently.'* (Thatcher, 1982) Lead and cadmium often occur together. Their concentrations in hair and blood show strong positive correlations and their overt symptoms of toxicity are not unalike. These similarities have led some researchers to the view that *'it is possible that some of the deleterious effects attributed to lead in correlation studies may instead be due to cadmium.'* They conducted a study on hair cadmium and lead levels in relation to cognitive functioning in children, in which the results showed that hair cadmium and lead levels were significantly correlated with intelligence tests and school achievement, but not with motor impairment scores. Statistical analysis suggested that *'cadmium has a stronger effect on verbal IQ than does lead and that lead has a stronger effect on performance IQ than does cadmium.'* (Thatcher, 1982)

Professor Bryce-Smith and his colleagues, aware of the inadequacies of single element studies, reviewed the levels of four elements, lead, cadmium, zinc and calcium, in stillbirths' bones and cartilage. They found that cadmium concentrates in the stillbirths were ten times greater than the levels normally found in human bones. Lead levels were also raised. Low calcium and zinc were sometimes associated with these marked elevations. (Bryce-Smith, 1977)

Research has shown that lead and cadmium can also cause problems for the neonate. A much larger study by Bryce-Smith and his colleagues studied 36 elements. In 1981, Professor Bryce-Smith reported that for most of the elements being studied, the levels in foetal and maternal blood were about the same. Only in lead levels was there a difference, with the foetal level about 95% of the maternal. He explained this thus:

'This means that the placenta passes all elements, both nutrients and toxins, to the fetus from the maternal circulation with little or no selectivity or filtering effect. We can see no evidence for a significant barrier to protect the fetus from inorganic toxins such as mercury, arsenic, and antimony; and there is only a slight, but significant ($p=0.01$) barrier in the case of lead for normal births only.' (Bryce-Smith, 1979)

Having begun by analysing nine tissues, including maternal and foetal (umbilical) cord whole blood and serum, amniotic fluid, placenta, and scalp hair from the mother and neonate, later on they decided that the placental element levels showed the clearest correlations with indices of foetal development for supposedly 'normal' births. Thus it was with this tissue that they continued the investigation.

In the first written report on the final 37 elements studied, the researchers observed highly significant negative relationships between placental cadmium/lead levels and birth weight, head circumference and placental weight: **the higher the level of cadmium and lead, the smaller the birth weight, head circumference and placental weight**. There was a statistically significant positive correlation between placental cadmium and lead levels where birth weights were less than 3,000g. For higher birth weights, the correlation, though still positive, was not significant. Placental zinc showed significant relationships with

97

birth weights up to 3,000g and head circumference of less than 34cm i.e. the lower the level of zinc, the lower the birth weight and the smaller the head circumference.

With respect to other elements, there was 'a weak positive correlation between placental iron and head circumference, and stronger but negative correlations for chlorine, vanadium, and lanthanum.' However, placental levels of iron did not correlate with birth weight, nor were the iron levels or birth weights significantly raised in those mothers receiving iron supplements. Indeed, the results in iron and zinc led the researchers to suggest that more emphasis should be given to zinc supplementation than to iron. The final point made in the paper states that, 'In cases of cadmium, lead, and zinc, biological, neurobehavioral, and biosocial studies in which the levels of all three elements are measured may prove more informative than those involving single elements.' (Ward, 1987)

Much the same conclusion was reached by the researchers who conducted further investigation into lead, cadmium, and cognitive functioning. Looking at the protective effects of zinc and calcium against toxic metals, they found that higher zinc levels seemed to protect against the effects of cadmium, while calcium did the same against lead. They concluded: *The results suggest that the effects of heavy metal pollutants on cognitive function cannot be adequately assessed without concurrently evaluating the status of essential nutrients with which these toxins are known to interact metabolically.* (Lester, 1986)

Detoxifying the body

The preferred method of detoxification must be nutritional since it does not have the same potential for harmful side effects as drugs. EDTA (ethylenediaminetetraacetic acid) is sometimes used by doctors in acute poisoning but it has disadvantages as it also removes many essential minerals at the same time.

Vitamin C and zinc supplements were used successfully in reducing blood lead levels of psychiatric outpatients in one study. The treatment was also found to reduce blood copper levels. Subjects included some hyperactive children. (Lester, 1986)

Vitamin C has also been shown to lower cadmium levels in birds. (Sohler, 1977)

Calcium helps prevent absorption, as well as removing lead from the tissues. Vitamin D is necessary for calcium metabolism and to help displace lead from the bones. Vitamin B1, taken with a B-complex, provides protection against lead damage. Lecithin can also help in protection, while vitamin A helps to activate the enzymes needed for detoxification. Trace elements that are protective, in addition to zinc, include chromium, selenium and manganese. In the diet, peas, lentils and beans act as detoxifiers. Algin, found in seaweeds, attracts lead in the gut and carries it out of the body. Yoghurt, garlic, onions, bananas and fruits such as apples and pears which contain pectin (especially the pips) help to reduce absorption, as well as detoxifying. (Spivey Fox, 1975) Vitamin E may also reduce lead poisoning. (Nutrition Search Inc., 1979) In animal studies exposure to sunlight has been found to help remove toxic metals. (Kime, 1980)

At Foresight, once they have found levels that need detoxifying, they give their cleansing capsule 'Vitamin C and Garlic', with nicotinamide. They also give the dietary advice as above, and after four months they retest to see if the levels of toxins have fallen to acceptable levels. If not, you and they will continue a little longer, until they have. This way, the sperm and ovum that make the future baby become ready to do so.

Vitamin C, garlic, milk thistle, vitamins B1 and B12 have been formulated as a cleansing tablet 'Vitamin C with Garlic'. This is usually used in conjunction with nicotinamide, to enhance liver function, and magnesium, zinc and other cleansing minerals.

The Foresight vitamins and minerals have been specially formulated by the Foresight nutritional advisers for preconception, pregnancy and lactation to provide a balance of essential nutrients. These may be used in conjunction with other supplements, where need is indicated by the test results. The organisation has had over 30 years of experience in trace mineral supplementation to restore optimum levels and cleanse the toxic metals.

Ruth's story:

Ruth had a fantastic job as a picture restorer at the Fitzwilliam Museum in Cambridge. She left her home in North London each morning at 5.30 am to drop Tom, her husband, at his job in the City, and then she would drive to Cambridge. They had been trying for a baby for two years, but she was exhausted. Her husband worked very long hours so Ruth was left doing everything in the house as well as having a full-time job. She realised that she was going to have to change her lifestyle and give up her job if she was to get pregnant.

For the next year Ruth rested during the day, did a few chores, cooked dinner and went to bed at 9.00 pm. After a year passed she concluded that she was not going to get pregnant naturally. She had a session of IUI and her FSH levels were so high that it was decided that she was going to have to have IVF. Two embryos were implanted and Beatrice was born.

Two years passed with no further conception. It was then that Ruth contacted the La Leche League, who suggested Foresight. Ruth's hair mineral analysis revealed that both she and Tom were very low in essential minerals, especially zinc, cobalt and iron. Both Ruth and Tom were PhD chemists from Oxford who thought they were pretty healthy. They did not smoke, drink or go out for late nights, yet it 'never occurred' to them to check their nutrition levels.

Ruth's diet was very good as she was still breastfeeding Beatrice and it was a huge relief to both of them to know that they were taking the right supplements. These were checked every three months and adjusted as changes in their nutritional status were revealed. Although Tom struggled, Ruth was very strict in taking her supplements. Knowing that she was on the Foresight programme and having some acupuncture meant that she could relax a little. Three months later Ruth conceived again, and gave birth to her first Foresight baby, a little boy.

With two healthy children they plan to be 'using the Foresight programme again very soon'.

The longer I live, the more I hate the cruelty of animal testing, but at the same time, the more I realise the benefits that we could gain, as a species, if we just took on board what all the researchers have uncovered for us. All the work and suffering should not be in vain. I just question why have we all had to wait for so long? The research in the last few chapters was all done in the 1970–80s. Why is everybody not tested as a matter of course before every pregnancy? How long is it going to take us to get it right?

We are able to test for lead and all the other toxic metals. We are able to eliminate them. Even those 'in high places' are prepared to cede that hair analysis is a useful guide to toxic metals. When we get the toxic metal levels to an acceptable level before the conception takes place, I believe we see the human child as he/she was meant to be. Our 'case histories' include chess players, musicians with exceptional ability, scholarship winners, 'little people' with sunny natures, robust health and a zest for life. As a species, we human adults make the environment so problematic – children have the right to expect we sort this out for them.

Read on...

Essential Minerals

This section includes a lot of the work from our previous book, as it comprises some of the excellent research that was done in the 1970s and early 1980s into the role of specific nutrients in reproduction. Here and there it has been updated, or commented upon by myself!

So many of you said to me in our telephone conversations: 'But is it all really important? How do you know?' 'Why does zinc deficiency matter?' 'What does selenium actually do?' 'Will it really help my husband's sperm count?' 'My mother thinks you are just making money out of us.' 'My husband is very sceptical, I'm afraid. He isn't going to do it.' And so on. I was not making money out of you. I worked voluntarily for 33 years! My motivation was to be sure that you all have healthy babies. **I love babies**. That is the momentum behind Foresight. Read on!

• Calcium

Calcium is needed for the formation of strong bones and teeth, and for controlling blood clotting mechanisms and proper nerve and muscle function. Other functions include assisting in muscle growth and strength, maintaining blood balance and acting as a catalyst in enzyme reactions. It is also said to help protect against allergies, viruses and tooth decay.

Calcium can sometimes run up very high. I find this usually relates directly to the level of calcium in the water or dust, so it is a natural happening rather than a metabolic fault. In the hair, the ratio of magnesium to calcium should be 1:10, so if the ratio of magnesium is lower than 1:10, we give some extra magnesium. This helps the body use the calcium as it should. High calcium without the balancing magnesium can be at a bit of a loose end in the body, and can form into kidney stones, gallstones etc. Magnesium will help to pack it into the bones, joints etc. where it is meant to be. This also helps to guard against arthritis, osteoporosis etc.

For pregnancy, we need plenty of calcium as we women are expected to build a little skeleton approximately 21–22 inches long ('unfolded', a newborn baby is approximately one third as tall as its mother), and a skull (containing a good working brain) of about 13–14 inches round (nearly two thirds the size of its mother's skull). All to be done in *nine months*! The deadline is absolute. It is not under our control.

So, calcium is vital for the growing of the foetus and the well-being of the mother. Davies recommends giving it, in conjunction with vitamin D, during labour to ease pain. It can ease leg cramps, and help sleeping. Calcium is lost from the bones during bed rest and also while on high protein diets. People affected will need to supplement the diet and to choose foods with high levels.

Lack of calcium can cause rickets, allergy, tooth decay, insomnia, back pain, osteoporosis, osteomalacia, irritability, nervousness, tension, uneven heartbeat, indigestion, stomach cramps and spasms, constipation, premenstrual tension, and cramping of the uterus (i.e. very painful periods). (Davies 1954, Davies 1974, Pitkin 1975, Nutrition Search Inc. 1979, Passwater 1983)

Unfortunately, due to modern farming practices and what is called 'increased efficiency in dairying', cows are now milked while they are pregnant. At this time, the milk contains the hormone that releases calcium from the bones, in order to give it to the growing calf they are gestating. This may make the milk less helpful as a source of calcium as once released, it can be excreted! We find that often people who consume a lot of dairy products are very low in calcium (and very surprised by this). Unfortunately, even people producing organic milk now use their cows in this way.

Foetal deficiency: Government documents state: 'signs of calcium deficiency are manifest in the bones and teeth of all young animal species, including humans. Effects include stunted growth, poor quality bones and teeth, and bone malformation.'

Rickets, tooth decay and a high raised palate. The high raised palate leads to cramping of the middle brain, possibly lessening the blood supply and subsequently leading to learning difficulties like dyslexia. (See Dr June Sharpe's study in Chapter 2)

Low levels in the baby are associated with low birth weight and low scores on developmental tests. Premature babies tend to have low levels.

Good sources: Dairy products, kelp, carob, bone broth, green vegetables, Brazil nuts, hazelnuts, almonds, dolomite, brewer's yeast.

Inhibitors: Foods containing oxalic acid (sesame seed hulls, rhubarb, spinach) and phytic acid (soda, unsoaked muesli and unleavened bread) can reduce availability.

Calcium is best taken with vitamins A, C, D, essential fatty acids, iron, magnesium and phosphorus. (Nutrition Search Inc., 1979)

- **Magnesium**

Magnesium is needed for the production and transfer of energy, muscle contraction, proper nerve function, protein synthesis, the functioning of many enzymes and the absorption and use of calcium.

Catherine's story:

In June, just two months after the wedding, they decided to start a family. By September, Catherine had lost her baby due to a 'blighted ovum'. Six months later, another miscarriage came at about seven weeks. Devastation, loss of confidence and a reluctance to get pregnant again gripped Catherine. As the months rolled on, Catherine read about Foresight, sent off for the Foresight Information Pack and, with her husband, went straight on to the programme.

The first hair mineral analysis revealed that her husband had raised levels of heavy metals aluminium, lead and mercury. His levels of zinc, calcium, magnesium and selenium were very low. Catherine's analysis revealed that she too had raised levels of lead and mercury and her magnesium levels were very low. A supplement programme was devised to rectify heavy metal toxicity and to increase the levels of important vitamins and minerals for each of them.

Six months later, after missing a period, a pregnancy test proved positive. Now she was scared – scared of miscarrying again and worried that the stress from being scared was affecting her pregnancy. She was too scared to be excited and too scared to feel pregnant until she got over the three-month barrier. Following the Foresight programme throughout the pregnancy, and having reflexology, the pregnancy held and a son was born weighing 6 lb 13 oz. He was followed a year or so later by a baby girl at 8 lb 7 oz.

'It made such sense. There was a reason for the miscarriages. I definitely felt healthy and I was actually doing something positive to ensure a safe pregnancy. If we were to have a third baby, I would definitely use Foresight again'.

Deficiencies cause involuntary muscle movements, such as spasms and twitching, convulsions, insomnia, panic attack, allergy, impaired protein synthesis, premenstrual tension, painful periods, poor memory, confusion, disorientation, hyperactivity, irritability, anxiety, nightmares, increased sensitivity to noise, irregular heartbeat, leg and foot cramps, bedwetting and depression. Pregnancy aggravates any deficiency.

A deficiency is said to contribute to painful uterine contractions at the end of pregnancy. It may also be associated with miscarriage or premature birth. Rats fed low-magnesium diets give birth to smaller pups with a higher rate of congenital deformities. They also develop calcium deposits and other abnormalities in the heart cells. Stones may form in the kidneys. Women with low levels tend to abort more or have low birth weight babies. (Pfeiffer 1978, Davis 1974, Hurley 1976, Spatling 1988) Magnesium deficiency is very common. (Nutrition Search Inc., 1979)

Foetal deficiency: Congenital abnormalities, calcium deposits, anorexia (failure to suck), convulsions and perinatal death. There is a condition, Williams syndrome, where calcium is found to be deposited in the brain, causing mental retardation. It would be interesting to know if this has been linked to lack of magnesium.

Good sources: Nuts, kelp, green vegetables, seafoods, eggs, milk, whole grains, dolomite. Epsom salts can be added to bath water to get absorption through the skin.

Magnesium is best taken with vitamins B6, C, D, calcium, phosphorus, protein. (Nutrition Search Inc., 1979)

• Potassium

Potassium is needed to regulate blood pH, to acidify urine, and for proper nerve and muscle functioning. It is involved in the utilisation of enzymes. It may be involved in bone calcification. Together with sodium, it maintains the fluid balance in the body and may help the transportation of nutrients into the cells. It is necessary for growth.

A deficiency causes disorientation, listlessness, low blood sugar, nervous irritability, insomnia, oedema, headaches, irregular heartbeat, bone and joint pain, constipation, cramping of muscles, weakness and fatigue. It is linked to poor sperm motility. In the embryo, it may cause abnormalities in the kidneys. Deficiency may result from too much sodium chloride (salt), too little fruit and vegetables, some diseases and some medical treatments.

Potassium chloride has been used successfully in the treatment of colic and diarrhoea in adults as well as children. (Passwater 1983, Nutrition Search Inc. 1979, Hurley 1976)

Foetal deficiency: Possibly low blood sugar, which will lead to disinclination to suck, and/or constipation in the newborn.

According to the EVM (Government) Report 2008, potassium exerts a beneficial effect on hypertension by lowering blood pressure. Potassium is a co-factor of many enzymes and is required for secretion of insulin by the pancreas. Most potassium is found in muscle and the skeleton. Also, there are high concentrations in the blood, central nervous system, intestine, liver, lungs and skin. Keeping levels steady may help to prevent diabetes.

Over-high levels of potassium and sodium together in the hair can indicate some interruption of liver and kidney function. We suggest checking for a urine infection when we see this. However, they will also be present if the liver and kidneys are stressed by clearing toxic metals, such as lead. If this is the cause, when the toxic metal has gone from the system, the potassium and sodium levels will settle back to normal. (Lodge-Rees, 1984)

Good sources: Brewer's yeast, wheat germ, whole grains, vegetables, fruit, nuts, milk, fish, shellfish, beef, chicken, turkey, liver. Potassium is best taken with vitamin B6 and sodium. (Nutrition Search Inc., 1979)

• Chromium

Chromium is needed for the regulation of the glucose tolerance factor, in combination with nicotinic acid and some proteins. Glucose is required for every bodily function – it is the body's fuel. Chromium is also necessary for the synthesis of fatty acids and cholesterol.

A deficiency may be linked with heart disease. (Passwater, 1983) It can lead to poor sugar handling, which can contribute to reactive hypoglycaemia, causing sugar cravings, which can lead to diabetes and/or obesity and/or alcoholism. Sugar and alcohol consumption will reduce chromium. Deficiency has also been linked to arteriosclerosis and hypertension.

Chromium is not easily absorbed, though it is readily removed from the body. Even a small deficiency will be serious.

Foetal deficiency: It has been linked to eye abnormalities, and possible later development of diabetes.

Good sources: Brewer's yeast, black pepper, liver, whole grains, wheat germ, vegetables, butter, molasses.

• Cobalt

Cobalt is an essential part of vitamin B12. There is a possible relationship between cobalt and iodine. It is necessary in B12 for the normal function of all cells, but especially red blood cells, and has been used in the treatment of pernicious anaemia. It activates some enzymes. Deficiency is associated with pernicious anaemia and maybe with slow growth and goitre. (Underwood 1977, Nutrition Search Inc. 1979) It can be present where there is a vitamin B12 deficiency in vegans and vegetarians, or in people eating a diet high in refined carbohydrates, or consuming much alcohol.

Cobalt is present in blue paints/colourings and high levels are sometimes seen in people using blue glasses and/or blue-patterned plates. We are not sure how much this matters, but usually advise them to change to another type of crockery or glassware in case it is harmful.

Good sources: Although it is said that cobalt can only be taken by humans in the form of vitamin B12, Underwood points out that organ meats and muscle meats each contain more than can be accounted for as a part of vitamin B12. Green leafy vegetables are a rich source if the soil they were grown in was rich; other sources include meats, brewer's yeast, seafood, nuts, fruit and whole grains.

Foresight supplements with B12 to enhance levels of cobalt. Cobalt is more effective when taken with copper, iron and zinc. (Nutrition Search Inc., 1979)

• Copper

Copper aids the development of brain, bones, nerves and connective tissue. It is involved in many enzyme systems, and is essential in the production of RNA. In practice it is the only necessary mineral that goes much above the normal value and has sometimes to be brought down. This is directly due to copper water pipes, or occasionally to the use of copper-containing algaecides in swimming pools. Use of the contraceptive pill (and other hormonal drugs) causes women to retain copper, so this compounds the hazards. Any of these factors may just overwhelm the normal homeostatic mechanisms and give the body more copper than it can cope with. The level of copper has to be brought back to normal before the start of the pregnancy or it can prevent conception, or cause miscarriage or premature birth.

It is, however, an essential mineral. Deficiency can cause porous bones, loss of hair, demyelination, heart damage and anaemia.

In the foetus of a number of animals, copper deficiency can result in depressed growth rate, de-pigmentation, anaemia, fine and fragile bones, ataxia, small brain and perinatal mortality. In rats, infertility has been noted. Skeletal and cardiovascular defects, central nervous system disorders, and steely wool hair (failure of melanin formation) have also been reported. (Nutrition Search Inc. 1979, Passwater 1983, Underwood 1977)

At this moment in time, 2013, however, copper deficiency is extremely rare, and copper in excess is common and can be toxic.

While copper water pipes are the norm, it is unlikely that copper deficiency will be seen. Copper excess is present in about 1 couple in 10 who come to Foresight. Almost always this can be corrected within four months to a year, although there have been two exceptions in couples where the drinking water level was exceptionally high. This can be due to the soil being very acidic, or due to corroding pipes that have been soldered together with a lead-containing solder. Heating water in an Ascot (or similar) water heater can add to the copper. If you have been using a water filter for several weeks and see the white contents of the cartridge change to bluish green, there is likely to be a significantly high level of copper and the water should be checked. Many people have excess copper in their bodies due to drinking or bathing in water with a very high level. When there is a blue-green stain on the surface where a tap has been dripping, this is verdigris and will indicate the water is quite high in copper. We normally suggest that tap water from all sources used is tested if either partner has a hair level of over 30 ppm. Then we can tell if any taps are the source and, if so, which ones. There are now so many different types of filter on the market, the best plan is to go on the internet and look for one that suits the problem. For example, in some cases a 'whole house' filter is needed, in other houses it may just be the shower or a single tap. If there are high levels of lead and copper together, then there may be a corroding pipe. This is usually due to a position where two pieces of copper piping are joined with a lead-containing solder, or the old lead connecting pipe running from the mains to new copper piping at the boundary stop-cock has been left in place. (This is illegal but quite often you find one still there!) You need a plumber to advise you.

However, as people become more aware of this, ABS plastic is being used. So we may need to be more aware of the symptoms of copper deficiency in the future, as the environment changes for certain people. Meanwhile we have to soldier on. There are stainless steel and fibreglass tanks available, along with ABS plastic pipes, which are hard plastic and are said not to leak dioxins into the water.

Copper kettles, pans and jewellery are occasionally other sources. There may be external contamination of hair samples by some henna dyes and rinses, and from swimming-pool water where the pool has been treated with a copper-containing algaecide. For an accurate hair reading cease the contamination for six weeks before having a hair mineral analysis.

Good sources: Shellfish, Brazil nuts, organ meats, dried legumes, dried stone fruits and green vegetables. It is best taken with cobalt, iron and zinc. (Nutrition Search Inc., 1979)

Important things to know: If you are a woman, the top level of copper you need in your drinking water – or bathing water – is 0.2 ppm. You absorb copper as you drink, and also when you bath. In women, copper can accumulate in the ovaries, where it is a stimulant. You do not need to be short of copper, as the ovary needs it to ovulate, but you do not want to **overload** it, as this can be a cause of cancer, particularly breast or ovarian cancer, or of failure to ovulate. I often see high copper in women struggling with obesity. As it could stimulate the ovaries to produce extra oestrogens, it could lie behind some cases of obesity. This needs further study. Many women find their weight rises, without changes in diet or exercise patterns, when they go on the pill, and after childbirth. This is all linked to the hormones being jiggled around, and high levels of copper may be relevant.

The legal limit for copper in the water was set at 3 ppm. This, I suspect, was to avoid any trouble for the water authorities! It is about 15 times what women really need. This all urgently needs to be studied and the limit to be revised. We suggest changes for the level not to be over 0.2 ppm.

As we said earlier, excessive levels of copper may be embryo-toxic or teratogenic (they can make the baby ill, cause a malformation or damage the brain). They are known to produce behavioural symptoms, such as uncontrollable rages, and are linked with pre-eclamptic toxaemia in the mother. Copper levels rise naturally during pregnancy, so if a woman conceives with a raised level she is at risk of overloading her body. This can lead to a premature birth. The ratio of copper to zinc in the blood is normally 1:14–17. (Carl Pfeiffer, New Jersey 1978 Bert Vallee, Harvard University Medical School 1965) Professor Bert Vallee, working with small rodents, found that in the third trimester of pregnancy the zinc was transferred into the placenta at an increasing rate, and therefore the ratio of copper to zinc increased in the circulating blood. Once the copper had risen to a certain level in relation to the zinc, then this stimulated the brain, and the phenomenon of birth started to take place.

Over the last 30 years we have confirmed that the level of copper rises in the hair as the pregnancy progresses. An 'old wives' tale' is that raspberry leaf tea will bring on labour if the baby is overdue. Raspberry leaf tea contains a lot of copper. (Old wives often knew a thing or two!) Another theory is that scrubbing and then sucking a copper coin will have an effect. Either/both are certainly worth a try before resorting to injections of hormones, pessaries, or having 'the waters' artificially broken.

Alison's story:

Any long-term debilitating illness is distressing, especially so when you are contemplating starting a family. Alison's injury had left her with damaged nerves in both arms and neck. How could she cope with a baby? Babies were so demanding and she was very ill.

A naturopath was consulted and suggested that her mercury fillings be removed and that she see a nutritional therapist. Although the mercury fillings removal did not make her feel much stronger, she and her husband decided to get on with starting a family.

The nutritional therapist, who happened to be a Foresight practitioner, put Alison on to the Foresight programme which included a diet that eliminated foods identified through a food intolerance test.

Hair mineral analysis revealed neither of them had any heavy metal toxicity but both husband and wife were generally low in most minerals. It took four hair tests before their mineral levels were good enough for Nim to advise them to go ahead. Alison conceived within a month and later gave birth to a beautiful baby girl weighing 7 lb 9.5 oz with an Apgar of 9.

'The birth was the most amazing thing. Everything and more than you could expect.'

'Advice given by Foresight was extremely professional and very friendly.'

Many girls with a high copper level and a history of infertility come to us at Foresight. As we increase the levels of zinc, manganese and selenium, the copper level tends to normalise. However, we do advise testing the tap water. Changing the pipes does sound a bit drastic, but believe me, anything is better than risking a very premature birth.

High copper levels in the woman can lead to post-partum depression, and have been linked to premature birth in a number of animal studies. Raised levels are associated with low levels of manganese and zinc, deficiencies of which are known to cause birth defects. (Elkington 1985, Pfeiffer 1978, Norwood 1980,

Vallee 1965) Foresight recommends a hair reading of no more than 18–24 ppm to start a pregnancy.

Copper is a brain stimulant. (Pfeiffer, Pfeiffer and la Mola, Pfeiffer and Hoffer) It can lead to feelings of euphoria, and heightened emotions of all descriptions. Anybody who has ever given birth will know we are all flying high for the first few hours after birth and this must be one of the reasons why a home birth must be such a blissful experience – for the baby as well, I would guess. Also, this was why the baby being taken to cry its little heart out at the far end of a long hospital corridor (as was the case 50 years ago) was such agony.

However, in the laboratories, rodents eat the placentas where all the zinc has been stored, and within 96 hours of birth, their copper/zinc levels are all back to normal balance. Evidently, nature reckons about four days of being high as a kite is enough to make sure of the mother-baby bonding, and that the long-term relationship is ensured.

It is interesting that the Native American culture allows the mother to spend 19 days in her own tepee, being waited on by female relatives, as a recovery/milk stabilising/baby bonding period.

I feel we could learn a lot from all of this. I think all new mothers would benefit enormously from the rebalancing of zinc levels. While we have copper water pipes I do not think this will happen automatically. So I would suggest, unless people are already on a comprehensive Foresight programme, they take at least 60 mg zinc a day for ten days following birth. This also helps to ensure good, satisfying breast milk, and then the baby sleeps well, which is always a mercy!

Post-partum depression is total exhaustion plus excess copper chasing much-needed zinc/manganese out of the system. Rat mothers who are short of zinc or manganese desert the scene, and go down to the far corner of the cage and roll up in a ball. They do not want to feed their pups, clean them up, or retrieve them if they fall out of the nest. If nobody intervenes, the pups are left to die. Presumably no lactation occurs.

Changes in 'fashion' and 'culture' are much more led by environmental factors impinging on brain biochemistry than by philosophers, politicians, writers or whoever. If the zinc galvanised plumbing on which we won the war had been left in place – what a different world we would be living in! *Think on,* all you young ones! And take more zinc!

• Iodine

Iodine is necessary for the formation of thyroxin and triiodothyronine, hormones produced by the thyroid. Thyroxin is necessary for growth, mental and physical development and the maintenance of health. Most people are aware that too little iodine can cause goitres, but a deficiency is also associated with fatigue, lethargy, susceptibility to cold, loss of interest in sex, slow development of the sex organs, anorexia, slow pulse, low blood pressure, rapid weight gain, high blood cholesterol, death from heart disease and cancer of the thyroid.

Deficiency in the pregnancy can result in cretinism in children, a congenital disease with mental and physical retardation. However, if iodine is given soon after birth, many of the symptoms are reversible. (Passwater 1983, Nutrition Search Inc. 1979, Davis 1974, Pharaoh 1971)

Good sources include water, iodised salt, watercress, onions, kelp, shellfish, and mushrooms and dark leafy vegetables if they are grown on soil rich in iodine.

Too much iodine can also have serious consequences for health. (Underwood 1977, Nutrition Search Inc. 1979)

• Iron

Iron is needed to make haemoglobin, the substance in the red blood cells, which carries oxygen in the blood. It also aids resistance to infection. It helps supply oxygen to the muscles. It helps in protein digestion and also in respiratory function.

Iron requirements increase in pregnancy because the number of red blood cells increases by 30%. Since it is thought that most women do not have a large enough store before pregnancy, many women are given supplements. This can be quite unsatisfactory if other nutrients are not given as well, since iron is not absorbed well without vitamin C and needs to work with other vitamins and minerals. Also, iron given alone can cause loss of other essential minerals, such as zinc, manganese, chromium, selenium and cobalt.

It is quite common for pregnant women to be 'diagnosed' as short of iron on the strength of a blood test, when this may not be the case. In early pregnancy, women are often very thirsty, and drink a lot of water. The blood is then quite diluted for a short while. Then the water is taken into the placenta and used to make 'the waters' (amniotic fluid). Then the blood will return to normal.

The huge doses of NHS iron (200 mg or 150 mg of ferrous sulphate) usually make women feel sick and make them horrendously constipated (which is hugely uncomfortable and difficult to manage in pregnancy). Ferrous sulphate is the least absorbable form of iron in any case. However, in 2008 NHS practices were being reviewed by the EVM and smaller doses of iron were being suggested. Possibly in the region of 60 mg. This is better, but still too high.

We find about half the people who come to us prior to pregnancy have some shortage of iron. We use our own tablets giving 7 mg iron amino acid chelate. Thus we can give 7 mg or 14 mg, according to what they need, and one of these doses will achieve adequate iron levels, without the side effects.

Shortage of iron can lead to weakness, excessive fatigue, depression, headache, pallor, lack of appetite, mental confusion and poor memory. Iron-deficient people will absorb two to three times more lead than non-deficient people. Deficiency can occur in women due to losses during menstruation. Deficiency is not quite so common in men, but it does occur. Also it is often present in children, particularly if they are eating a diet which includes white flour and white sugar.

In the foetus, severe iron deficiency can cause eye defects, slow growth, bone defects, brain defects and neonatal mortality. (Nutrition Search Inc. 1979, Pitkin 1972, Gibbs 1980, Lesser 1980, Passwater 1983, Davis 1974, Watson 1980, Oberleas 1972)

Blood donors of both sexes are at risk of iron deficiency, so giving blood when you are planning a pregnancy should be avoided.

The usual test for iron is using blood. However, since the body will draw on its stores from the tissues and bone to maintain the amount circulating in the body, blood is not the best way of checking levels, so Foresight prefers to use hair samples.

Good sources: Organ meats, kelp, brewer's yeast, molasses, wheat germ, beans, nuts, dried fruit, poultry, fish, almonds, parsley, egg yolk, lean meats, whole grains, vegetables. The iron of egg yolk is poorly absorbed unless taken with a food containing vitamin C. Thus, a glass of fresh orange juice with an egg makes it a good source of iron. (Nutrition Search Inc., 1979)

- **Manganese**

Manganese is needed for numerous enzyme reactions, bone growth and development, lipid metabolism, and nerve function. It is necessary in the formation of thyroxin (see iodine) and in blood clotting. It has been found to contribute to a mother's maternal instincts and love, through its role in certain enzymes. A deficiency has been found to cause epilepsy, depression and schizophrenia. (Pfeiffer & La Mola)

Manganese is sometimes very high, often in combination with highish lead. Usually this will be from scraping down paint. The powers-that-be made lead in paint illegal in the 1960s, and replaced it with manganese. This was a good development but older houses stayed full of lead paint, of course, and evidently it is not yet all scraped off nationwide! Therefore, we quite often see high levels of lead and manganese together in the hair of DIY enthusiasts! Manganese is not a toxic metal, but I am never too happy about something being wildly out of the average range, so I would always wear a mask and rubber gloves when you scrape off, whatever you are uncovering!

Nonetheless, deficiency is the more serious hazard, and more usual.

Although the function of manganese in reproduction is not understood, there is no doubt that a deficiency can affect foetal development. In a study of hair levels of manganese, babies with congenital malformations had significantly lower levels of manganese than babies without malformation. (Saner, 1985) There were also similarly significant differences in the mineral levels of the mothers' hair. (Underwood, O & C)

In rats it has been shown that in the least severe stage of deficiency, there is an increase in the number of offspring born with ataxia. In the second, more serious stage, the young are born dead or die shortly after birth, while in the third, most serious stage, the animal will not mate, and sterility results. This is also seen in hens. In the male rat and rabbit with severe deficiency there is sterility, and also absence of sex drive, in association with degeneration of the seminal tubes and lack of spermatozoa. In the young there may be faulty cartilage and bone matrix formation, and heart and neural function problems. Animals from mothers who are deficient show difficulty with behavioural tasks. (Williams 1973, Pfeiffer 1978, Underwood 1977, Oberleas 1972, Saner 1985, Riopelle and Hubard)

Foetal deficiency: Malformation of the inner ear (impaired hearing), impaired balance, ataxia, bone malformation, lack of coordination, head retraction, tremor, lack of righting reflex, epilepsy.

It was also noted by Pfeiffer, and by Oberleas and Caldwell, that lack of manganese could lead to rejection of the baby by the mother. This is too often overlooked. It has a major bearing on post-partum depression. It needs to be remembered that **organophosphate pesticides can inhibit the uptake of manganese by the blood**, due to their inhibition of function of the choline-containing enzymes which are necessary for the transfer of manganese from the gut to the blood. It is therefore **particularly important** to avoid these noxious chemicals during pregnancy and around the time of birth.

Unfortunately a lot of shop-bought cut flowers are rather heavily treated with bug-killers. We are trying to encourage people to grow their own, and florists to stock those that are organically grown. Beware of you and the baby being surrounded by commercially grown floral tributes, however lovingly presented!

Try to raise awareness of the dangers of pesticides. As new parents, you are particularly likely to be getting together a new home with new carpets, furnishings and perhaps even bedding. It is possible to get these chemical-free from places such as Healthy House, Green Fibres, Blendworth and others. People need to know this. Other manufacturers need to be informed so that organic becomes the norm.

Manganese is the only trace element that carries oxygen to the mitochondria of the brain cell. The mitochondria form the small inner part of the cell that organises how it works. Without oxygen this does not function properly. It seems likely that the widespread use of OPs on our food (as well as aluminium contamination) is at least partially responsible for the huge rise in cases of Alzheimer's disease. This does need further research urgently. Meanwhile, those of us who **think** buy organic food!

Good sources: Nuts, whole grains, seeds, leafy green vegetables, brewer's yeast, egg, liver, parsley, thyme, cloves, ginger, tea.

It is best taken with vitamins B1, E, calcium, phosphorus and choline. (Nutrition Search Inc., 1979)

- **Nickel**

Nickel is found in high concentrations in DNA and RNA and in all the body's tissues and fluids. Most of the work on it has been focused on animals. It is needed for the action in the enzyme urease. In studies, deficiencies have been linked with reproductive failures, early infant deaths, and growth problems. In the rat, it is associated with the metabolism of copper and manganese. It may have a role in hormonal control and as an enzyme co-factor. High levels are found in the blood of patients who have suffered heart attacks. It is thought that the damaged heart muscles release the nickel. Levels are decreased in those with cirrhosis of the liver or chronic uraemia. Deficiency is found to have a negative influence on growth and life expectancy and to impair iron metabolism. (Underwood 1977, Pfeiffer 1975, Neilson 1984, Anke undated, Pfeiffer 1978, Spears 1984)

Foetal deficiency: (in animal studies) Heart defects, kidney defects, liver defects, neonatal death. (Nielson, Anke) EVM

(Government) papers say deficiency is associated with reduced growth, impaired reproductive function and reduced haematopoiesis. As lambs and piglets with nickel deficiency were seen to die early, it may be associated with cot death.

Good sources include organ meats, dry beans, lentils, nuts, buckwheat, grains and vegetables and kelp supplements.

Nickel jewellery is occasionally found to cause dermatitis.

• Phosphorus

Phosphorus is the second most abundant mineral in the body, being found in every cell. As it functions with calcium, both being the main constituents of bone, it is important that its balance with calcium be maintained. It plays a part in almost every chemical reaction in the body, in the utilisation of carbohydrates, proteins and fats, in muscle and nerve function, digestion, kidney function, and proper skeletal growth. It is found in important substances called phospholipids, which break up and transport fats and fatty acids. Among their many functions is regulating the promotion of the secretion of glandular hormones.

Deficiency is rare, since it is found in artificial fertilisers. It is also a common ingredient in many food additives and soft drinks. The right way to ensure that it is balanced with calcium and other minerals is to obtain it from the whole foods. (Pfeiffer 1978, Nutrition Search Inc. 1979, Davis 1974)

Good sources: Brewer's yeast, whole grains, bread, cereals, meat, fish, poultry, eggs, seeds, nuts.

Phosphorus is best absorbed when it is eaten as part of food containing vitamins A, D, essential fatty acids, calcium, iron, manganese and protein. (Nutrition Search Inc., 1979)

• Selenium

Selenium, like vitamin E, with which it is associated in some functions, is a powerful anti-oxidant which helps to prevent chromosomal damage in tissue culture. Such damage is associated with birth defects and cancers. It is a vital part of an important enzyme which helps the body to fight infections. In animals and chickens, deficiencies are associated with slow growth, cataracts, infertility, loss of hair and feathers, degeneration, nutritional muscular dystrophy, swelling and haemorrhages, pancreatic atrophy, and liver necrosis. Also seen is increased sensitivity to inhaled allergens, linked to asthma and rhinitis. It is also linked with muscle weakness. In human cell culture selenium is required for growth, so it will be necessary for normal growth. Selenium will combine with toxic metals such as cadmium to remove them from the body, so it is useful for detoxifying. It may be important in preventing cot deaths. In the USA in the 1970s about a quarter of the babies who died each year were found to be deficient in selenium and/or vitamin E. Most of them were bottle-fed. (Pfeiffer 1978, Underwood 1977) Fluoride is known to be antagonistic to selenium. The EVM report states that there are beneficial effects of selenium intake on AIDS symptoms, male fertility, skin disorders, anxiety and asthma.

When I heard of this experiment I took from my files the hair analyses of the youngest three Down's syndrome children I had tested (Ages 11 months to 2 ½ years). All three had no measurable selenium in the hair. I then looked at the hair analyses of three mothers who had previously given birth to Down's Syndrome babies. Two had almost no measurable selenium; the third had a low level of selenium, but her child was by then 7 years old, so she had possibly had time to make up some of the deficiency.

Another finding we seem to make quite consistently with the Down's Syndrome children, when tiny, is that they have a high level of toxic metals. This is usually lead, cadmium or aluminium, but I have seen one over-high copper. Any of these metals, if way out of line, could use up the selenium, as the body uses selenium to clear the toxic metals.

I have heard of three half-Chinese Merseyside children with Down's Syndrome whose Chinese fathers all came from a part of China where the soil is lacking in selenium. The mothers in each case were English.

This evidence is anecdotal, but all points to the involvement of selenium deficiency compounded/caused by a high level of toxic metal in the body.

American research has linked low selenium in the mother with increased risk of chromosomal damage, which can lead to Down's syndrome, Patau syndrome or Edwards syndrome in the baby. For this reason we are meticulous in obtaining an optimum level of selenium prior to conception, especially in our older mothers. As fluoride is antagonistic to selenium, we also suggest using fluoride-free toothpaste, and not drinking the tap water if it has been fluoridated. Adequate selenium levels have been found to be essential to sperm development.

Anti-dandruff selenium-containing shampoos, however, if used in the bath, or more often than the makers recommend, can produce an excess of selenium in the body which can drive down other needed minerals. For this reason they should be used with caution. They are also liable to confuse the hair analysis, so we often have to reject the findings and ask for another sample in eight weeks' time, when the hair has grown sufficiently to give us an uncontaminated sample. This can be very frustrating for keen prospective parents!

The upside of this is that a footbath with a selenium shampoo in it can help to raise the levels if they are low in the hair (but do not use on the hair as this will confuse the analysis!) It is possible that some Xerox copying machines can also produce selenium in the atmosphere.

Good sources: Butter, smoked herring, wheat germ, Brazil nuts, brewer's yeast, whole grains, garlic, fish offal, eggs, cereal and liver. For the baby, human milk is said to be an excellent source.

Selenium is most effective when taken with vitamin E. (Nutrition Search Inc., 1979)

- **Silicon**

Silicon is critical in the formation of connective tissues, bones, the placenta, arteries and skin, keeping it impermeable. It has been found to be essential for growth and skeletal development in rats and chickens. (Underwood 1977, Passwater 1973)

Good sources: whole grains, wholemeal bread, alfalfa, vegetables (especially the skins), pectin and hard water.

- **Vanadium**

Vanadium is present in most tissues in the body and is rapidly excreted into urine. It is thought to exert some influence on lipid metabolism by inhibiting cholesterol formation. It is part of the natural circulatory regulation system. Deficiency in animals results in impaired bone development, reduced growth, disturbance of blood metabolism, decreased reproduction and increased perinatal mortality, and reduced fertility in subsequent generations. (Underwood 1977, Nielson 1984)

Good sources: Buckwheat, parsley, eggs, sunflower seed oil, olive oil, olives, rice, green beans, vegetables.

- **Zinc**

Zinc is needed for the health and maintenance of hormone levels, bones, muscles, sperm and ova, also eyes, organs and teeth. It is important in healing. It is needed for the functioning of at least 200 enzymes. It is an important component of semen. It is necessary to stabilise RNA. It is needed in vitamin A metabolism. It is essential for brain development and function. Caldwell and Oberleas have shown in rats that *'even a mild zinc deficiency has a potential influence on behaviour, despite an apparently adequate protein level in the diet.'*

Zinc can increase the size of the penis and testes in growing boys. It also increases sperm motility and helps to prevent impotence. Zinc-deficient sperm are unable to penetrate the ova.

Lack of zinc is associated with loss of the senses of taste and smell, both of which affect appetite. This can be a major contributing cause of anorexia, also 'food fighting' in toddlers. Probably a wise strategy of nature's to prevent the child eating food for which the digestive tract does not have the required enzymes. Each enzyme needs a co-factor to 'make it work', and many different enzymes need zinc (I believe it is over 200). The intestine is lined with alkaline phosphatase, which is a zinc-dependent enzyme. It is not a good idea to try to force children to eat – it is upsetting for both parties and causes tension at mealtimes, which prolongs the problem. It is better to give them zinc and B-complex vitamins, (in drops) and let the natural appetite return.

In animals who have lacked zinc in the womb, eye problems, high rates of miscarriage (resorption), and, in the surviving babies, brain malformation, cleft palate, cleft lip, club feet, stillbirth and urinary-genital abnormalities have been found. Low levels in maternal rats have been associated with learning problems and behavioural problems in their offspring (i.e. they cannot find their way out of mazes, and become aggressive and panicky). With all the concern about a general weakening of the immune system, it is worrying to note that in an experiment with mice, damage occurred to the immune system of offspring whose mothers were zinc-deficient. The damage persisted even when supplements of zinc were given.

Low zinc status in the female rat can result in lack of ovulation and menstruation. In humans it is a factor in infertility, and low birth weight. Low plasma levels of zinc in mid-pregnancy have been associated with more complications at delivery and a high incidence of malformations.

Deficiency also inhibits vitamin A metabolism. Due to this there is inhibition of the immune system, and children will suffer more allergies and more infections, and infections will be more serious. Deficiencies have been found in children with learning disabilities, especially dyslexia and hyperactivity. Low levels of zinc were found in the hair of children suffering from anorexia, poor growth and hypogeusia (loss of taste). (Sandstead 1984, Pfeiffer 1978, Crosby 1977, Crawford 1975, Caldwell 1969, Bryce-Smith 1986, Hurley 1969, Jameson 1984, Ward 1987, Lazebnik 1988, Grant 1985, Hambidge 1972, Nutrition Search Inc. 1979) We always see low levels of zinc and manganese in children suffering from autism. The condition improves as these are corrected. The response varies, but in most cases, it is well worth the effort involved.

The EVM report stated: Zinc is an essential constituent of more than 200 metalo-enzymes. Zinc deficiency results in poor prenatal development, growth retardation, impaired nerve conduction, and nerve damage, reproductive failure, dermatitis, hair loss, diarrhoea, loss of appetite, loss of taste and smell, anaemia, susceptibility to infections, delayed wound healing and macular degeneration (which will lead to impaired sight). (NB: Despite the above, no recommendations were given for national testing or supplementation!)

Zinc supplementation will help with lowering excess levels of copper and lead. As mentioned before, these are very commonly seen due to copper plumbing soldered together with a solder containing lead. Although this is now illegal, the joins were never removed from houses where this had been done. So, by now, the pipes have corroded and are releasing both lead and copper into the water.

When these minerals appear together in the hair (which we see several times a week, or sometimes it is just high copper), we advise they test the water from all over the house. Sometimes it is just the shower – it is useful to know what is coming from where. We found one high copper level was due to a kettle with a copper element. (If it is copper alone it is sometimes from a swimming pool, due to the copper-containing algaecide.) Wherever it is coming from, this needs to be detected and corrected, or it will not be possible to get the zinc level to rise sufficiently. Copper and lead contamination will continually lower it again.

Filters can be obtained and fitted. Pipes can be changed to ABS plastics. The zinc/copper balance is the most important factor in restoring menstruation or ovulation, and also in raising the sperm count to a viable level. I often say to couples, 'You don't need a doctor, you need a plumber!'

If the ovaries have been idle for a long time, however, in order to remind them what they are there for, it is often a good idea to have some reflexology. The combination of nourishment, freedom from toxins, and stimulation is often successful. I have heard that acupuncture can also be helpful. We find most people prefer reflexology, however.

Good sources: Oysters, whole grains, meat, brewer's yeast, wheat germ, fruit, vegetables, nuts, fish, poultry, shellfish.

Zinc is best taken with vitamin A, calcium, copper and phosphorus. (Nutrition Search Inc., 1979) Also, manganese and vitamin B6. (Pfeiffer)

Multi-element studies

Multi-element studies are few. One such study was the Foresight research conducted at the University of Surrey (1993). This confirmed that the mineral status in the female and male is closely linked to their reproductive ability. Of special importance in relation to problems in conception were calcium, magnesium, potassium, iron, zinc, chromium, manganese and selenium. Raised levels of lead, cadmium, aluminium and possibly mercury inhibited reproductive success. Sperm problems were most notably associated with lower levels of zinc and possibly selenium, and with high levels of lead and cadmium, especially for malformed sperm. Poor motility was linked with low levels of calcium, magnesium and potassium (also mobile phone use!).

In females there were significant differences between those who had had normal births and those showing previous problems related to pregnancy, including infertility, miscarriage, therapeutic terminations, stillbirths, small-for-date or low birth weight and malformations. The data demonstrated that, in general, those having malformed babies or stillbirths showed high levels of toxic metals and low levels of essential elements. Dr Neil Ward found that those women with no previous problems had higher zinc levels than those with previous problems. (Ward, 1993)

In another study, zinc levels were tested in women suffering from post-partum depression, and in a control population. The zinc levels of all those with depression were very significantly less than for the ones who did not suffer depression. This study was conducted by Dr John Nichols, MD, of Guildford, Surrey.

Good zinc levels contribute very significantly to quick and clean healing of birth abrasions of the vagina. They lessen the chances of painful engorgement, and encourage abundant lactation. They also significantly lessen the fatigue due to broken nights, as the baby sleeps better, and they also lessen the chances of cracked nipples and picking up an infection.

Zinc is the king of all the nutrients, in my estimation, but it is not the only one. As you have seen from the above bona-fide, scientific research from all over the world, keeping up the levels of nutrients can make the difference between a joyful birth, babyhood and childhood, and an anxious, miserable one beset with a whole host of physical and mental problems.

You now have the knowledge, so you can now make the best possible choice!

Onwards!

CHAPTER 4
Voluntary social poisons

This chapter is about what I call the VOSPs, the voluntary social poisons we choose to make ourselves ill with, because we enjoy it (at least in the early stages!) – the ones we are encouraged to use because it feels unsophisticated or 'do-goody' to be seen without them.

Smoked and pickled old journalists rumble on about the 'nanny state'. The 'method' schools of acting teach vomiting as an advanced level of thespianism (we went through a period when you hardly dared turn on the television without laying out the newspapers in front of it!). Latterly, this seems to have died down a bit, but the theme seems to have been taken up enthusiastically by teenage revellers in town centres. Excess is 'in', sanity is 'out'.

Smoking

How much harm does smoking really do either at a national level or to our own tiny baby son or daughter (albeit that they may, as yet, just be a sperm with a twinkle in his tail, and an ovum with a forming game plan)?

There are two ways of looking at 'national'. Firstly, looking at the approximately one out of three adults who smoke, and secondly at the rest of the country – the hapless taxpayers who have to shell out, year on year, to pay for the costs of the first group's illnesses and absenteeism from work. 'Hey,' you can hear the smokers yell, 'we pay plenty of money in taxes on our cigarettes.' However, I gather there are reliable figures to show that this does not cover the costs that are inflicted on the NHS – and thus on the rest of us.

The truth is that the time has come when we have to learn to look at illness in a different way. Fifty years ago it was all looked upon as 'just bad luck'. You were shunted off to hospital (nice, clean, caring hospital) and visited by friends with cards and flowers, grapes and sympathy, and in due course, those who emerged fully repaired would rejoin the human race and get on with their lives. That was then. Not too many people were ill, and by and large the NHS could cope. Not so many people were **volunteering for illness**, at younger and younger ages. Not so many people were made ill before they were even born. It was containable!

Now, as the rate of illness has increased, year on year, the NHS is on its knees. Bigger and bigger hospitals have been built. Many are so tall the windows have to be made so that they do not open, as we are told that changes in the air pressure could put undue strain on the structure. Far be it from me to wish to see the whole thing fall to the ground, but I feel uneasy about an entire building full of sick people hermetically sealed in with the so-called 'air conditioning' blowing smells and germs from one place to another...

I am also unsure as to whether the modern young woman, with all the education and opportunities made available to her, wants to become a nurse or 'carer', and devote her life to coping with sickness, dementia and double incontinence. Think about it.

I hear the anguish of those who have left their beloved relatives in this situation and have watched them lose their life to C-diff or MRSA, in very un-ideal conditions. They may complain to their MP and we may hear a lot of rhetoric from the green benches, or from Dimbleby's *Question Time*. However, have any of 'those in power' ever faced one week of coping with these scenarios close up? I think not.

The days of the Nightingale-inspired saints and the devout and devoted nuns are over. They are unlikely to come back. So the point of all this is simple – we need to learn how to keep ourselves well and, above all, sane, if humanly possible, and we need to bring the next generation into the world fit. Happily, it is actually not as difficult as it may sound.

What the body needs is to have the nutrients to build and repair itself – good food, required supplements, clean water, fresh air – and to be free from the toxic factors that destroy human cells – namely, what I term 'drugs, bugs and plugs' (VOSPs, medical drugs, exogenous hormones, infections, infestations and rogue radiation). This is perfectly achievable with a bit of effort, and it is becoming even more necessary.

Now it is well known that smokers' children are much more likely to smoke than non-smokers', so if you *are* a smoker it is probably not your fault. Your parents maybe set you up for your habit. But, for exactly the same reason, you can see how vital it is that you stop now, so this huge disadvantage is not passed on and on by succeeding generations. It is in your hands.

There is a lot of scientific evidence out there that smoking causes abnormal pregnancies, illness, handicap and deformity in the babies. On average, the babies of smoking mothers are about half a pound (226 g) lighter than they would have been if their mother had not smoked.

Both the nicotine and the lack of oxygen affect the growth of the baby, as they reduce the blood flow to the placenta and the uptake of protein.

Researchers have also reported large areas of dead tissue in the placentas of smoking mothers. The baby is totally dependent on the placenta for his 'support services', so this short-changes the baby while he is in a position where he cannot complain about it or walk out and find a better situation elsewhere.

Cadmium, which as we know can damage the brain and kidneys in the newborn child, is present in large quantities in smokers' babies. The damage inflicted is not reversible.

There is a greater risk of the baby being stillborn, miscarriage, cleft palate and hare lip and central nervous system malformations. When you have waited as long for this precious little person as so many of you have, stillbirth or miscarriage is the very last thing you could bear. Never do anything that appreciably increases the risk. Cleft lips or palates are reversible by surgery but it is a long and arduous process, more so for the baby than for the parents. For a tiny baby, surgery is terrifying as well as painful as you cannot explain to them what is going on (I have been through this five times, and I cannot bear it.) Some of those with a bad cleft have lifetime problems with diction and a few have some permanent disfigurement. Central nervous system aberrations can include spina bifida and mental retardation.

Many smokers' babies will be born small and early which is agony if they have to be left behind in hospital in Special Care. This, good as many of the SCBUs are, can never be as special as being with mother, as love is everything at this age. If you are breastfeeding, getting through the traffic to get back to your child every three hours can become a Herculean task (I know one mother who had to do this through the Christmas traffic for the whole of one December). Being held up in traffic when you know your tiny person may be crying for you, and getting more and more miserable when you do not appear, is a nightmare. Prematurity is to be avoided at all costs, any mother who has been through it will tell you.

Ectopic pregnancies (where the embryo implants outside the womb, almost always in one of the fallopian tubes) are more common in smokers. This can often lead to a tube being removed. This does not necessarily impede future fertility significantly, so long as the remaining tube is viable, but it usually means emergency surgery with all the panic and pain that that entails. In addition you lose the hope of that baby.

Last but not least, poor little smokers' children have been shown to have 'poorer learning abilities'. This is not their fault but, when they come home with a report at the end of term saying they are near the bottom of the class and full of phrases like 'could try harder' and 'does not pay attention', it is very depressing for them as well as for their parents.

The old-fashioned view was that the parents should then 'give them a good talking to'. Hopefully we have now moved into a more understanding era. However I would guess a lot of teenage 'switching off' (girls) or bravado (boys) in class, and later sick notes and truancy, comes down to a biochemically disadvantaged brain stemming from before birth, whether through smoking, alcohol, deficiencies, food additives, pesticides etc. It can make for a miserable little life.

As if all these disadvantages were not hard enough for the poor little baby, if the mother continues smoking after birth, things get even more disappointing, as smoking has been shown to adversely affect milk production. It has also been shown that physical and emotional development is slower. This can be permanent.

So far we seem to have concentrated on the smoking mother. However, the adverse effects on the sperm can be just as heavy. Smoking can lower testosterone and affect numbers of sperm, their health (normal forms) and their motility – i.e. their keenness to do their job and reach the ovum. In other words, there are fewer sperm and they are not fit for purpose.

Furthermore a study from Germany showed that the children of **smoking fathers** were two and a half times more likely to have a deformity. Another study found facial defects to be related to paternal smoking. Yet another study has shown a smoking father to be a much increased cancer risk to their children.

On the Foresight website, the work of Tuula Tuormaa goes into all the disadvantages in detail and is backed by 155 scientific references. She leaves us in no doubt!

So what do we do?

Firstly, you need the motivation. You need to take in all of the previous pages and realise how your future child could be significantly better-looking, probably taller, certainly brighter academically, and that crucial but difficult to define area, 'more together' generally. They will also be much less prone to illness. A huge amount of influence on their future lies in your hands.

The women I talk to usually tell me that the men won't give up alcohol, and they (the women) can't give up smoking which is quite an interesting lesson in psychology. It appears that the belief is that the men are in command and will make their own decisions. The women are in submission, even to their bullying 'you-want-me' cigarettes. So let's disprove that last bit, and show the little brutes who is in charge!

Some people find it easiest to just throw the pack away, tell their friends what they are doing and ask for their support. If two or three of you can decide to do it together, the moral support will be helpful.

For health practitioners who wish to give talks about smoking and fertility/pregnancy, Foresight have a PowerPoint presentation.

The Bad News

- Smoking is the greatest single cause of ill health and premature death in the UK.
- Smokers have a 1 in 2 risk of getting ill and dying early from smoking.
- Smoking kills 120,000 people each year in the UK, compared to 5,000 killed in road accidents.
- Thirteen people die each hour from smoking.
- Over 80% of all lung cancer deaths are caused by smoking.

SOURCE: DEPARTMENT OF HEALTH, 2002

Some Chemicals Found in Tobacco Smoke

Acetone	Widely used solvent, for example in nail polish remover
Ammonia	Found in strong cleaning fluids
Arsenic	A deadly poison used in insecticides
Benzene	Used as a solvent in fuel and chemical manufacture
Formaldehyde	Highly poisonous, used to preserve dead bodies

So, how can you give up? The following are some ideas that have been successful for some people:

- Firstly, giving up caffeine at the same time (coffee, tea and chocolate) is said to lessen the cravings. Yes, really, although I hear a few groans!

- Homoeopaths can give you what they call a remedy or nosode, comprising a minute amount of tobacco potentised in such a way it helps to remove tobacco residues from the system. These are obtainable from Ainsworths Homoeopathic Chemists (see Useful Addresses list in the back of the book).

- I have been told by one successful 30-a-day quitter that you leave out one cigarette every few days, and say to yourself, 'later', starting with the first one of the day, and giving up one at a time. I think it took her four to five months but it was a 'lasting quit'. She also put the money she saved in a jam jar in the kitchen and looked at it at intervals. I think in those days it was about 11 pence a cigarette but now it is more. She found it encouraging and useful!

- Eat little protein or fruit snacks throughout the day: nuts, hard-boiled eggs, fruit, mustard and cress, cheese cubes (white goat's cheese is lovely, so is organic Cheddar), celery, carrots, muesli bars (not as fattening as chocolate, cake, biscuits etc!)

- You have a hair analysis and get a Foresight programme. Tell them you are quitting and they will structure your programme to help as much as they can.

- See your local NHS 'stop smoking nurse' and have a lung capacity test. This is very motivating, I am told. It shows you how your lungs are struggling! They also offer nicotine chewing gum (I am told it doesn't work and it stains your teeth), nicotine inhaler (I am told this does help) and nicotine patches (I am told they help. They gradually reduce the amount in the patch so that it tails off...).

- Helping people to stop smoking is usually a cooperative effort. Just half an hour reading through all the misfortunes that can plague smokers' children is very convincing. The most usual response is, 'I have been meaning to give up for ages, and this has really made my mind up.'

- Quitters say it is helpful to occupy your hands and your brain cells: So: embroidery, sewing, knitting, cross pointe, crochet – they have the advantage that you could make some money at it! There is also watercolour painting if you have a little talent, this could become another money-spinner! I guess you could write a novel, design gardens, make new curtains and make new clothes? Anything to let the emerging entrepreneur take over from the addict! Think of yourself as a butterfly emerging from a chrysalis. Good luck!

> **60 mg of pure nicotine placed on a person's tongue would kill within minutes.**
> Source: Department of Health, 2002

I have recently read with a feeling of doom that Indian women are enjoying the newfound 'freedom' of the contraceptive pill and cigarettes. I would say this is not liberation, but commercial exploitation.

Way back in 1980, I was rung up by a very intelligent young man from Teeside University. 'I've got some students needing to do a study,' he said. 'Is there anything we can do to help you?'

'Can you make a rat smoke a cigarette?' I asked him.

'No problem,' came the reply. 'You want me to get the effects of tobacco on pregnant rats, then?'

'No, on the father.'

'The father – you think it affects the mate?'

'Well, that's what I need you to find out for us.'

'I see... well... yes... all right.'

A year later, the following study emerged. It was with mice, not rats, and, as you see, it tells us a great deal. God bless Teeside University, and Dr Barry Hemsworth.

Teeside Study

Male mice were given daily injections of nicotine. This was calculated according to body weight and blood volume so that the amount of nicotine in their blood equated to that of a fully grown man smoking 20 cigarettes a day. Spermatogenesis in the mouse takes 11 days.

After 5 weeks of 'moderate smoking' the first cohort of mice were mated. The female mice from these matings suffered a 16.4% in utero death rate (equivalent to human miscarriage but with litter animals the remains are resorbed). This worked out at approximately one pup in six being lost. Of the remainder, 4.8% suffered limb reduction deformities. This was a 21.2% major disaster rate.

133

A second cohort of males were then allowed off their nicotine injections for a week and then mated. As spermatogenesis in a mouse takes only 11 days, this was roughly the equivalent of a 'one third contaminated' sperm population, compared with the previous group. The resultant matings from this group produced a 13.1% in utero death rate, and a 1.6% limb reduction deformity rate: exactly one third the number of pups with malformed limbs from the first group. A 14.7% major disaster rate which was a considerable improvement, although some nicotine was still present.

The final cohort was mated after 3 weeks entirely free from nicotine. The mothers then suffered only 3.8% in utero losses, and there were no malformed limbs. Only a 3.8% disaster rate. To show this more graphically:

Resorbed/Miscarried

Nicotine +	16.4%
Nicotine ½	13.1%
Nicotine -	3.8%

Malformed (Limb reduction deformity or missing limbs)

Nicotine +	4.8%
Nicotine ½	1.6%
Nicotine -	0%

[Hemsworth, BN, *'Deformation of the mouse fetus after ingestion of nicotine by the male'*. IRCS Medical Science: Anatomy and Human Biology; Biochemistry: Developmental Biology and Medicine: Drug metabolism and Toxicology: Pathology: Pharmacology: Physiology: Reproduction: Obstetrics and Gynaecology. 1981. 9, 727–9]

This study is interesting for two reasons. It demonstrates that although a reduction in nicotine smoking does give some help, it is not enough. The whole process of spermatogenesis needs to take place free from this noxious element completely; we can see from the second group how early in spermatogenesis the sperm can be damaged. It also poses the question, **what could be achieved worldwide by healthy fatherhood?**

Currently, 1 in 4 or 5 (20–25%) of all babies in the UK are miscarried. If those born alive are 600,000 (approximate figures), then in the region of 37,500 babies perish in the womb every year. How many of these family tragedies are down to non-viable sperm?

Over 5,000 babies are born every year with limb reduction deformity: 1 child in 120. How much of this could be prevented by no parental smoking?

At the very least, this should all be considered urgent for further research. However, to obtain this research, a lot of pressure will have to be brought to bear by the general public, as the wealth, and therefore the influence, of the alcohol and tobacco firms is immense. So we are unlikely to hear any more about this; just make up your own minds and protect your own children. Good Luck!

Alcohol

Alcohol, however, is a much more frequent problem. If I had one pound for every time I've heard, 'My husband definitely won't give up his beer, no way!' I would be a very rich woman.

The most usual argument is that our mother or father drank and we are fine! Well, maybe, but probably they ate better food – less processed and less intensively farmed, so the probability is that they were much better banked up with essential vitamins and minerals. However, even so, if their offspring find they are unable to give up alcohol, this is indicative of unstable blood sugar, so it was not really an unqualified success! You could do even better for your children!

Well, as with the smoking, there are a lot of good reasons for giving the baby a level playing field. Foetal Alcohol Syndrome, FAS, has been well documented in the last 30 years. More recently in the USA, they have studied the effects of quite small amounts of alcohol, and have identified a new category of lesser disadvantages they have called FAE (Foetal Alcohol Effects).

135

More recently still, it has been queried whether a grandparent's past drinking is affecting the grandchildren. In one way this sounds like very bad news. But, on the other hand, we can stand this on its head, and say that, by abstaining now you could be benefiting not only your own children, but even your future grandchildren!

In the Bible we are told *'the sins of the fathers will be visited upon the sons, even until the 10th generation'*. This is usually looked upon as a particularly dire, almost vindictive, threat. But I think in reality it was a warning. As with most biblical pointers, it was pertinent and intended to be helpful, so we may as well take it on board. Think about it. Grab a calculator. If each generation multiplies by only two, by abstaining now you will be helping 2,046 of your descendants to have a better life. Formidable, really!

As people so often come to Foresight when they have one very much loved, but damaged little person, I am all the time hearing:

'He is very hyperactive, he never stops all day, or all night really, we haven't had a full night's sleep since he arrived, we take it in turns…'

'My little girl is covered in eczema, hardly anywhere on her body is not affected…'

'One of my children is autistic. I have help with him during the day, but it is very hard…'

'My little boy has asthma. It is quite frightening sometimes. We have had to rush him to hospital for oxygen more than once…'

And so on. They all wanted to know **one thing**: is there anything we can do to stop it happening again? They are coping manfully, but the cry is, 'We just couldn't manage with two of them like this.'

Well, yes, we do manage to produce one without problems with their cooperation and the help of the full Foresight programme. We also help the original little one with his or her problems, looking for food and other allergies, for mineral deficiencies (zinc, manganese, selenium and magnesium will be low). Often copper or a toxic metal will be high, there may be a urinary tract infection, a bed in a position vulnerable to geophysical stress and so on.

But recently, I have started to ask: 'I hope you don't mind this question, and of course you need not answer me if you do not want to, but was there, by any chance, any quite heavy consumption of alcohol in any of the grandparents?' And I have been very interested by how many times I have heard:

'Oh my God yes, permanently awash.'

'Grandfather, yes, very much so, I'm afraid.'

'Yes, indeed, yes. What we went through...'

'Don't mind you asking, no, but why? Are you finding out something? Is it connected to the problems with the kids? I always thought it might be.'

'Alcohol, oh my dear yes, very heavy, very heavy indeed, I think you could say.'

And so on. Not too surprising really.

a) alcohol dehydrogenase is a zinc-dependent enzyme. So consumption of alcohol removes zinc from the system big-time.
b) essential fatty acids, and most particularly omega-3, are also used up.
c) B-complex vitamins are squandered.

If the sperm and/or the ova that create the child are short of these elements (and a host of others also, no doubt) then the resultant babies will also be deficient. But the fascinating, but daunting, follow-through is that their minute ova and their tiny testicles may also be short, and, unless this is addressed and rectified before they start to reproduce, some of their future offspring may also suffer (I hope some really switched-on scientists will do a study on this before too long).

One thing we do know is that when the mineral imbalances etc are addressed and fully corrected before conception, the children come through very well. They are intelligent and often with surprising bonuses, such as a talent for music, or chess, or drawing... whatever.

Research has shown unequivocal answers. In one study, male mice were given alcohol for 26 days and then sobered up for two days prior to mating. The litter size was halved, and of those who were born, 88% died within a month. Another study proved that alcohol had a specific effect on the chromosomes. This would have implications for many miscarriages, as well as physical and mental handicaps.

Effects on male fertility are dire – in heavy drinkers, the sperm have been noticed to have no tails. This would, of course, mean they cannot reach the ovum and do the deed. Russian research has found abnormalities in the sperm of alcoholic men which they believe could cause abnormalities in any children they produced.

Another study in 1975 found alcohol-induced testicular atrophy. Yet other studies have linked alcohol to problems with the production of testosterone and the function of the testicles.

It seems to me extremely likely that this is a brilliant design mechanism of nature. If the sperm are likely to produce a physically or mentally afflicted baby, nature does her level best to ensure they cannot reach the egg and thus cannot fertilise. So many lifelong tragedies may have been averted by this excellent mechanism.

This is why, once the intake of alcohol has been temporarily interrupted, after about four months we get the ecstatic phone call we so love to hear, 'Would you believe it, I'm pregnant!'

Sperm take approximately 116 days to 'make', so this is often the timescale between 'he says he will give up alcohol' and the magic moment.

The direct opposite to this is the IVF scenario where the sperm are taken by force, manhandled into a saucer, made to do their duty (against their better judgement) and then the tears because the 'treatment' has failed or later because there has been a miscarriage.

People come to us constantly having had three, four, five failed IUIs, IVFs, ICSIs and so on. The man drinking a 'normal' amount, 18 to 25 units a week, says, 'Nobody ever told us it mattered. Does it really? Will it make a difference?' Often they have spent £12,000 to £20,000 and there is still no baby (probably fortunately).

Typically, foetal alcohol syndrome (FAS) is described thus: growth retardation, meaning low birth weight, failure to thrive and subsequent short stature, although at puberty there may be weight gain, particularly in the girls, who tend, later in life, to be short but obese.

There are facial characteristics which include a low nasal bridge, back-tilted nose, 'exaggerated epicanthic folds' (sides of nose to corner of mouth), a flat philtrum (space between nose and mouth) and a very little vermillion for the upper lip. The openings for the eyes tend to be rather short, giving a 'round-eyed' kittenish appearance, and there may be a squint. The ears tend to be unusual in form, sometimes simple and sometimes with the top folded down lower than normal on one or both ears.

There are often (in about 40% of cases) some muscle and skeleton defects such as bent fingers and hip or rib cage abnormalities. Psychologically, as well as physically, the worst effects can be the genital abnormalities where it is hard to tell if a child is a boy or a girl. Some kidney abnormalities have also been detected. Nearly one in three will have a heart defect of some kind, often requiring surgery, which is sometimes fatal.

Defects of the central nervous system can range from poor hand-eye coordination, resulting in excessive clumsiness, to seizures and mental retardation. As infants, they may be fretful and have difficulty suckling and feeding, making them very unsettled and difficult to rear.

The average IQ of children born with FAS is 65, well below the national average of 100. FAS is the leading known cause of mental retardation. About 70% of the children with the syndrome are hyperactive, and are prone to rocking and head banging.

When they arrive at school age there are serious problems with behaviour and quite severe learning difficulties.

The problems do not abate with age, but it would appear that they become more severe, with difficulties with acquiring skills, keeping jobs, managing money affairs and retaining relationships.

The work of Dr Ann Streissguth of the USA, who followed the lives of her little FAS children through to adulthood, makes for very sad reading. According to her, the FAS child, although sometimes a bright, chirpy, giggly little thing at the outset, upon coming to the challenges of real school will find life very stressful, be prone to tears and tantrums, disappointment and resentment, as his limitations become exposed and possibly his friends become scornful about his lack of ability. As school continues, his inability to organise himself and fully take in everything around him becomes more and more of a burden to him. He may clown his way through or he may become deeply depressed.

Dr Streissguth followed her little FAS patients through to maturity, and she found them more prone to alcoholism, drug-taking, living off benefits, mental illness and suicide. They found it difficult to stay in a job or a relationship. Many became destitute despite their best intentions, and the support of family and friends. These were the frank FAS children.

FAE (Foetal Alcohol Effects) is the term for the children less severely affected, but not untouched by their background. The effects can be less severe, but nonetheless, the child's life can be limited and his ability diminished. Do we want to inflict this on them? No, we don't.

Reading the research, it is obvious that we would be living in a very different world if no unborn baby were affected by alcohol. In the Foresight booklet 'The Adverse Effects of Alcohol on Reproduction', Tuula Tuormaa sums up the problems. She wrote with such dedication and such clarity that I felt I could not better it, and so I have asked her to let me use it to show you how widespread and how damaging the problems are. Parts of the booklet are reproduced at the end of this chapter.

For the most part, I find that once the possible consequences of drinking prior to/during pregnancy and during breastfeeding are explained to women, they are immediately able to take in the implications. After a lot of explanation and persuasion, almost all of the men who contact us are also convinced! Stratagems we find helpful with those who find it really hard to give up include:

- **Combating reactive hypoglycaemia.** This occurs when the pancreas is functioning at a less than optimal level. This may be because of heavy alcohol or sugar consumption in previous generations (we do not yet know this, but it would be worthy of study). This could have meant the pancreas was small or weak (poorly functioning) at birth. Or it could just be because of a childhood diet high in sugar, possibly white sugar and flour. This would have meant the pancreas was overused and undernourished.

  The pancreas needs the trace minerals chromium, manganese and zinc, and plenty of the B-complex vitamins, especially pantothenate and the essential fatty acids, to function properly.

  If the pancreas is somewhat exhausted, the person will crave sugar, or alcohol. Indeed, they will feel unable to function adequately without a boost.

  Once the alcohol (or chocolate, coffee etc) kicks in, this causes a rise in the blood sugar, and creates a 'high'. If the alcohol intake is considerable there will be feelings of boundless energy, infallibility, and elation. If things have not gone 'over the top', for a period, the drinker will function well, physically or intellectually.

  This will, however, be followed by a commensurate fall in blood sugar, and (in overt alcoholism at least) the 'fall' period will be filled with fatigue, muddle, depression – sometimes with self-doubt and despair – sometimes with self-pity, feelings of being exploited and righteous indignation! All not easy to live with for the long suffering relatives and colleagues! This is a pattern that may also be mirrored at a milder level in the more modest imbiber!

- **Hair analysis is a helpful measure, plus a tailor-made programme of supplements**, which would include B-complex vitamins, chromium, zinc, manganese and omega-3 supplements to restore optimum nutrient status. Also vitamin

C, garlic, milk thistle and nicotinamide to help cleanse the liver and kidneys. Drinking plenty of water and having a good wholefood diet will help.

- **Increase the intake of omega-3 oils.** They are present in oily fish and in supplements of specific fish oils, or in flaxseed oil such as High Barn Oil. Although it is said that absorption from flaxseed oil can be more difficult, as it requires the body to take one more step in the conversion, I feel there are advantages in High Barn Oils as they are more reasonably priced. They are less likely to be contaminated with heavy metals than oils from deep sea fish (the oceans are becoming depressingly polluted). Subjectively, I also find they do not give me a headache, and I often find the fish oils do. I am sometimes told by Foresight people that they find this too.

If you get the oil capsules you can bite them, chew them for a minute to obtain all the oil, and then spit out the capsules and throw them away, which saves you having to digest the gelatine.

- **Attention to possible allergies:** Dr Theron Randolph, an American doctor with a keen interest in allergies, found that some regular drinkers had a craving for alcohol made from a substance to which they were allergic. I think it is permissible to wonder which came first – the heavy intake of the fermented substance or the allergy to the basic foodstuff? Be that as it may, it is worth taking his theory on board, if there are difficulties. It has the merit of being completely harmless and not costing anything!

Whisky cravings: eliminate grains (wheat, barley and rye).
Vodka cravings: eliminate potatoes etc, as above.
Wine cravings: eliminate the grape.
Cider cravings: eliminate the apple.

I admit to feeling somewhat nonplussed regarding gin. Do we eat any relative of the juniper berry? My botany does not stretch to this, but I am very anxious to learn. Help welcomed.

It is worth noting at this point that, when giving up alcohol, your use of cigarettes, coffee, chocolate and sugar will make the situation *worse*. They will all tweak at the pancreas, which is already somewhat fed up.

It is possible to drink a huge range of other substances, so long as you are not allergic to them. Alcohol-free wines and beers are an option as long as they do not set off any cravings again.

There are endless hot or cold milk drinks if you are not allergic to milk. If you are, you may be okay on goat's milk, rice milk or nut milks such as almond milk.

There are herbal teas, fruit juices, smoothies in huge varieties. There is Marmite (if you are not yeast-allergic) and, if you are not grain-allergic, beef or chicken Bovril, also Tesco's 'Beefy' which is gluten-free. Soya milk has become a bit suspect as they may be allowing in GM soya. However, as long as you are not a whisky craver, there is a lovely milk called Oatly.

The 'Land of Milk and Honey' was, of course, the land of goat's milk and honey, and this is very possible to achieve these days, as even the most modest little corner shop sells goat's milk. Maple syrup can be another idea to alternate with honey. Probably clean water is the best of the lot, and it is almost certainly the most helpful to fertility!

It is an excellent idea to take more care of the pancreas and the liver with B-complex vitamins, zinc, manganese and magnesium. As the whole digestive system starts to function better, the blood sugar, and thus the brain function, becomes more stable. Caffeine and sugar need to be avoided. Protein, fruit and vegetables, with some complex carbohydrates (which means brown bread and brown rice, or foods made with brown flour), can be taken on board. All this, plus plenty of clean water and plenty of fresh air, will help.

- **Leisure time:** we all need time for music, good books, planting things in the garden, art, writing, the gym or sport? How about making clothes, embroidery and tapestry – just doing something creative. These things provide a 'mood-lift' because they are satisfying. I believe these could be more helpful than anything else.

I believe that we don't spend enough time outdoors. We should be freer, more in tune with nature and less tied to routine and schedules and much more joyful about what we do! Isn't loneliness or boredom somewhere at the root of addiction in many cases? Contact with animals teaches us empathy and helps develop our basic instincts. We seem to listen too much and sing too little; walk too much and dance too little. We do not spend enough time with little children. If we took into ourselves more of that which makes us happy in the long term, and much less of the stuff that makes us happy for a couple of hours and then cantankerous and dreary in the long term, the world would be a better place!

- As with smoking, Foresight have put an excellent summary of 124 papers on alcohol and fertility compiled by Tuula Tuormaa on their website. They also have a PowerPoint to help any bold pioneers who will try to help the cause by going out there and giving talks. They need help from all of you.

If only we can rescue the next generation by seeing that they are properly nourished from the ovum and sperm stage to birth, that the birth is accomplished with as little drug use as possible and they are then breastfed by a drug-free mum – I think we have every hope of beating the evil of drugs. Teenagers who have had too little energy and zest for life all through their childhood are vulnerable to the myth of substances they are told will give them new and exciting experiences and make them more trendy and alluring.

I recently had a Christmas card from the mother of our first ever pair of twins. One had just done his PhD and two universities were after him for research into environmental issues. His twin sister had just been out to Africa to help build a school! The excitement and the fulfilment of hopes and dreams is on offer out there – the young ones just need to be well enough and bright enough to take up the challenges!

Onwards!

HEART DEFECTS ACCOMPANY FAS

In the history of 24 patients with FAS, 13 (54.2%) had a heart defect. (sic)

- ♥ 7 congenital heart disease
- ♥ 2 ventricular septal defect
- ♥ 1 patent ductus arterioscus
- ♥ 4 heart murmurs (later spontaneously corrected)

(NB: there appear to be 14 (58.3%) from the script)

Accompanied by typical growth retardation, development delay and facial anomalies.

JAMA May 1976

BMJ Vol. 286. January 1983
Alcohol & Advice to the Pregnant Woman

Californian study of 32,000 pregnancies:
In women taking 1–2 drinks daily the risk of miscarriage doubled when compared with non-drinkers.

New York study of women who drank twice weekly, only 2 drinks per occasion, had miscarriage rate of 25%

Seattle study on congenital abnormalities:
4 drinks per day, 19% abnormalities
2–4 drinks per day, 11% abnormalities
Fewer than 2 drinks per day, 2% abnormalities
Some criticism due to maternal age in some cases

The United States Surgeon General 'advises women who are pregnant (or considering pregnancy) not to drink alcoholic beverages and to be aware of the alcoholic content of food and drugs.'

Nutrition Reviews. February 1982

Average Birth Weights:

In mothers consuming alcohol throughout pregnancy:
2,786 g ± 485 g (6 lb 2 oz)

In mothers who drank previously, but abandoned alcohol upon becoming pregnant:
3,137 g ± 466 g (6 lb 15 oz)

In mothers who did not drink alcohol:
3,520 g ± 419 g (7 lb 12 oz)

CAFFEINE AND MISCARRIAGES

Drinking 3 or more cups of tea or coffee a day is associated with increased risk of miscarriage. (American Journal of Epidemiology 1996)

Caffeine during pregnancy can increase the probability of chromosomal abnormality which could lead to a miscarriage. (American Journal of Obstetrics and Gynaecology 1985)

Since 1980, the US Food and Drug Administration has advised pregnant women to minimise caffeine intake, citing the dangers of possible miscarriage or having a mentally retarded baby.

Even de-caffeinated coffee is linked to an increased risk of miscarriage. (American Journal of Epidemiology 1996)

Excerpts from 'The Adverse Effects of Alcohol on Reproduction' by Tuula E Tuormaa – published in the International Journal of Biosocial & Medical Research issue 14.2 1994. (Original obtainable from Foresight)

It was not until 1967, in France, that Lemoine and his team first described in scientific terms a group of children affected by maternal alcohol abuse, which included defective intra-uterine and post-partum growth, unusual facial features, congenital malformations, such as cardiac defects, cleft palate etc. combined with mental sub-normality.

These findings in France and, five years later, independent observations by Dr Jones and his colleagues from the United States, led finally to a recognition of a distinct dysmorphic condition associated with maternal gestational alcoholism named as Foetal Alcohol Syndrome (FAS), which has since become a clearly established clinical entity.

Foetal Alcohol Syndrome (FAS):

The most common characteristics of children born with FAS are as follows:

Growth abnormalities: Prenatal growth deficiency can be significant and includes all three of the following parameters of growth: weight, length and head circumference.

Frequently the growth deficiencies are so severe that the newborn has to be hospitalised because of obvious failure to thrive.[20] Postnatal growth and weight retardation is also significant and this continues for life despite the infant being reared in an ideal nutritional and social environment.

Craniofacial abnormalities: The eyes of the affected children are often small with exaggerated inner epicanthic folds, and squints are common in later years. The nasal bridge is usually poorly formed, giving the nose a small 'retroussé' appearance. The vertical groove running from the nose down to the upper lip tends to be shallow or absent, and the upper lip itself is often narrow. The ears tend to be large and somewhat simple in form. Cleft palate may also be present.

Musculoskeletal abnormalities: Variable musculoskeletal and limb defects are found in approximately 40% of cases, ranging in severity from minor problems such as contractures of the finger joints to more severe lesions, such as congenital hip dislocations and thoracic cage abnormalities. Genital abnormalities are also frequent, such as undescended testes and malformations of the lower wall of the urethra in males and hypoplastic labia in females. Minor kidney abnormalities have also been detected.

Cardiac abnormalities: Congenital heart disease is found in 29–50% of reported cases. They are commonly atrical or ventricular septal defects, but also complex and sometimes lethal cardiac abnormalities can occur.

Nervous system abnormalities: When first delivered, the affected infants may show clear evidence of alcohol withdrawal. They are often fretful, tremulous, have a weak grasp, poor eye-hand coordination and frequently a great difficulty with sucking and feeding. Cerebellar damage is also common, resulting later on in excessive clumsiness and even in recurrent seizures.

Neuro-developmental delay or mental deficiency: The average IQ in children born with FAS is around 65, indicating moderate mental handicap. Mental retardation also occurs frequently in varying degrees. In fact FAS is now recognised as the leading known cause of mental retardation, surpassing Down's syndrome and spina bifida. Around 70% of children with FAS are severely hyperactive, frequently engaging in body rocking, head banging or head rolling. Without exception all children with FAS suffer from severe developmental disabilities. With the onset of school, these severe IQ and attention deficits, combined with various behavioural problems, emerge as serious intellectual and learning disabilities.

Adolescents/adults with FAS: The natural history of FAS has now been traced into adulthood. The short stature and microcephaly seem to be permanent. The average academic functioning of these adolescents and adults does not ever seem to develop beyond early school grade level, even though in one sample of 61 studied, 42% had IQ levels above 70 and all had received constant remedial help at school. A particular deficit was found in arithmetic skills and extreme difficulties with abstractions like time and space, cause and effect, as well as generalising from one situation to another. The most noticeable behaviour problems were found to be with comprehension, judgement and attention skills, causing these adults born with FAS to experience major psychosocial and adjustment problems for the rest of their lives.

The effects can induce foetal malformations both at the earliest and at the lowest level of intake, its effectiveness spreading differentially over the whole spectrum of reproduction, affecting the developing foetus in varying degrees, in both extent and severity, depending on the dosage and timing.

This explains also why maternal alcohol consumption can affect the offspring through all gradations of teratogenesis, ranging from moderately affected right up to the full blown Foetal Alcohol Syndrome.

Alcohol is quite capable of crossing the placental barrier and entering the foetus, causing the level of alcohol in the foetus to be approximate to that of the mother. In the first 21 days of the foetal development the preliminary cell organisation of the embryo begins to take place. If an excessive amount of alcohol is consumed before the blastocyst is embedded in the uterus, the impact can be so severe that the foetus is miscarried. By the end of the 36th day, often long before the woman even realises that she is pregnant, the neural tube is clearly present and open, and most of the rudimentary organs have already been formed, such as limbs, heart, brain, eyes, mouth, digestive tract etc.

It is therefore obvious that if a teratogenic substance such as alcohol is consumed during critical days this can result in various forms of malformation in the newborn, such as defective heart, musculoskeletal abnormalities, mental handicap etc., without any specific outward signs of FAS.

Even though it is considered that the first three months of gestation is the most critical period for alcohol-induced malformations to occur, both human and animal experiments have been able to demonstrate that the teratogenic effects of alcohol continue throughout the whole gestational period, affecting at the later stage particularly the brain development and function.

Foetal Alcohol Effects:

The teratogenic effects of alcohol spread differentially over the whole spectrum of reproduction, varying only in the extent and degree. At one end of the spectrum are the children warranting a firm diagnosis of FAS, and at the other end of the spectrum are the children who lack the common physical characteristics of FAS but who, nevertheless, have some subtle or marked physical and/or mental deficiencies from being exposed to varying amounts of alcohol in utero.

It is now widely accepted that the classical diagnosis of FAS is totally inadequate, as for every child born with FAS there are thousands of others whose lives are partially handicapped, or limited, by being exposed to alcohol during gestational development. These children, without sufficient physical stigmata for firm diagnosis of FAS, are now identified as suffering from Foetal Alcohol Effects (FAE).

On the second day of life, compared to a child without FAE, they had a longer latency to begin sucking and had a weaker suck as measured on a pressure transducer with non-nutritive nipple. They also suffered from disrupted sleep patterns, low level of arousal, unusual body orientation, abnormal reflexes, hypotonia and excessive mouthing.

By eight months, and then onwards, these infants seemed to suffer from disrupted sleep-wake patterns; poorer balance and motor control; longer latency to respond; poorer attention, visual recognition and memory; decrements in mental development, spoken language and verbal comprehension, including lower IQ scores.

The conclusion of the above findings was that two maternal alcohol use patterns have now been identified as being particularly detrimental to the offspring: two or more drinks on average per day during pregnancy, and a 'binge-pattern' of alcohol consumption, e.g. five or more drinks on any occasion, particularly when consumed in the month or so before pregnancy recognition, as both can lead to marked behavioural and learning disabilities in school-age children.

It was also concluded that these alcohol-related behaviour and attention decrements seemed to have been already clearly observable from an early infancy, long before academic learning had even occurred.

This wide pattern of performance deficits uniformly occurred despite the presence of average IQ, suggesting that maternal alcohol-induced behaviour decrements in the offspring seem to be a more sensitive indicator of central nervous system damage than the IQ scale itself. The study concluded that maternal social drinking seemed to result in the offspring having consequences similar to, but less severe than those seen in children born with FAS, indicating in both cases *the clear occurrence of alcohol-induced permanent central nervous system damage* during critical stages of foetal development.

FAE in adolescents and adults: As with children born with FAS, population-based studies carried out on the offspring born to socially drinking mothers have shown that, on maturation, these children can still show subtle and permanent alcohol-related neurobehavioral deficits, IQ and achievement decrements, combined with various attention, memory and learning problems.

Alcohol and Male Reproduction:

Alcohol is a direct testicular toxin. It causes atrophy of seminiferous tubules, loss of sperm cells, and an increase in abnormal sperms. Alcohol is also known to be a strong Leydig cell toxin, and it can have an adverse effect on the synthesis and secretion of testosterone. Alcohol can cause significant deterioration in sperm concentration, sperm output and motility. Semen samples of men consuming excessive amounts of alcohol have shown distinct morphological abnormalities. It has been also established that approximately 80% of chronic alcoholic men are sterile and, furthermore, that alcohol is one of the most common causes of male impotence.

Summary:

There is now an ever-increasing recognition that alcohol is the most common chemical teratogen presently causing malformations and mental deficiency in the human offspring.

In 1977 the following statement was made by Dr Ernest Noble, Director of the National Institute of Alcohol Abuse and Alcoholism of the United States: 'The Fetal Alcohol Syndrome is the third leading cause of mental retardation and neurological problems in infants, ranking after Down's syndrome and spina bifida.' Several other investigators have also recognised maternal alcohol abuse as being one of the leading causes for the occurrence of mental retardation in children in the Western world.

In addition, it has been estimated that maternal alcoholism may be responsible for over 10% of all infant congenital malformations.

As stated previously, alcohol is a poison at all levels, and therefore no totally safe level of alcohol use during pregnancy can be established. Alcohol-related damage to the foetus has been linked with every form of drinking pattern, from heavy drinking to intermittent as well as moderate social drinking, i.e. one or two drinks daily most days during pregnancy, and from very infrequent, but relatively heavy, drinking to one single drinking binge prior to pregnancy recognition.

The teratogenic effects of maternal 'social drinking' are considered less detrimental to the foetus than those of abusive drinking, but social drinking can still nevertheless affect the infant, maybe in a less serious but much more subtle manner.

The infant may be born with lighter weight, suffer from difficulties with habituation, feeding, and disrupted sleep-wake patterns. By eight months onwards to young school age, the children born to social drinkers seem to show poorer balance, motor control, attention, visual recognition, memory, sleep patterns and mental development than infants born to non-drinking mothers. When at school, the academic performance and IQ of these children seem to be generally below average. In addition, overall classroom behaviour of these children has been found to be negatively related to: cooperation, retention of information, comprehension of words, memory, impulsiveness, tactfulness, word recall, organisation, as well as attention skills, all indicating increased risk in learning abilities.

On maturation and as adults, these children born to social drinkers show still subtle, but permanent, alcohol-related neurobehavioral deficits, including IQ and achievement decrements, as well as attention, memory and learning difficulties.

In summary, it now seems to be evident that maternal social drinking results in the offspring suffering consequences similar to, but less severe than, those seen in children born with Foetal Alcohol Syndrome. This finding is not unexpected, as the toxic effect of alcohol can damage the foetus permanently and irreversibly through all gradations of teratogenesis.

During the 1990 Betty Ford Lecture Dr Streissguth stated: 'In summary, every community should know the following about alcohol and pregnancy: There is no known safe level of alcohol consumption during pregnancy. Pregnant women should be advised to abstain from drinking during pregnancy and when they are planning a pregnancy.'

The most salient point that can be made about alcohol-induced foetal damage is that it is totally preventable, and by informing both prospective parents of the potential dangers of alcohol consumption before conception, and particularly all women during pregnancy, we can hope to control the problem. It is frightening to realise how long the knowledge has been there that alcohol indeed damages the unborn child, without anyone seemingly worrying about it.

Drugs

Regarding other drugs such as cannabis, we are so lucky to be in touch with Mrs Mary Brett, a wonderful teacher who is the British representative in Europe regarding the control of drug use. She really has her pupils' best interests at heart and has been spreading the word about the dangers of street drugs for many years.

She has been kind and generous enough to say we can use her material to give you the very best information available and has given her article to us free of charge. She is a wonderful woman and we should all help her to spread the word.

• Cannabis – the facts (Mary Brett)

Cannabis (marijuana, pot, grass, weed, joints, spliff, hashish, blow) is a hallucinogen, a depressant and our commonest illegal drug.

How drugs work in the brain

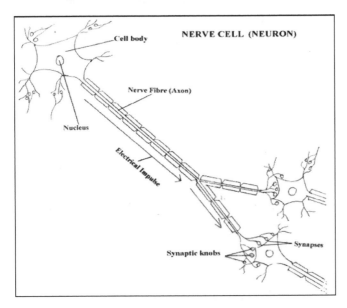

100 billion nerve cells (neurons) may have up to 10,000 connections to other neurons in the vast brain network. Messages pass along the nerve fibres as electrical impulses, then cross the

gap between the neurons (the synapse) in the form of chemicals – neurotransmitters – the brain's natural drugs. Each neurotransmitter molecule has a particular shape to fit into its receptor site on the next neuron as a key fits into a lock.

Mind-altering drugs like cannabis or more specifically THC (tetrahydrocannabinol), the ingredient that gives the 'high', mimic the shape of these neurotransmitters so the brain is 'fooled'. Cannabis mimics anandamide and also interferes with the transmission of the other neurotransmitters because THC dissolves in the fatty cell membranes and persists. Fifty per cent of the THC is still there after a week and ten per cent a month later. Traces are still detectable in hair and urine for weeks after that.

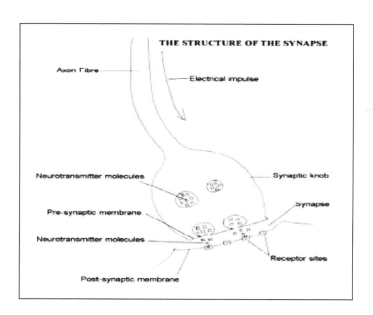

The immediate effects

Taken for euphoria, usually smoked with or without tobacco, or eaten in 'hash' cakes (but enhances the mood you're in so you may well feel worse).

An intoxicant, like alcohol, so people should not be driving. If you have a joint today you should not be driving tomorrow eg airline pilots on flight simulators could not 'land' their planes properly

155

even 24 hours and more after a joint and had no idea anything was wrong!

One 20 mg joint has the same effect as being just over the legal alcohol-driving limit. The combination of cannabis and alcohol is 16 times more dangerous when driving than taking either drug alone.

Panic attacks and paranoia can occur immediately after a joint.

The long-term effects

Just one joint per week or even one a month will ensure a permanent presence of THC. Since the other neurotransmitters are affected, new nerve connections cannot be made properly. Concentration, learning and memory are all badly affected. School grades fall, some students miss out on university places. A cannabis personality develops. Users become inflexible, can't plan their days properly, can't take criticism and struggle to express themselves. They feel lonely, miserable and misunderstood. Apathy, amotivation and dropping out are all common.

Few children using cannabis, even occasionally, will achieve their full potential.

Dependence:

Psychological addiction, the craving for cannabis is very strong.

Physical addiction occurs. As more and more THC is consumed, more receptor sites are made, tolerance builds as more THC is needed to get the same effect. All the receptor sites need to be satisfied – this is physical addiction. Withdrawal symptoms are not so dramatic as they are for heroin as THC persists in the body. More young people now are treated in the USA for marijuana than alcohol dependence.

There is no foolproof cure for any type of addiction.

Mental health:

Cannabis psychosis has been reported in scientific papers for decades. Cannabis causes far more mental illness than drugs like heroin.

156

The increased risk factors for psychosis, anxiety and depression range from 3 to 5. Schizophrenia is triggered or worsened by its use – it may even be caused. Cannabis increases the amount of the neurotransmitter dopamine in the brain. Schizophrenics have an excess of dopamine in the brain; sufferers of Parkinson's disease, too little. One in four of us carries a faulty gene which controls the release of dopamine. If a child inherits a copy of the gene from each parent, and if they then use cannabis, the chance that they will develop schizophrenia rises from 1 or 2%, the norm in the population, to 15%. The presence of one gene increases the risk by 5 to 6 times.

Violence and suicide: A Swedish study found more suicides among pot users than among those who used alcohol, amphetamines or heroin. The manner of death was more violent. A study in 2001 from Dunedin found that young male cannabis users were nearly five times more likely to be violent than non-users – the risk for alcohol users was around three. Violence seems to occur with the psychosis or during withdrawal.

Other effects on the body

Cannabis contains more cancer-causing substances than tobacco – its smoke deposits three to four times as much tar in the lungs and airways. Cases of lung cancer, bronchitis and emphysema have been reported. Rare head and neck cancers are now being found in young pot smokers. The average age for these conditions in tobacco smokers is 64.

The immune system is damaged. Fewer white blood cells are produced – many are abnormal and can't fight off infections. People are more vulnerable to disease, their illness is more severe and they stay sick longer.

Sperm production is decreased. Infertility and even impotence have been reported.

Babies born to cannabis-using mothers are smaller, hyperactive, have behaviour and learning problems and are 10 times more likely to develop leukaemia.

THC interferes with the production of new cells being made in an adult body – white blood cells, sperm and foetal cells. It causes faulty copying of DNA and hastens cell death.

Blood pressure and heart rates rise to the levels of real stress. Heart attacks have been reported. Two teenagers had strokes and died after bingeing on cannabis, another was left paralysed.

Cannabis as a gateway drug?

Tobacco, alcohol and cannabis can all act as gateway drugs. A recent New Zealand study showed that weekly cannabis users were 60 times more likely to progress to 'harder' drugs. The more they use, the greater the risk. Almost 100% of heroin users started on pot. New research suggests that cannabis can 'prime' the brain for the use of other drugs.

Relaxing the law

Holland turned a blind eye to cannabis in 1987 and is now the crime capital of Europe. The country is awash with dealers and it is a major producer and exporter of drugs, especially ecstasy.

Health and social problems have escalated and the amount allowed for personal possession has been reduced from 30g to 5g. The present Dutch government wants to close all the coffee shops. Many have gone.

Since down-classification in 2001 in the UK, regular cannabis use is still rising among 11- to 12-year-old boys – older teens seem to have progressed to cocaine.

Strength

In the sixties and seventies, the average THC content of herbal cannabis was just 0.5–1%. Today's specially bred varieties from Holland, such as skunk and nederweed, have THC contents of anything from 9–27%. These strong types are now commonly grown in the UK and are thought to account for 60% of the cannabis consumed here.

The rest of the cannabis used here is cannabis resin with a THC content of around 4 to 5%.

Drug testing

More and more employers are testing for drugs in the workplace; cannabis will show up for weeks and a conviction would prevent someone from getting a visa for the USA.

Quotations from the experts

Mental illness:

'Five years ago, 95% of psychiatrists would have said that cannabis doesn't cause psychosis. Now I would estimate that 95% say it does.' (Professor Robin Murray, Director, Institute of Psychiatry, London, October 2006)

'The mistake was that in its 2002 report, The Advisory Council on the Misuse of Drugs denied that cannabis was a contributory cause of schizophrenia, continued to deny this for the next two years and thus mislead ministers into repeatedly stating that there was no causal link between cannabis and psychosis.' (Professor Robin Murray, letter to The Guardian, 19/01/06)

Personality:

'If the development of identity does not progress, the teenager remains at a childish level of development characterised by both a lack of independence and a deficient integration in the adult world.' (Swedish researcher Jan Ranstrom, 2003)

Academic performance:

'Use more often than twice per week for even a short period of time, or use for 5 years or more at the level of even once per month, may each lead to a compromised ability to function to their full mental capacity, and could possibly result in lasting impairments.' (Dr Nadia Solowij, Cannabis and Cognitive Functioning, 1998)

The warning on Nabilone reads:

'THC encourages both physical and psychological dependence and is highly abusable. It causes mood changes, loss of memory, psychoses, impairment of coordination and perception, and complicates pregnancy.'

Dr Robert Dupont, founder of NIDA (National Institute for Drug Abuse) in the USA, said, *'I have been apologising to the American people for the last 10 years for promoting the decriminalisation of cannabis. I made a mistake. Marijuana combines the worst effects of alcohol and tobacco and has other ill effects that neither of these two have.'* He added, *'In all of history, no young people have ever taken marijuana regularly on a mass scale. Therefore our youngsters are in effect making themselves guinea pigs in a tragic experiment. Thus far our research clearly suggests we will see horrendous results.'*

Mary Brett, Former Head of Health Education, Dr Challoner's Grammar School (boys), Amersham, Bucks.
UK spokesman for EURAD (Europe against Drugs).
References can be found in *'Cannabis – a general view of its harmful effects'* by Mary Brett on the *'Talking about Cannabis'* website (www.talkingaboutcannabis.com) June 2007.

STREET DRUGS

Marijuana – pot, cannabis
4 times more dangerous than cigarette smoking
3 times more tar in the lungs and 5 times more carbon monoxide

Psychoactive substance is tetrahydrocannabinol (THC) – steroid structure found in the sex hormones and in certain hormones of the adrenal glands.
THC accumulates in the ovaries and testes.

Women – upsets menstrual cycle, tolerated and then restored.
Men – lowers blood testosterone, lowers sperm count, greater than usual impotency and diminished libido. Sperm motility affected and an increase in number of abnormal sperm.
Effects the synthesis of DNA. In animals linked with increased foetal deaths and malformations.

Cocaine & Crack
In mice – teratogenic even at non-toxic levels.
Humans – decrease in weight of foetus, higher malformation rate and increased stillbirth rate.

Crack is a cocaine derivative which is purer than cocaine.
Withdrawal symptoms in the new born are severe.
Heroin
Heroin and other opiate narcotics such as opium, morphine and codeine are all extremely addictive.

Decreased fertility and atrophy of the male accessory sex organs, decreased testosterone.

3 times more stillbirths
4 times more premature births
6 times more growth problems

Babies are born addicted to the drug and have to endure withdrawal.

CHAPTER 5
Contraception, including the Pill

Margaret's story:

They married quite young as their love had been kindled when they were school children. Their life was ahead of them, a house, their careers and children. They both loved children but were careful – Margaret was on the pill. There was time for children later.

When they decided to start a family, Margaret came off the pill but it didn't happen. Her menstrual cycles stopped, and they were deeply distressed that there was a problem. A previous illness had left Margaret underweight, which contributed to their situation.

A family friend, a paediatric consultant at a local hospital, suggested that they contact Foresight – as it was Foresight who had previously helped the consultant with her own fertility issues. Both Margaret and her husband were put on the Foresight programme. Hair was sent for analysis, the diet was tidied up, alcohol and tobacco were dropped.

The hair analysis revealed that there were high levels of mercury in both their samples, which was a result of eating a lot of tuna. Once this was addressed, their mercury levels dropped and previously low zinc levels began to rise. The periods returned quickly!

For 18 months they followed the programme. Their GP told them that they could try Clomid but that 'it doesn't always work' and they would have to try IVF. This would have taken longer than they wanted to wait, but they stayed on the Foresight programme, with six months of Clomid, and Margaret conceived and her baby daughter was born weighing 8lb 7 oz.

Margaret has continued on the programme as 'it kept me healthy'. Now, as they are looking to enlarge their family, both husband and wife are back on the programme.

About Foresight, Margaret said, 'Excellent.'

For information on risks associated with the pill, Dr Paavo Airola, a world authority on nutrition and biological medicine, has listed the risks under two headings: the less serious, which are still bothersome and those which cause serious complications. We could argue with his divisions – depression and increased susceptibility to vaginal and bladder infections are hardly 'less serious' – but taking both lists together, we can gauge the detrimental effects on female health. His lists include:

'Less serious, although bothersome'

Increased susceptibility to vaginal and bladder infections
Lowered resistance to all infections
Cramps
Dry, blotchy skin. Mouth ulcers
Dry, falling hair and baldness
Premature wrinkling
Acne
Sleep disturbances
Inability to concentrate
Migraine headaches
Depression, moodiness, irritability
Darkening of the skin of upper lip and lower eyelids
Sore breasts
Nausea
Weight gain and body distortion due to disproportional distribution of fat
Chronic fatigue
Increase in dental cavities
Swollen and bleeding gums
Greatly increased or decreased sex drive
Visual disturbances
Amenorrhoea (no periods)
Blood sugar level disturbances which complicate diabetes or hypoglycaemia

'More serious complications'

Eczema
Gallbladder problems

Hyperlipemia (excess fat in the blood)
Intolerance to carbohydrates leading to 'steroid diabetes', which can lead to clinical diabetes
Strokes
Seven to ten times greater risk of death due to blood clots
Jaundice
Epilepsy
High blood pressure
Kidney failure
Oedema (swelling)
Permanent infertility
Varicose veins
Thrombophlebitis and pulmonary embolism
Heart attacks
Cancer of the breast, uterus, liver, and pituitary gland

To this list Foresight can add:

Vitamin and mineral imbalances
Ectopic pregnancy
Miscarriage of later pregnancies
Food allergies
Genitourinary disease, including cervicitis
Congenital malformations in later babies
Osteoporosis
Ovarian and lung cancer
Fungal infections

The items that are in bold are the ones for which there are specific warnings on the instructions which come with all packets of the pill. Obviously, for most women, this is where they will get their information and it is, therefore, very important that it is not misleading.

There was a brief trial of men being put on a male version of the pill. However, this was very soon abandoned as the men complained of headaches and shrunken testicles. The experiment was instantly halted and has not been repeated!

Shirlayne's story:

They had decided that they would like to get their future sorted out in terms of job security etc before starting a family. So, for nine years, Shirlayne was on the pill. In 2002, they decided to start planning for pregnancy.

She stopped the pill and used the Persona method of natural family planning so that her body could adjust itself after years on the pill. In 2003 it was time to start a family and Shirlayne conceived almost straight away. Due to constant bleeding, four scans were performed at the Early Pregnancy Clinic between weeks 4 and 6, by which time a miscarriage was confirmed. A second conception took place, but this was also miscarried at ten weeks.

Flicking through a magazine, Shirlayne found Foresight. She contacted them immediately and went on the programme. Her husband, short of hair, just couldn't, on numerous occasions, get enough hair for the laboratory. Shirlayne's analysis revealed high copper levels which were addressed straight away. Within two months she conceived and again bled. Undeterred, Shirlayne continued with the Foresight programme and a Foresight baby girl was born at 43 weeks weighing 7lb 13oz, Apgar 10.

Not wanting a large gap between babies, once back on the programme, Shirlayne fell pregnant again and this time bled for only one week. Her pregnancy was very easy with no nausea at all. Foresight Baby Girl 2 was born weighing 8lb 11oz, Apgar 10. Whilst the recent baby was on both mixed breastfeeding and solids, Foresight Baby 3 was conceived. The first two babies had been born by caesarean section but the scar had begun to rupture so Foresight Baby Girl 3 was also born by caesarean section at 36 weeks, 6lb 1oz.

Shirlayne says: 'Why is Foresight not known about more? It's a shame people only contact Foresight when they find it difficult to get pregnant. Such good and sensible advice.'

Children born after pill use are more prone to birthmarks, skeletal abnormalities (deformities of the skeleton such as cleft palate and spina bifida), reduced IQ, and learning difficulties such as dyslexia and ADHD. These problems will be mainly due to the fact that the pill raises the level of copper in the body and lowers the level of zinc, manganese and B6.

As is discussed elsewhere in this book, these deficiencies can be righted in time by the full Foresight programme. However, every problem we examine does make us realise how very much at risk the general population is, and how it is no wonder that we have a generation of children riddled with deficiency, allergic illness, behavioural problems and inability to learn.

So what are my own feelings about the development of life for women since the advent of the pill? I was part of the pre-pill generation and I have watched life unfold over the last 80-odd years.

The line we were all sold over the pill was that it 'heralded a new deal for women', a brighter era had dawned. Family size could be limited to manageable, as there would be choice about how many children you had in your family. You would decide, in view of the mother's health and the financial viability, exactly when you had your babies. 'Every child a wanted child' was the battle cry (every pill a profit to the industry concerned, of course!).

The public believed this was the end of poverty as everything would be under control. The household budgets would be manageable, women would no longer be exhausted, harassed, and strapped for cash – it would be a land of happiness and plenty.

So far, so good (it could have been if they had gone for natural family planning, of course, but more on this later...)

Fast-forward to what has actually happened. Let's face it, the 'libertarians' rushed forward with what they called 'free love'. This meant, in reality, sex free from love. Men then felt free to seduce their secretaries or their friends' wives or anyone else. Let's face it, there were many more deserted wives, loveless unions, and single mothers left to fend for themselves and do most of the upbringing of one or more children on their own.

Jane's story:

Not long after trying for a baby, Jane conceived, but the joy was short-lived when at around 12 weeks bleeding began. A chromosome 22 was detected and a termination was organised. Determined, they approached a fertility specialist who organised an IUI. When that failed, both Jane and her husband were told not to worry, to forget about it. 'It will work out all right.'

Three years later they went for IVF; this too failed. At 37 years old they travelled abroad for another IVF but sadly nothing happened.

On their return to the UK, Jane, as determined as ever, began to search for information on pregnancy and came across Foresight listed in the back of one of the books that she had read. Foresight was contacted and both of them began the programme.

Painful periods led her to get information on herbs and to try acupuncture. She got involved in natural products, changed her diet and bought organic food where possible. Both followed the programme for the next three years, taking their supplements, including lots of zinc. They didn't worry any more, exercised regularly and generally went on with their lives.

Being aware of her cycle, Jane found that she was late. She had gone on to day 44. She took two tries at a pregnancy test because she couldn't believe her eyes! When she spoke to her husband, he already knew. 'I told you so!' was what he said!

A baby boy, 9 lb 3 oz and 57 cm long, was safely delivered. 'He's into everything, very determined, growing fast and loves his food. We prayed, people in church prayed. I am nearly 40 years old. He is our miracle baby.'

It had taken ten years!

So much for less hardship and less exhaustion! On the heels of this sad little revolution comes the era of teenagers and older people sleeping around, living alone or cohabiting without bothering with marriage. Lots of sexually transmitted disease, lots of girls and women ill with the side effects and without even having the information about where the PMT and the explosive mood changes are coming from! Also lots of babies born out of wedlock, and, if no babies at an early stage, later a Holocaust of broken dreams, with the infertility and/or miscarriage, the premature births and infants who aren't quite right. Again, the lost hopes of the women who tried to wait to have their children until the marriage that never came, or came too late, the panic and the tears and sometimes the bitter disappointment.

'You can have it all,' the girls are told. 'You have your career, and when you are well established, you will have a double income household and will be able to afford childcare'. It is an artificial damming-up of the natural flow of love and maternal feelings that everyone appears to accept as 'part and parcel' of the deal. Their blandishments, the manipulation of the hormones that control emotional development, and the whole feminist movement seem to have confused an entire generation of young women. They are encouraged to suppress their natural instincts – then the chemicals in the pill take over and more brutally do this for them.

To fall in love, to marry, to have your children, to love your house and garden and love looking after your family – that is doing what comes naturally. The joy grows inside you as your body matures and natural hopes and desires play like music in every cell of your body.

Babies are wonderful. The happiest and the most joyfully chaotic days of your entire life will be spent bringing up a young family! It is a huge, growing, developing, loving experience for everyone. It is what a young woman's body wants to do. To make love, get pregnant, have babies and breastfeed and nurture them until they grow up. Every animal in the wild is doing the same!

So what have the problems been? Why has loving and laughing gone out of fashion with so many people? Because, given the chance, hormones develop naturally in growing women and are the secret orchestra that plays their body music for them – and all their thoughts and dreams and future plans dance to their body music.

So what happens when you switch the music off? Initially, the hormones given in the first pill were very strong. Women I knew told me they felt sick all the time, like pregnancy sickness. Another side-effect was that it reduced the libido. Not a happy effect at the beginning of married life. Those who realised the connection complained...

Then a small amount of male testosterone was added to the pill. Just to 'switch the libido on again'. The effects were gradual and subtle but the change was tangible after a time. Women journalists 'dared' to say that they were not enjoying motherhood – that it was getting in the way of their careers. It became fashionable to abandon the idea of having babies.

The DINKYs started to appear. 'Double income, no kids yet', the estate agents chorused with joy. The truth is that instead of women marrying, and happily starting their families when they wished to (as envisaged at the outset of the pill era), they are harassed, exploited, overworked and cash-strapped as seldom before!

They are forced to become wage earners for the best fertile years of their young lives. They have to chemically crush their natural fertility and all the precious dreams and the thrust and excitement that goes with it. Many of them have to sit tapping away at a computer all day long to get enough money to pay for a much smaller house or flat than a previous generation had for far less money. Many are having to put their children and even very young babies into childcare whether they want to or not. It takes a couple's combined efforts to pay the astronomical mortgage and all the other bills which have risen too, as all the country's other employees also have to keep a roof over their heads!

Some women are deeply unhappy about having to hand over their beloved babies into the care of strangers and most of them find it stressful. A few years ago, the National Council of Women did a survey and found that 94% of women who had small children and were doing a job were finding it stressful and almost all of them would have preferred to be at home with their children – 94% of women not as happy as they could be and dare I say 100% of children not very happy either.

When mother and child are apart all day, the maternal/baby bond does not develop as love should develop. Many of the children are disoriented and unhappy and gradually they become unmanageable. It is not normal or natural for a tiny child to be parted from its own mother. Anyone who has been with animals will tell you how a lamb will bleat for its mother, how a foal will whinny to be returned to the mare etc – this is normal and natural. When I was a child in Wales, the way you took a cow and a calf to market was to put the calf in the pony trap, and get in and trot off. The cow would trot behind as she would never let the calf be taken out of her sight.

We do not want to lose this instinct. Love is what life is all about. It is indefinably precious and far-reaching. It fuels family love, it fuels understanding of others, it fuels all positive emotions. It is the basis of how a parent can influence a child. This is called 'up-bringing'. I fear that the pill cocktail with its testosterone fillip just puts this age-old instinct right off!

Women are finding fertility hard. Far too many cannot have the baby of their dreams. Many have found previous pregnancies hard and have had many health complications, followed by a long and difficult labour. Sometimes they have the baby successfully but the milk does not come in. I was told about their struggles with previous pregnancies, every day. In many cases, a baby has been born prematurely and some, tragically, do not survive and some have lifelong disabilities.

Many of these sad happenings are directly due to the fact that the contraceptive pill induces copper to rise in the body and due to the imbalance, the elements zinc and manganese fall. Copper and zinc/manganese are biochemical antagonists, and as one rises, the others will fall. (Pfeiffer, Bryce-Smith, Grant)

Lack of both zinc and manganese has been found to eliminate the maternal instinct in laboratory animals. (Carl Pfeiffer and Oberleas and Caldwell) Rat mothers deprived of zinc have a long and difficult labour, which is otherwise unusual in rodents. (They have litters of young, and so in the normal way the young are commensurately smaller and easier to produce.) After the birth, if she is deficient, the rat mother will go down to the far corner of the cage and curl up in a ball, pull her tail over her nose and switch off. She will not go near the litter to feed them, clean them up or pull them back into the nest if they fall out. All the usual loving attention a mother rat instinctively gives to her babies is entirely absent.

The same thing happens exactly if she is kept short of manganese. The rat pups are left to die – unless the laboratory assistant finds them a foster mother. It is interesting that, even when the offspring are given a replete foster mother, this exercise is not very successful. Zinc/manganese-deficient youngsters are poor suckers and their general development is much slower than rats who received sufficient zinc/manganese in the womb. Their coats are sparse, they are slow to gain weight, late to cut their teeth and slow to leave the nest. I think we can conclude that life is a struggle for them.

The work of Professor Bert Vallee of Harvard University Medical School, again researching with rats and rabbits etc, showed that zinc deficiency/copper excess could lead to premature birth. He demonstrated that in the third trimester of pregnancy, the copper rose in the body and the zinc was all gathered in from the bloodstream and given to the placenta. As the copper (which is a brain stimulant) rose and the zinc fell to a certain ratio, the phenomenon of birth was started and the labour went ahead. The rodents then ate their placentas immediately after giving birth. As the placentas were so rich in zinc, within 96 hours, the copper/zinc balance was restored in the blood. As the zinc level rose in the milk, the rat pups became calmer and were more easily satisfied and settled to sleep better.

Professor Derek Bryce-Smith, when he was at Reading University, tested a large number of human placentas and found the zinc content was between 350 and 600 mg. At Foresight, we are usually giving about 60 mg a day at the time of birth – we find this prevents any depression and means the milk comes in very well. The milk is satisfying and this means a happy baby as well!

We find non-Foresight mothers with post-partum depression, recover in three to four days when adequate zinc – 100 mg a day –

is given. This will filter through to the milk also, in the quantities required, and then the baby will settle to sleep.

The combination of zinc/copper imbalances resulting from copper in the drinking water (coming from copper water pipes), and the contraceptive pill causing the woman's body to retain it, is all a major modern woman's health hazard and it can affect all areas of her life.

These problems, and the fact that the zinc lost in the placenta is not replaced (unless supplemented at the time), lead to a whole range of mental illnesses in women. This may lead, in some cases, to being put on Benzodiazepine, Valium, Prozac etc. Much long-term mental illness, abandonment of children, breaking up of marriages etc stems from this.

A lot of conditions in children born after pill use, such as eczema and asthma, are partly due to lack of zinc (in asthma, lack of selenium and essential oils is also involved) and epilepsy can often be due to lack of zinc, magnesium and manganese. (Underwood, Pfeiffer, Brostoff, Passswater & Cranton, Saner, Underwood, Ward, Williams)

We constantly do hair analysis for the previous children of couples who come to us where there are problems. The imbalances in the children reflect those in their parents but they are usually more severe in the children and are often producing chronic illnesses and/or aberrant behaviour.

Conditions such as dyslexia and ADHD always show up with low hair zinc. It is since the pill and copper water pipes (also mass vaccination) that these problems have suddenly appeared, having virtually not been there in previous generations. They will continue to escalate, unless we take steps to reverse them. Each generation will suffer more severely than the previous one. (Grant, Bell, Bennett & Neil)

It is almost certainly due to this huge prevalence of zinc-deficient children that the vaccinations are causing such appalling problems. Zinc is needed to fire up the immune system. Therefore introducing foreign substances into the bloodstream will call for more and more zinc every time it happens.

These events can result in the immune system making huge and sudden demands for zinc leading to flare-ups of eczema, so it has now been suggested that overtly eczematous children be excused vaccination. However some whose poor zinc levels are manifesting in other ways, or whose levels are borderline, will still be vaccinated, and will still suffer (parents should know that they can refuse vaccination, and should do so).

The small intestine is normally covered with a lining that is rich in an enzyme called alkaline phosphatase. This is a zinc-dependent enzyme, i.e. it needs a zinc co-factor. Enzymes all have a co-factor, which is usually, although not always, a mineral. The co-factor, apparently, is like the outboard motor on a dinghy – without it, the enzyme 'does not work'.

With zinc deficiency, therefore, the working of the small intestine is deprived of alkaline phosphatase and is usually severely compromised. Hence, if the vaccines do not cause the body to call in the zinc from the skin, giving the poor little child the nightmare of itching eczema, it will call for zinc from the alkaline phosphatase in the gut and the poor little mite will have diarrhoea.

The diarrhoea will give the body a shortage of **every** essential nutrient before too long. So about a couple of weeks after vaccination, the child's development will start to regress. The child will also feel desperately ill, exhausted and distraught, and will have what are described as 'tantrums', 'night terrors', etc. The parents will find the child 'difficult'; the child may just continue to regress into autism or sometimes, in the most tragic cases about 16 days after the event, into 'cot death'.

Dr Viera Scheibner, PhD, Principal Research Scientist (Rtd) Brataslava University has noticed that the adverse reaction to vaccination has a measurable rhythm to it. The children were worse on the 3rd, 6th, 11th and 16th day after the jab. It seems each time the body called for the zinc (and possibly other nutrients we know less about, very possibly vitamin A or C) the response took a little longer.

The skin, the intestine, and probably the brain itself, would need to relinquish zinc it could ill afford. The immune system acts on the rest of the body rather like a poor relation who keeps suffering 'bad luck' and unfortunately keeps having to be 'sustained' until the long-suffering family are driven slowly bankrupt! Hence the huge increases in many diverse childhood conditions in the last couple of generations. Too much is demanded from a tiny body for the amount of nutrients there are to go round. Part of the story is the pill having created at least part of the paucity in the first place.

There is another aspect of this much-trumpeted 'freedom' for women that is not all unadulterated benefit. Abortion. 'The woman's (or man's) right to choose' – to destroy her baby. We need to think about this more than we do. Most women love their baby from the moment they know it is there and for many, having to have their baby removed from their body by force, is a cruel and devastating experience. This may not be a very modern way to look at it but women are not modern inventions – they go back a long way. They have very deep feelings that are not entirely obliterated either by present-day 'culture' or by the hormonal manipulation provided by the pill. Rather like dyeing the hair – the surface changes in appearance, but the real stuff still grows out!

Write and tell me if I am wrong, but most of the women who talk to me when they have been through this experience are still sad that it happened, even many years on.

Some fear that the womb was damaged and this is why they are having problems conceiving now and many are still lonely for the baby they lost. If they are aware that their child is alive in the life to come, they miss them and are deeply frustrated not to have been able to know and love them. They are often aware of how old the child would be and know the 'birthdays' and so on. My own belief is that most abortion is the product of love-free sex which is usually deeply disappointing for a woman. However we are entitled to wonder and you are all entitled to rethink many aspects of life on behalf of your own generation, and those to come.

Yet another aspect of the pill-promoted 'culture' is the influence the little dollops of testosterone have had on the maternal instinct and the way this has been perceived by the male psychiatrist.

Overlaying the normal hormonal ebb and flow around the cycle with a daily clobbering of hormones from outside the body (be they from another animal or manufactured in a laboratory) is bound to change the mood. You cannot 'turn off' the role of the ovaries and the uterus without 'turning off' or drastically altering a large portion of the woman's emotions.

'Mood swings' is even acknowledged on the list of side effects put on the pill box! What exactly is a 'mood'? Is it the amount you love, the way you handle relationships, the way you care, the way you react? The feelings behind everything you do? If you are in minute-by-minute contact with someone who is so dependent and needs your love as a baby or small child does, how does this affect his and your emotional development together? Have the 'scientists' ever thought of this one?

Then we have the psychiatrists telling us that all mass-murderers had terrible mothers who gave them no affection and ruined their emotional lives, causing them to erupt into violence they were unable to contain. Yes, well. I would go back a lot further than that. What affected the mothers so badly – the pill, lack of zinc (remember how the zinc-deficient rats treated their litters)? Maybe the mothers too had smoking, alcohol-drinking and pesticide-contaminated parents? Maybe during their infancy, their brains were bashed by a thiomersal cocktail (vaccine) every few months? Copper water pipes (in certain areas) have a lot to answer for as do food additives, medications, fluoride, vaccinations etc etc.

Let's understand where it all comes from. Let's stop the blame game and let's just put it all right for the next generation. Let's try and tidy everything up for them, so they start with a clean slate. It is a lot of effort but it's not too expensive or impossible.

So what do we do?

Well, Foresight has worked out a programme that it is offering to you, that can reverse the damage. It provides information on diet to make it replete in all the vitamins and trace minerals.

Get shot of tobacco, alcohol, caffeine and street drugs.

How to avoid the plague of the contraceptive pill and the copper coil! Learn natural family planning (NFP) from Colleen Norman so you need never risk using them again.

Colleen will tell you how to reliably control your fertility without the need for the pill. She has an excellent website where you will find everything you want, including, hopefully, the name of your nearest natural family planning teacher.

This, in Colleen's own words, is how she describes her approach for us:

Natural Family Planning
Fertility control by education, not intervention.

There are basically two approaches to fertility control. The standard clinical approach has been to encourage couples to believe they are permanently fertile and insist that a method of contraception be in use every time they make love. This 'continuous contraceptive approach' is certainly effective but there is a price to be paid in health risks with some methods, and reduction of satisfaction levels with others. Since in fact there are only a few days in each monthly cycle when a woman is fertile, many couples regret this 'blunderbuss' approach of continuous contraception, where each day is treated as highly fertile, and are seeking alternatives.

The alternative approach which is therefore enjoying increasing publicity and demand is to offer couples a programme of education in fertility awareness, teaching them to identify accurately those few fertile days in each cycle. The couple can then build a natural loving sexual relationship around the fertility cycle, including at the fertile days if they wish to plan a pregnancy, and avoiding them if pregnancy is not desired at that moment. It provides an efficient means of fertility control which is non-invasive and therefore free of side-effects and health hazards. This can be termed the 'ecological approach', otherwise known as the fertility awareness method, or natural family planning.

Past myths

The main objection to this second approach has been its reputed unreliability. The reasons for the high failure rates associated with the old 'calendar rhythm method' need to be understood, but it must not be confused with modern techniques of natural family planning, which on WHO statistics has a biological failure rate of virtually zero. Back in the 1940s when the rhythm method was developed, the accepted fertility facts were that a woman always ovulated 14 days before the onset of her next period, that her egg lived for three days, and that sperm also lived for up to three days (none of these facts is actually correct!). A woman was required to calculate the date of her next period, then count back 14 days to her estimated day of ovulation. To avoid pregnancy, couples were told to avoid intercourse for four days before and after that date.

The reasons for the high failure rate (declared in all studies to be 33%) are obvious – irregular cycles, and misinformation.

The egg, in fact, is fertilisable for only 8–24 hours, but sperm can live up to six days given certain circumstances. The luteal phase (the time between ovulation and menstruation) is not a fixed gap of 14 days but can be as short as 10 days for some women and as long as 16 days for others. How does a woman know which one she has? No calculation method could embrace so many variables.

Yet despite all that, it is amazing how many couples have used this method with success. I am meeting them all the time in NFP clinics! The old-fashioned calendar calculation method, with all its inaccuracies, is of course still used in most sub-fertility clinics, where couples are told to have intercourse 14 days before the period is due, which is too late for some, and too early for others.

New knowledge

A step forward in the identification of ovulation came in the 1950s with the introduction of the temperature method, perfected by Prof. John Marshall, a consultant neurologist in London. If a woman was prepared to take her temperature for a few mornings each month, before getting up and at approximately the same time, with a special fertility thermometer, she would find that her body temperature was at a lower level until she ovulated.

After ovulation her temperature would rise and stay at a higher level for the next two weeks. If she had conceived, her temperature would continue to stay up, providing her with a free proof of pregnancy. If she had not conceived, her temperature would fall with the onset of her period and a new fertility cycle would start, repeating each time this biphasic temperature pattern. Prof. Marshall's studies showed that if a couple waited till three high temperatures had been recorded after ovulation, the failure rate for the rest of the luteal phase was very low. In the 1970s Prof. Tietze in his international review of all methods of contraception ranked the temperature method (post-ovulation only) as a 'highly efficient' method of contraception, 'comparable to sterilisation or a high-dose pill'.

The limitations of the method were that, though it accurately confirmed the event of ovulation and released nearly half the average cycle for infertile intercourse, it gave no warning of an approaching ovulation. When couples had intercourse based on calendar rhythm calculations before ovulation, the failure rate jumped from virtually zero to 19%! The temperature method is also used in sub-fertility clinics but its benefits are often lost when couples are told to have intercourse when the temperature dips and again when it rises. The temperature could 'dip' on any day if she took it earlier than usual. If she waits till the rise, hormone assays have shown that the rise can be delayed up to 48 hours after ovulation. Since the egg is fertilisable for as little as 8–24 hours, it could well be a case of closing the door after the horse has bolted!

What was needed, both to plan and to avoid pregnancy successfully, was a sign obvious to a woman that her egg was ripening in her ovary. Here we are indebted to a team of doctors and researchers in Western Australia, headed by Drs John and Evelyn Billings, who began to study the pattern of vaginal discharge in women. After years of double-checking their work with hormone assays, this is what they learnt:

As the egg-sac (follicle) starts ripening in the ovary, a hormone called estrogen is produced, which stimulates glands in the neck of the womb (cervix) to produce a wet, slippery, relatively clear mucus discharge. This mucus is alkaline and neutralises the acidity in the vagina, enabling sperms to survive in it. It is also rich in nutrients which attract and feed the sperm prolonging their life for several days. Its thin watery nature has a molecular structure that produces a swimming lane structure through which sperm can migrate out of the vagina and into the cervix at incredible speed, and thereafter upwards towards the ripening egg. The mucus increases in flow for approximately the 6 days that the follicle takes to fully ripen. It produces a sensation of wetness and lubrication at the external opening of the vagina which most women cannot fail to notice. When ovulation is imminent, the wet slippery mucus can become so clear that it looks like raw egg-white. This mucus is vital for sperm, which can live minutes or hours at most without it. But once in this mucus, the sperm can live for 3–6 days inside the neck of the womb.

As the egg is released, the mucus, having done its work, dries up and forms a plug in the neck of the womb to prevent the passage of any more sperm upwards. In that way the womb cavity is kept clear ready to receive the baby down the fallopian tube should it be conceived. The womb lining becomes very thick and spongy, ready for the baby to implant into it. However, some 10 to 16 days after ovulation, if there is no baby implanted in that lining, then the lining is washed away in menstruation, and a new fertility cycle starts. For this reason many older midwives used to speak of the menstruation as 'the weeping of the disappointed womb'.

The accuracy of the mucus symptom as an indicator of ovulation is beyond doubt. The hormone assays of James Brown in Melbourne, now supported by ultrasound studies in many centres, my own included, have all shown that the subjective observations of simple women (even those with minimal education levels in developing countries) are as accurate in identifying ovulation as tests for LH peak. When these observations of mucus patterns are combined with minimal use of the temperature method, the biological failure rate of natural family planning is virtually zero. The user failure rate, as with all methods, can be higher. So whenever I am asked the question 'How successful is NFP in preventing pregnancy?' my answer is the same: 'It is as successful as you make it. If you stick with the rules, it works. If you take risks, the failure rate is high because you are using the potentially fertile days.'

It goes without saying that mucus observation is vital to couples experiencing sub-fertility. It frees them from inaccurate calculations and temperature charts that are only useful in retrospect. Instead it allows them to identify their potentially fertile phase, no matter how short or inadequate it may be, and enables them to maximise their chances of conception.

Couples in all other aspects of their lives are usually trying to live in harmony with nature rather that in destructive conflict. Yet they often come up against a brick wall when seeking a natural solution to the most intimate area of their lives, their sexual relationship and the control of their fertility. There are at last several good books on the subject and simplified charting systems to help couples use the method successfully. Having used natural methods over 25 years of marriage, I am convinced of the benefits of NFP for modern society. I hope I have given you food for thought and dispelled some of the prejudice against natural methods.

If you would like further information about charting the fertility cycle, please contact Colleen enclosing cheque or PO for £4 and she will send you literature and the address of your nearest NFP teacher.

Mrs Colleen Norman
218 Heathwood Road
Heath, Cardiff
CF4 4BS
Tel: 02920 754628
www.fertilityet.org.uk

We all owe a huge debt of gratitude to Colleen. She is totally dedicated and has worked for most of her life to bring NFP to those who need and wish to use it.

One more thing: Colleen is constantly in need of new people to train as Natural Family Planning teachers. On her website Colleen advertises where and when these courses will be taking place. She will be absolutely delighted to hear from you, if you would like to attend one.

Colleen's way of doing things is the right one. The likelihood of unintentional pregnancy using the method she describes is down to about one baby per hundred.

However, I do know that some of you will find the five days of abstinence very hard. So, as a Black Protestant (as we were called in Tudor times), I am happy to suggest the cap or the diaphragm, used with a little manuka honey, at these times. Honey has a natural anti-candida agent. It also seems a little more sperm-friendly.

It has to be understood that this adapted approach is probably a little less sure of success than Colleen's stricter regime, but then again I always think another baby is the happiest thing that can happen in any family! Another huge advantage of taking on board Colleen's knowledge is, of course, that when you intend to conceive you can use your expertise to make sure you do so as soon as possible! Yet another huge advantage is that your life is entirely under your own control. Your moods, your dreams, your hopes, your loves are your own. You are not being altered and manipulated by some little white pill, made somewhere miles away by somebody who does not even know you!

Yet another advantage: the hormones from your urine entering the water table are not polluting the planet, and perhaps inadvertently causing infertility to wildlife – or PMT or cancer, migraine, premature birth – who knows? We do not know what we are doing, do we?

We all need to wonder what this huge uncontrolled dose of extra hormones is doing to our own species. There is the pill, then fertility drugs, then HRT, and since all of this has been pouring into the biosphere there has been such a huge increase in paedophilia and exchange of pornography on the internet. Children are being abducted and murdered and all sorts of chillingly aberrant sexuality seems to be on the increase. Why? Do we know how much in the way of aberrant hormones accidentally found their way into these strange, troubled minds? Was their mother on the pill for many years before they were conceived? Were they fed on breast milk laced with pill-hormones? Were they fed on beef-burgers from American steers fed 'growth hormones'? Was their drinking water awash with female hormones? Was it in the fish which were fished out of similarly suspect river water with very damaged genitalia? Are we eating fish that have had similar problems?

Do you ever feel we can be over-educated, and under-loved with too much sitting at a school desk and then an office computer, too much paperwork, too little humour and too little interaction with other people? It seems that we are all being 'trained' to chuff along the rails and make a contribution to some great amorphous commercial giant organisation rather than enjoying our own family? Are we all being 'trained' to live a life we do not really enjoy living?

What is going on? Do we need to rethink our lives? Let's all of us try to struggle back onto the road to 'Natural'. We have no idea what we are doing otherwise. Life should be lived much more by instinct – the eternal wisdom we carry inside us like the birds and animals etc. Remember, there is a Supreme Love that can make a butterfly sperm that can effortlessly reproduce the resplendent wing colours every time... Let's put more faith in our own natural instincts and help the planet to remain a normal, cheerfully fertile spinning miracle!

Onwards!

CHAPTER 6
Genitourinary and Other Infections

This chapter is about the health disruptors that can undermine, in some cases, your general feeling of 'wellness', and, as we know, anything that does this can also be undermining your fertility.

Any type of illness causes you to activate the immune system. This calls for vitamins A and B2, folic acid, zinc, manganese etc. All the good guys who work for us tirelessly around the clock are squandered as they chase armies of unnecessary bugs.

The genitourinary infections are known as GUI. Things like chlamydia, which everybody has now heard of, are alarmingly prevalent, and the damage they do to couples and their babies' health seems to be catastrophically under-estimated.

During World War II, we were left in no doubt about the danger of venereal disease (VD), as it was then called. Every post office, train station, public convenience or bus stop had posters in A3 size, listing the symptoms and advising on the whereabouts of the nearest VD clinic. The government recognised that they could not afford to be coy about it, as many of the service men would be bringing home 'a packet' and the women needed help on what to do.

Today the prevalence is likely to be much greater than in yesteryear but what is out there and what it does, remains, in essence, exactly the same. My advice on how to tackle it would be:

(a) Ring your local large hospital and ask if they have a genitourinary medicine (GUM) clinic. They probably do, but if they do not, they will be able to tell you where the nearest one is. You may also find family planning and sexual health clinics in telephone directories. There is also a helpline: 0845 310 1334. Make an appointment and if possible both of you should go. If one partner is reluctant, then the other should go. If the partner who attends is clear, then it is more likely that the other one will be, but this is not infallible. Do your best. If the partner who attends has an infection, then it is extremely likely that you both do. At least get the second partner to take the treatment.

(b) Once you have the diagnosis, you can take the antibiotic given by the clinic or you can consult a homoeopath for a homoeopathic remedy. Ainsworths Homoeopathic Chemist, in London (see Useful Addresses), has remedies for many conditions, ready and waiting. Whatever the case, you should **both** take the remedy.

(c) Once you have taken the solution of your choice, leave it for three weeks, then return to the clinic to check that this has solved it. If not, repeat the remedy and recheck again.

(d) At the same time (or directly afterwards if your homoeopath thinks this is preferable), take 3 gms of vitamin C and 100 mg of zinc for a couple of weeks (plus 5,000 iu of vitamin A for three days while you have your period).

If you have had the infection for a while, it may later be advisable to have the patency of your fallopian tubes checked, as if the bugs have travelled up the tubes this can cause blockages. Sometimes an experienced reflexologist can tell if the tubes are not in a good state. Sometimes they can increase the peristaltic action a little bit, to get them to evacuate mucus and pus, and this way it may be possible to clear them. For this reason I would make reflexology your third port of call, after a diagnosis and obtaining the remedy.

Now for all the detailed scientific information.

For the scientific nitty-gritty, I think I can do no better than to reproduce Gail's excellent chapter of 1994, which also includes other infections that could affect the course of the pregnancy and the outcome.

Gail Bradley's Chapter:

We have long recognised that certain diseases can adversely affect the foetus (e.g. German measles), or cause sterility (e.g. mumps). But we often overlook the importance of genitourinary infections, which include sexually transmitted diseases. Clearly, any infection in the baby at the start of its life is serious. We have seen that stress increases the need for nutrients – nutrients which are needed for the development of the sperm, egg or foetus. Thus, infection can indirectly affect the development. It may, of course, have direct effects, causing sight problems (eye infections) or brain damage (as in some meningitis cases).

In this chapter we review some of the literature on genitourinary and other infections.

Toxoplasmosis (not a GUI but important nonetheless)

This is an infection which may result from eating raw or insufficiently cooked meat and raw fish, or from contact with cat faeces or cat litter, or from eating foods soiled by animal carriers of Toxoplasma gondii, the organism which causes toxoplasmosis. (Ideally you should be screened before becoming pregnant.) If it is contracted in the first half of pregnancy, it may cause the baby to suffer from hydrocephalus, eye problems, psychomotor retardation, convulsions, microphthalmia, and intracerebral calcifications (calcium deposits in the brain). In the second half of pregnancy, the damage it may cause to the foetus is likely to be less severe. If diagnosed early, toxoplasmosis can be treated with antibiotics which do not harm the baby. If you think you may be carrying the organism or if you have flu-like symptoms then you should see your doctor immediately. You may have to convince your doctor of the necessity of a test since not all GPs think the test is reliable and not all know that the infection can be treated.

Cytomegalovirus (CMV)

Caused by one of the herpes viruses, this can have serious problems for men, women and infants. It is linked with low sperm count and inflammation of the testicle. Prenatally, it can cause miscarriage. Some 3,000 babies are estimated to be infected each year, 300 of them being left with a subsequent handicap. It is the most commonly known viral cause of mental retardation, though it may also be responsible for other conditions. These include microcephaly, psychomotor retardation, developmental abnormalities and progressive hearing impairment, respiratory illness, jaundice, small size for gestational age, failure to thrive and eye infections.

Mumps

For the fertile male, mumps can cause inflammation of the various parts of the sex organs, leading to eventual sterility in some cases. But it can also affect the foetus. An excess of diabetes was found among people exposed to the infection in the mother's womb in the first three months of pregnancy. By the age of 30 years, researchers had found a 15-fold increased risk of developing diabetes. (NB: This will almost certainly have been due to the loss of vitamins and minerals caused. Any infection causes significant over-use of nutrients. Foresight would compensate and problems would be much less likely.)

Listeriosis

Listeriosis infection is caused by Listeria monocytogenes, an organism widely distributed in the environment. The most likely source of the infection for humans is food. Pregnant women are advised to avoid eating soft, ripened cheeses (Brie, Camembert and blue-veined types). All cook-chill meals and ready-to-eat poultry should be heated until very hot. They should never be eaten cold. In 1988, out of 291 reported cases, 115 were associated with pregnancy. Among these were 11 miscarriages, 9 stillbirths and 6 neonatal deaths. Abortion, stillbirth or premature labour may occur soon after signs of maternal infection. Congenital listeriosis and acquired neonatal infection may present as pneumonia, septicaemia or meningitis. Studies suggest *'up to a third of neonates may die and a third suffer long-term neurological damage.'* Another paper has reported about a 50% mortality rate if listeriosis infection occurs in the newborn, period. (NB So we avoid insufficiently heated 'ready meals' by avoiding 'ready meals' *anyway*, and we give a wide berth to blue cheeses, which can cause candida anyway!)

Influenza

There is some debate about whether prenatal exposure to influenza is associated with an increased risk of later schizophrenia. Some studies show no risk, while others show an association. In one study on 3,827 schizophrenic patients born in England and Wales between 1938 and 1965, the researchers found that females, but not males, exposed to influenza five months before birth can have a significantly greater rate of adult schizophrenia. They cannot explain the gender difference.

(NB Well, we, I think, can: mothers would have used up zinc, fighting off the flu. The male foetuses, who need much more zinc, would have died or been miscarried. If the females survived, they would have been zinc-deficient. Carl Pfeiffer's work shows zinc deficiency to be a major factor in schizophrenia).

Genitourinary Infections

Sadly, the number of people suffering from genitourinary problems continues to rise. There are many reasons – increased use of the pill and IUD, poor nutritional status leading to a weak immune system, and earlier sexual activity, to mention but a few. Greater sexual freedom, leading to more partners, has certainly increased the risk of infections, though some genitourinary conditions occur even among couples who are completely faithful to each other (e.g. candidiasis and E. coli).

Most of the infections can have dire consequences for fertility and the foetus, not to mention the general health of the sufferer. If you think there is any chance, whatsoever, that you may have an infection, especially if you have an unpleasant or coloured discharge, you should visit your local genitourinary medicine clinic. The only normal vaginal bacteria known is lactobacillus.

Urinary tract infections

Bacteriuria infections include cystitis, pyelonephritis and asymptomatic bacteriuria. Bacteriuria are detected in 2–10% of pregnant women, a similar number to that in non-pregnant women. In non-pregnant women these infections frequently clear up spontaneously, but this is not so in pregnant women, where the clear-up rate is lower. If not cleared with medical help, such infections can lead to spontaneous miscarriage. (NB: They will steal zinc, once again, so check out **before** the conception.)

Common sexually transmitted diseases:	
VIRUSES	Wart (HPV)
	Herpes
	Cytomegalovirus*
	Hepatitis B*
	AIDS
MYCOPLASMA	Mycoplasma hominis*
	Ureaplasma urealyticum*
BACTERIA	Chlamydia trachomatis
	Gonorrhoea
	E. coli*
	Entercocci
	B. streptococci
	Gardnerella
	Bacteroides)
	Mixed anaerobes) Anaerobes
	Syphilis
	Haem influenzae
	Haem strep
	Staph aureus
	Strep milleri
FLAGELLATES	Trichomonas
FUNGI	Candida – thrush*

*Indicates the condition is not exclusively sexually transmitted in adults.

Candidiasis (thrush)

The yeast candida albicans occurs naturally in the body, and in healthy people it causes no problems. It is well known as the cause of thrush, both oral, which is common in babies, and vaginal. But it is now recognised that an overgrowth of the yeast can be a contributory factor in many other conditions. In some cases this may arise as a condition secondary to viral or bacterial infections which thrive because of a weakened immune system. The use of antibiotics kills off both good and bad organisms in the gut and other mucous membranes, allowing the yeasts, which are not killed off, to proliferate. Symptoms of chronic candidiasis are many.

Those such as allergies and sensitivity to food and/or chemicals, cravings for refined carbohydrates and/or alcohol, and alcohol intolerance, irritable bowel syndrome, and iron or zinc deficiency can affect nutritional status and may therefore compromise reproductive outcomes (though any symptom which shows an adverse state of health could do this). One authority has said that there was a doubling of new cases of genital candidiasis reported between 1971 and 1975. Such candidiasis may also cause painful intercourse and possibly provide a hostile environment for the sperm. With treatment for both partners, which includes anti-fungal agents and nutritional therapy, most of the symptoms can be relieved. Short courses of vitamin A, which protects the mucous membranes, have been found to be helpful, as has the local application of yoghurt. (N.B. You should take up to a maximum of 20,000 iu of vitamin A for three days; this should be reduced to 2,000 iu before conception. The larger dose should be taken during menstruation to be certain pregnancy has not occurred. Then, postpone conception for a couple of months, to be sure your level is safe).

Chlamydia

Chlamydia trachomatis is a nasty pathogen (disease-carrying organism) which is thought to be the most common sexually transmitted pathogen in the Western industrialised world. It is responsible for a great deal of sexually transmitted infection, as well as infertility, and ill health in infants. **Since the symptoms are not always obvious, the woman may not even realise she has it, until her health is very much undermined.**

In men, chlamydia, as it is usually called, causes between one-third and half of non-gonococcal urethritis, although it often occurs together with gonorrhoea. It can also cause inflammation of the prostate tubes, a painful and potentially sterilising effect, or even of the rectum, testes and *vas deferens*. In women, it is a major cause of pelvic inflammatory disease (see below), cervicitis, cervical cell dysplasia and urethral syndrome. When it spreads from the cervix to the womb lining, it may induce endometriosis.

If it goes on to the fallopian tubes, it can cause salpingitis, which can result in blocked tubes and infertility. If the tubes are partially blocked there is a risk of an ectopic pregnancy, which can be fatal for the baby. More antibodies are found in infertile couples than in fertile ones.

One study has shown an incidence of 1.9% among 7,305 pregnant women. However, when the sample was restricted to women under 25 years of age who had at least one risk factor as identified in the study (young age or nulliparity or a new sexual partner in the last year), 81.7% were positive. The authors suggest that pre-screening criteria could optimise the use of specific diagnostic tests. (No, just screen **everybody!**)

For women coming for abortions, the researchers concluded that 'Estimated costs of hospital admissions for complications of chlamydial infection were more than double the cost of providing a routine Chlamydia screening programme and prophylactic treatment.'

In children, at least 50% of infants born to chlamydia-positive women are likely to develop infections. One study quoted a 61% rate of infection, with a 44% rate of clinical disease in infants born to infected mothers. Prematurity may result, and other main problems are conjunctivitis, found in 25–50% of exposed infants, and pneumonia in 10–20%. Rhinitis, otitis media, proctitis and vulvitis have also been reported. For example, in one study, exposed infants had twice the rate of pneumonitis and recurrent otitis media (which can lead to hearing defects) in their first six months of life. Those who had pneumonitis had higher subsequent rates of gastroenteritis. The researchers concluded: *'These results suggest that appreciable outpatient infant mortality may be associated with maternal infection with chlamydia trachomatis and that it may either cause or promote the occurrence of early recurrent otitis media and gastroenteritis.'* Another study found chlamydia trachomatis in the infant's pharynx and conjunctiva, the mother's cervix and the father's urethra. The researchers recommended searching for chlamydial infections in preterm infants with atypical respiratory disease even if delivered by caesarean section. (NB: Yes, but this is too late, isn't it? Search for it in prospective parents and *stop this happening* in the future.)

Gonorrhoea

Caused by the bacteria *Neisseria gonorrhoea-gonococcus*, this is one of the most contagious diseases there is. Often symptoms pass unnoticed, but if it is not treated, it can have very serious consequences for men, women and infants.

In men it can lead to sterility and low sperm counts. In the female, it is a major cause of pelvic inflammatory disease, which may lead to sterility. It also seems to leave her more vulnerable to chlamydial infections.

If a woman has suffered from gonorrhoea, she is likely to be tested during pregnancy (NB: though with good preconception care, she should be free from infection before conceiving). At least one researcher has found that prolonged rupture of the membranes and later chorioamniocentesis in infected women predisposes the baby to acquire the infection. There are also risks of prematurity with infected women.

Infections in the newborn are common if the mother is infected, as the bacteria are passed to the baby during its passage through the birth canal. Conjunctivitis is the most common problem, as the conjunctiva comes into contact with the infected cervix during birth – this can lead to a serious discharge with risks to sight, including blindness. Other parts of the body may also suffer, with infections of the umbilicus, the anogenital area, or the nose and throat. There may be arthritis or meningitis.

Herpes

There are various types of herpes virus, causing a number of conditions, some of which we have already mentioned. However, it is the herpes simplex virus which causes the condition known commonly as 'herpes'. There are two similar types. Type 1 causes sores around the mouth and nose, often referred to as 'cold sores', and, more rarely, in the eyes or genital or anal area. Type 2 causes sores in the genital and anal area and, more rarely, on the mouth. Genital infections caused by Type 2 are more severe. Small sores appear which can be quite painful. There may be

191

itching or pain on urinating. The symptoms clear but further attacks usually occur.

It is very important for a woman to tell her doctor if she has or has had genital herpes as it could affect the birth procedure. A caesarean section may be advised where there is an active sore in the vagina or on the cervix. If the waters break, a path is created for the virus to reach the baby, so a caesarean section should be done quickly. The virus may also be passed to the baby after birth by kissing if one has a cold sore or if there are sores on the breasts during breastfeeding. It is rare for the foetus to be infected in the womb and this would generally result in a miscarriage.

Researchers have concluded that herpes 'can result in spontaneous abortion, congenital and perinatal infections in the infant, or disseminated infection and death in the mother'. The frequency of risk factors is unknown. In their study there was a 40% incidence of serious perinatal disease or illness. Some of the infants whose mothers became infected in the last three months of pregnancy had perinatal morbidity such as prematurity, intrauterine growth retardation, and neonatal infections with herpes Type 2.

The main problem is the baby's immature immune system may not be able to cope with the virus and this can lead to an overwhelming infection, resulting in encephalitis with consequent brain damage, or eye infections, with eye damage. There may be jaundice, pneumonia with breathing difficulties, or even spells with no breathing at all. Microcephaly, microphthalmia and intracranial calcification have also been reported. There have been reports of physical impotence in men who suffered from herpes and proctitis, which then resulted in nerve inflammation.

Syphilis

This is a very dangerous infection although now, thankfully, comparatively rare. Fortunately it responds to *early* treatment. In both sexes it can lead to sterility and damage to many vital organs, including the heart and brain. The brain damage leads to psychiatric problems.

Syphilis is transmitted from the mother to the foetus via the placenta, thus making it prenatal rather than congenital, though in the child it is usually referred to as 'congenital syphilis'. It only occurs when the mother's syphilis is not diagnosed and treated, making it now comparatively rare as most women's blood is screened at the antenatal stage. (N.B. Of course, if you have followed the Foresight programme you will have been screened before conception.)

Without treatment one third of the babies will be born healthy, one third will be aborted or stillborn, and one third will have congenital syphilis. Stillbirth will occur if the maternal infection is present very early in pregnancy and if there is so great a dose of the organism responsible that the foetus succumbs to infection.

The baby suffering from congenital syphilis may appear healthy at birth, though occasionally there may be a rash. However, failure to thrive and gain weight, often the first clinical signs of early congenital syphilis, becomes apparent two to eight weeks after birth. There may be weight loss and often the baby has a wizened appearance, like an old man. Other symptoms include skin lesions, mucous membrane lesions, visceral lesions, enlarged liver and/or spleen, abdominal swelling, meningitis, and bone lesions.

Mycoplasmas, including Ureaplasma urealyticum

These organisms are the smallest free-living pathogens, capable of causing a wide range of problems in humans. In the reproductive system, Mycoplasma hominis and Ureaplasma urealyticum are the most commonly cultured. A direct relation between the frequency of venereal infection and serum antibody levels has been found. One authority writes: 'Mycoplasmas, which commonly reproduce when the subject's health is impaired, can cause attacks of vulvovaginitis, genital irritation and urinary frequency. Symptoms may persist for twenty years or even longer.'

In men, Ureaplasma urealyticum is a major cause of non-gonococcal urethritis, which can lead to infertility, non-specific urethritis (NSU), and prostate and kidney disease. Higher concentrations have been found in the genital tracts of sterile couples than in fertile couples. In women, pelvic inflammatory disease can result if the mycoplasmas, including Ureaplasma urealyticum, are allowed to proliferate. Scarring may lead to infertility. Miscarriage and premature birth are also associated with mycoplasmas. Of the common organisms Ureaplasma urealyticum is the most frequently implicated in repetitive abortions.[61]

Genital mycoplasma infection is difficult to eradicate and prospective parents who have such a condition may have to be patient. Women need local treatment of the cervix.

Pelvic inflammatory disease

This can be gonococcal, chlamydial, or non-gonococcal, non-chlamydial in type. It is sometimes misdiagnosed, so tests for all types should always be conducted. Treatment for one type may be ineffective against another. For example, antibiotics for gonorrhoea do not cure chlamydia.

One study found a high incidence of non-gonococcal infection among the male partners of women with PID. Over three-quarters of the males were showing no symptoms. (N.B. The men never admit to symptoms in any case. It does not mean they do not need to attend a clinic).

The consequence of untreated PID include sub-fertility, sterility, menstrual difficulties, chronic abdominal pain and ectopic pregnancy. The risks of tubal infection leading to infertility seem to be related to the number of types and infection. In one study, even after treatment with antibiotics, a single tubal infection, including chlamydia, produced a 12.8% infertility rate; two infections produced a 35.5% infertility rate, while for three it was a 75% rate. Catterall reports that: 'If the statistics are correct there is a 50 per cent chance of relapse ... a one in three chance of being sterile, a 25 per cent chance of dyspareunia (painful intercourse) and a 10 per cent chance of ectopic pregnancy.'

Genital warts – condyloma acuminata

These are caused by a virus called 'papillomavirus'. The symptoms may only be warty nodules which may not be readily apparent. Some types of the virus have been linked with cervical cancer and may therefore affect reproduction. By 1987, one in six women attending Islington family planning clinics had a positive smear.

One in three had cell abnormalities and/or the cancer wart-virus. (It is not clear, though, how representative a group this is, compared with the general population.)

Trichomoniasis

This condition is caused by the organism Trichomonas vaginalis. Women may suffer from excessive and itchy vaginal discharge, while the newborn may have fever, be irritable and fail to thrive.

Hepatitis B

Hepatitis means 'inflammation of the liver'. Type B, one of three types, can be spread through sexual contact or contact with body fluids, such as blood, urine and saliva, so it is not just sexually transmitted. Like chlamydia and gonorrhoea, it is possible to have it without any symptoms. Treatment may be slow, being bed rest and nutritional therapy. Vaccination is available to some people, although at least one authority has advocated screening for everyone, with vaccination as appropriate, because it is a serious condition leading to neonatal deaths. It can also lead to an increase in food and chemical sensitivities in the mother, which may affect a baby who is being breastfed. At least one authority has argued that 'the cost-benefit of screening is difficult to assess, but it is likely to be substantial'. (N.B.Need we always be so obsessed with cost? How about mother-benefit and baby-benefit? The health benefit would pay off handsomely, surely?)

AIDS (Acquired Immune Deficiency Syndrome)

AIDS was first recognised as a distinct syndrome in 1981; the human immunodeficiency virus (HIV) which is generally thought to cause it was identified in 1983. By September 1993, 20,590 people in the UK had tested HIV positive. Since 1982, 8,115 people have been diagnosed as having AIDS, of whom 5,553 have died. These figures are acknowledged to be under-estimates. Treatments have now improved so that HIV-positive people, if treated early, may find there is a delay in the onset of symptoms. Even 8–10 years of health is possible in the West.

There is some debate as to whether or not pregnancy will increase the risk of developing AIDS-related complex or the risk of the baby being infected in the womb.

(NB: This was written in 1994. This is not an area that we have a great deal of knowledge about, so it may not be as accurate now as it was then. I have the greatest sympathy for anybody burdened with this terrible disease, but would suggest you think again about the idea of pregnancy, as for a baby to lose his parent in 1–9 years of life would be a devastating loss).

Gardnerella

There has been some debate about whether or not the presence of anaerobic bacteria, including Gardnerella, in such abnormal amounts as to cause the condition bacterial vaginosis, can have an adverse outcome in pregnancy. Researchers at Northwick Park Hospital found that 'late miscarriage and preterm delivery are associated with the presence of bacterial vaginosis in early pregnancy. This is independent of recognised risk factors such as previous preterm delivery.'

Gail Bradley's conclusions

Many infections can be damaging, whether to the reproductive tract, the sperm, the ova or the foetus. We have written about the most common infections individually, but unfortunately they often occur in combination, and this multiplies the risks of damage. In one study, Mycoplasma hominis was found in 30–50% of vaginal cultures of sexually active women, with Ureaplasma urealyticum in 60–80% of cultures. Another study looked at the incidence of sex infections in pregnant adolescents. They were aged 13–17 years, all from very poor socio-economic backgrounds and in their third trimester. The results showed that only five appeared to be free from all the infections being considered, while 34% had trichomonas, 38% candidiasis, 70% Mycoplasma homini and 90% Ureaplasma urealyticum. Chlamydia trachomatis was found in 37% of 115 specimens. Gonorrhoea was originally present in 12 subjects early in pregnancy, but only in one in the third trimester. Three had evidence of genital herpes infection and three others evidence of papillomavirus infection.

A survey of 109 patients attending a Hertfordshire Foresight doctor for preconception care confirmed the importance of screening. Of 32 men tested between 1989 and 1991, 15 had one or more infections. These included B streptococci, chlamydia, ureaplasma, enteroccus, Staph aureus, candida, E. coli, Klebsiella, anaerobic bacteria, Haem influenzae and Strep milleri. 77 women were tested, showing a total of 39 positive cervical swabs and 22 positive chlamydia antibodies. Infections identified included B streptococci, ureaplasma, mycoplasma, anaerobic bacteria, candida, Gardnerella, E. coli, Strep millerii, Staph aureus.

A study of 400 women attending another clinic for abortion revealed 28% had anaerobic bacteria, 24% candida, 32% chlamydia, 0.75% trichomonas and 0.25% gonorrhoea.

While the immune system may cope with one mild infection, if there are multiple infections, it is likely to be unable to withstand such an onslaught. There is also the risk that not all infections will be treated, even if symptoms persist. Comprehensive screening is vital and it is sensible that, where possible, a colposcope should be used as it is a superior technique for at least one condition and thought to be a better technique for others. If you suspect that you may have an infection, attend a genitourinary medicine clinic for a full examination with the appropriate swabs taken and the use of a colposcope. This may mean travelling a bit. However, in view of the many adverse effects of genitourinary infections, it is worth making an effort to get the best treatment available.

Any infections or cell abnormalities on the cervix should be diagnosed and treated *before pregnancy* as the rise in hormones during pregnancy increases these problems. The extra artificial hormone stimulation given to infertile women is especially likely to cause a flare-up of cervical or pelvic infection.

Checklist regarding GUIs:

1. Always ask for a genitourinary examination if you suspect any infection or if you are having difficulty conceiving. For a woman this should involve the use of a colposcope.

2. If a genitourinary infection is diagnosed it is vital that both partners receive treatment and follow-up checks.

3. The male partner should have his semen and/or prostatic fluid checked for infection. Urine screening alone is inadequate.

My conclusion

As many infections are symptomless they therefore may be unsuspected. However, we now know what devastation and long-term damage they can cause to the baby. Just get checked out, **whatever!**

Onwards!

CHAPTER 7
Allergies and Intestinal Parasites

Food Allergy is any adverse reaction to food in which the immune system is demonstrably involved.

False Food Allergy denotes a special kind of non-immunological reaction, seen with particular foods in which the food triggers the mast cells directly. The immune system is not at fault and the body does not overproduce IgE but the end result is with symptoms the same as allergy.

Food Intolerance means any adverse reaction to food, other than false food allergy, in which the involvement of the immune system is unproven because skin-prick tests and other allergy tests are negative. This does not exclude the possibility of immune reactions being involved in some way, but they are unlikely to be the major factor producing the symptoms.

Food Sensitivity is employed as the umbrella term for all non-psychological adverse reactions to food.

Food Aversion means the dislike and avoidance of a particular food for purely psychological reasons.

Jonathan Brostoff, 1989

The incidence of allergic illness in children has risen enormously in the last 50 years. We all need to examine the many possible contributing reasons for this if we are going to be effective in reversing this trend. Do not believe officialdom's suave explanations, *'We are now better at diagnosis.'* Rubbish! The problems were not there to *be* diagnosed until the environment became so problematic and vaccination so universal that a lot of illness was created.

In my school of over 200 girls in wartime Britain (1940s), I remember only one person who had any form of allergy – she reacted to strawberries by coming out in a rash. In my nursery nursing days, we had well over 100 children in the nursery, many from very less-than-ideal backgrounds, but the allergic illness etc. was not around. In the 1950s I worked in a prep school, and over the years knew about 180 boys. Only one, who had been born very prematurely, had a very occasional attack of asthma. All the boys ate well, but there was no obesity, nor hyperactivity, dyslexia, eczema, epilepsy, asthma, and so on.

So what has changed so much that we now *accept* that one in four children have learning difficulties, one in seven carry an inhaler in case of an asthma attack, and many carry a syringe in case of threatened anaphylaxis? We know that 2,000 die each year as the result of asthma. We are also told one in five have eczema.

Way back in the 1990s, when Gail and I first wrote the book, *Planning for a Healthy Baby*, we said: 'We are now seeing an escalation of diet-related diseases. There have, for example, been increases in the incidence of allergic illness, anorexia/bulimia and mental disorders.' Now the problem has escalated even more, rather than receded. Is it due to lack of nutrients? Is it due to pesticides and food additives? Is it due to vaccination? Why?

As we mentioned earlier, maintaining optimum health in the modern environment is a challenge but a large area we need to study particularly is how to produce an allergy-free generation! So what are the possible causes of this huge influx of illness which has only arrived in the last 40–50 years? There has to be an answer.

The 21st century environment is high in toxins. These are:

(a) **inhaled**: such as traffic effluent, cigarette smoke, organophosphate pesticides – both from agriculture and from indoor uses such as indoor plants, moth-proofing and fire-retardants, also flea drops for pets, house dust mites' faeces, pets' dandruff, good old pollen etc.

(b) **ingested**: such as hazardous food additives, pesticides on food, fluoride from water, alcohol, caffeine, aluminium, artificial hormones, growth promoters, the pill, fertility drugs and medicines.

(c) **inflicted**: such as by vaccines and immunisations, bacteria and viruses (albeit supposedly more or less dead) with the carriers such as the bullock's lymph, monkey lymph and sheep, hen, mouse, guinea-pig fluids or peanut oil they are floated in, or

200

thimerosal they are preserved with. Also there are injections of antibiotics, and mercury amalgam fillings in our teeth.

All, or any, of these may result in an over-responsive immune system.

At the time we wrote our last book, we did not link allergic illness/behavioural problems very closely with vaccination. The hazards of the bug/animal lymph/mercury cocktail had not become so apparent. It should have been obvious that its effect on zinc levels in children would be catastrophic. But the impact had not really been felt as it has today. However, after Neil Ward's work, in particular, the link was clearer – when zinc goes down, for whatever reason, behavioural problems arise.

Children's brains and central nervous systems cannot cope without zinc. In the mid-1950s the country started to recognise dyslexia, hyperactivity and cot death. This has led on to effects from lethal allergic reactions, such as death due to asthma or anaphylaxis, to fits and ADHD, and into full-blown autism.

Do we now have 'subclinical autism'? Children so out of control that they are knifing each other, alcoholic in their teens, and so many on drugs, even from so-called 'middle-class' families? Is the present deterioration of behaviour down to what is loosely termed 'allergic reaction'?

It has been recently discovered that a group of macaque monkeys were given the whole programme of immunisations/vaccinations normally given to American children, and they became hyperactive and violently aggressive. Not typical monkey-moods at all.

The MMR was started in this county in 1988. Children aged one at that time are now 26 years old. Is this the age group where the knife-carrying, binge drinking into oblivion, the drugging, the gangs, the children now described by the press as 'feral', all started? I think so.

The Government should not be considering fining the parents – it should be compensating the entire family. Blaming 'absent fathers' is a red herring. During the Second World War, almost all fathers were 'absent' but no children behaved in this way. I know, I was there.

The present-day unborn child is deficient, allergic and full of toxic substances as never before. Remember the 287 toxic substances reported in the press as found in amniotic fluid a short while ago? However, we can work away to keep our children safe from all of the possible hazards and persuade our friends!

There are also the problems of nutrient deficiencies, and the hazards of early weaning.

Many problems can be due to deficiencies of needed nutrients, such as vitamin A, B vitamins, zinc, chromium, manganese, selenium and others. These are required as co-factors for enzymes. The co-factor is rather like an outboard motor on a dinghy – it makes it 'go'! Without it the enzyme that is needed to protect the skin, linings of the lungs etc, and/or to digest and process the food, can't function properly.

Why should babies and small children be short of these essential nutrients? Partly because so much modern food is lacking in nutrients and partly because of a lack of much needed information at crucial times. This meant the parents were short of these nutrients:

Firstly, during the pre-conception period when the egg was 'ripening' or getting ready to be shed, and the sperm were being formed and matured ready to get down to business.

Secondly, during the pregnancy, when mistakenly mothers can be persuaded to totally forgo vitamin A, and when pregnancy sickness can be an additional problem.

Thirdly, while breastfeeding, when possibly the mother is very busy and may be too tired to cook, especially if she is short of nutrients in the first place, which exacerbates the fatigue. This is a very usual scenario with the modern baby, where there has been no Foresight help with preparation.

Sometimes a hair analysis and a comprehensive nutrient programme – vitamins given with zinc, manganese and selenium, and with omega-3 oils – can be all that's needed to improve the health of both mother and baby and to nip things in the bud.

Our mothers' hard work on the Foresight programme can usually pre-empt these and a whole host of other problems (especially exhaustion in the mother, and allergies leading to much vocal complaining by the baby!). This means breastfeeding will go ahead happily, and much cow's milk allergy can be avoided.

If early weaning has been necessary, this again can be a factor that starts allergy off. If a baby is weaned on to cow's milk formula this will often be the start of eczema, wheezing, colic, vomiting and/or diarrhoea. I have known of cases where this has all continued throughout childhood, with no end of medical drugs being taken to try to prevent the allergic symptoms and the vomiting (NB As seen in the papers recently, not until the child was 16 years old, in one case, and 23 years in another, was the cow's milk stopped and the vomiting brought to an end).

Breast milk is the natural food for a human baby and cow's milk is the food that is perfectly constituted for the calf. Although cow's milk is now available modified and adapted to some degree, it is still less than perfect for the human baby. This could mean that each successive generation finds it less easy to handle. 'Bottle feeding' has by now been around for about 100 years, so we need to give this some thought.

Then again, with cow's milk itself, there have been some very dramatic alterations in its production since the World War II days. Then we used to milk by hand into a galvanised bucket and pour it into the individual enamel billy-cans at the farm gate. We never heard of 'milk allergy' in the village in those days. Now, cows are machine-milked. There are long lengths of rubber tubing (does this give off PCBs?). This is cleaned with Milton, which is a bug-destroyer. The milk then goes into tankers, which are cleaned with another germicide. Do these bug-bugging chemicals end up in the milk? In what quantity? If so, what effect do they have on human intestinal flora? Are enzymes or vitamins destroyed in the milk? (We do know that when milk is pasteurised, this destroys lysine, which is a useful protein.)

We know that these days cows are not fed exclusively on grass, hay and mangelwurzel tops, as was the case 60 years ago, but are partly fed on cow-cake which contains grains. Are the grains full of pesticides? Some cows seem to manage on this but some have projectile diarrhoea (and you don't want to be standing behind them when this occurs!). Is this a sort of bovine coeliac condition? Has this any link to the fact that some coeliacs cannot take cow's milk?

We also know that cows are now milked when they are pregnant. This means there are different hormones released into the cow's blood and hence into the milk. During the War, in Wales, this never happened. The cow was 'dried off' and rested for eight weeks before being taken to the bull again. It was believed that the milk was 'unwholesome' if the cow was pregnant. The cows lived long and productive lives. I remember one cow who was still being milked aged 22 years. We held them all in great affection. Now they are slaughtered at five years. They are just regarded as milk machines.

In the War, all the young men had gone away 'to fight' and it was just the old men and the children and the women left at home. The old men I knew could not read or write as they used to bring things into the house for my mother to read to them. But they were so wise, so compassionate, so strong, so gentle, so humorous, so kind to everybody and so good to the animals. Nobody was allergic to their farm's milk.

In addition to what may be in the milk, we have recently been told that babies' plastic feeding bottles give off bisphenol A, a by-product of the plastic, and furthermore some babies are allergic to latex (the teats are made of latex). So one way and another, it is hard to win through with bottle-feeding – especially if you are the baby.

For optimum breastfeeding, I would stick to the full Foresight programme – the breast milk is likely to be more plentiful and breastfeeding will be less tiring. Breastfeeding mums put a lot of their precious nutrients into the milk. The 2am feed usually goes on for about six to eight weeks before the babies' little tummies are big enough for them to tank up and sleep a bit longer. This is quite tiring enough without running short of nutrients!

'Lactation failure', as the medics call it, is just tired mothers with too little of the B-complex vitamins, zinc etc to keep them on top of things. Experimental rats fed on very well nutrient-prepared 'Rat Purina Chow' were fine. They had litters of 12–14 babies and they all thrived. The poor deprived rat mothers with low zinc etc were the ones that opted out of motherhood and made a run for it. They retreated into the far corner of the cage and curled up with their tail over their nose. Presumably this was 'post-partum depression' plus 'lactation failure' or they would have gone back to the nest. Nutrients to keep things going do not get the positive press they deserve but they can be the golden solution for avoiding much maternal misery and allergy in the children.

To return to the matter in hand, other major allergens are the gluten grains (wheat, oats, barley and rye). Many more people are now being diagnosed with either wheat intolerance or coeliac condition. This, in one way, is rather good news for those of us, like myself, who are coeliac! Providing gluten-free food is now a growing industry, and all the supermarkets have a thriving gluten-free section and the products are delicious! Waiters are sympathetic when you dine out, and even some fish and chip shops provide gluten-free batter! Progress! However, for all that, it would certainly be a benefit to most people not to have this particular bugbear.

Nevertheless, if you suffer 'irritable bowel syndrome' and are constantly told it is 'stress' or 'nerves' (the fashionable non-diagnosis) I would try going onto a gluten and/or milk-free diet for a few months so see if things clear up. There is nothing to lose, the alternative food is good and you will come to no harm. If this does not help, then it could be candida or intestinal parasites – keep on searching until you have the answer!

On the whole, milk allergics are tired, heavy, lethargic, have black rings under their eyes, and are prone to fatigue, bloating and diarrhoea, also to catarrh and snoring.

Gluten allergics also suffer diarrhoea, and tend to be a bit hyperactive, argumentative and thin (sometimes to the point of emaciation) with itchy eyes, irritable skin and poor sleeping patterns, possibly up and down all night to urinate, sometimes 'workaholics'.

Some evidence has recently arisen that there may be alcoholic parents or grandparents behind coeliac disease. I have known at least five or six families where this applies. However, whether the alcoholism caused such zinc-deficiency in the dependants that this precipitated the allergic condition, or whether the person with the alcoholism was an undiagnosed coeliac, it is hard to say. I would be very interested to have any feedback on this one.

Be that as it may, if allergy seems likely to be in your family for whatever reason, I would avoid eating much gluten or dairy in the preconception period and during pregnancy and breastfeeding. I would also leave it until at least 9–10 months before introducing it, very cautiously, to the baby. 'Rice Dream with Calcium' is a good milk substitute for the pregnant or breastfeeding mother. Or goat's or sheep's milk, both of which appear to be less allergenic to many people.

Other very common intolerances are caffeine (in coffee, tea, chocolate and cola) and sugar. The unborn babies are better if these are kept right to a minimum. Caffeine has been closely linked to increased risk of miscarriage and sugar could be the trigger to gestational diabetes.

One cheerful hot drink is Marmite (but not too strong so as not to give too much salt) and also, if you are not gluten intolerant, Bovril, both beef and chicken flavoured. Or Tesco's 'Beefy' which is gluten-free. The green/herb tea unit in the supermarket seems to grow every week and it is possible to grow mint, sage, basil, dill, fennel etc in pots or in the garden, and make your own herb teas. For cold drinks, juice, smoothies, goat's milk, Rice Dream, Provamel, Oatly, almond milk and others are out there if you are milk-allergic. Horlicks, Ovaltine etc are a bonus for those who are neither gluten- nor milk-allergic – lucky them!

We should note here that some herbs are contraindicated during pregnancy, for example:

- Saw Palmetto – when used orally, has hormonal activity

206

- Goldenseal – when used orally may cross the placenta
- Dong Quai – when used orally, due to uterine stimulant and relaxant effects
- Ephedra – when used orally
- Yohimbe – when used orally
- Pau d'Arco – when used orally in large doses
- Passion Flower – when used orally
- Black Cohosh – when used orally in pregnant women who are not at term
- Blue Cohosh – when used orally; uterine stimulant and can induce labour
- Roman Chamomile – when used orally in medicinal amounts
- Pennyroyal – when used orally or topically
- Red Raspberry Leaf – there is some controversy about whether this should be used throughout pregnancy or just in the second and third trimester. Many health care providers will remain cautious and only recommend using it after the first trimester. I think maybe just at the very end, as it contains copper which can bring on early contractions, which could mean premature birth.

It would be wise to check the internet yourself for current thinking on all herbal teas.

Some people are allergic to citrus fruits and this can cause diarrhoea, sneezing, skin problems – from a vague 'little itch' which seems to have no visible origin – to full-blown eczema, and even arthritis. Some people react to just orange or just lemon etc. Some are allergic to any citrus fruit.

Some react to the 'belladonna' family which consists of tomatoes, potatoes, peppers and aubergines. Tomato ketchup may start a reaction, or baked beans in tomato sauce. Again, some people may just react to one of them, some to the whole family.

Another huge source of 'allergies', using the word in its broadest sense, are the ubiquitous 'food additives' which seem to lurk in everything you pick up unless it is straight raw food. To cut a long story short, the Hyperactive Children's Support Group (run by Sally Bunday and, until her death, her wonderful old mother, Vicky Colquhoun) and Foresight have been campaigning about the E numbers for over 30 years. At v-e-r-y long last, there seem to be faint stirrings at government level (Spring 2008: six were banned!).

In 1984 Foresight brought out *FIND OUT*, a little booklet pointing out the numbers and names and the reactions the additives produced: asthma, eczema, diarrhoea, epilepsy, migraine, cancer and so on. In 2003 *FIND OUT* was updated. Alas, none of the dangerous ones had been banned. However more dubious ones had been introduced and a few of the ones about which there had been 'conflicting reports' had now been confirmed as health hazards. In 2004 *FIND OUT* was translated into French and Spanish by a very enterprising multilingual Frenchwoman, and over 140,000 copies have been sold on the Continent to date!

Many of these additives produce hyperactivity which can ruin the life of the child, and cause much disappointment and anxiety to the whole family.

Since the banning of the six 'worst offenders' (tartrazine, sunset yellow etc.) in the 2008 government initiative, those allowed in the UK include:

- 48 which cause hyperactivity
- 82 which cause digestive disorders
- 54 which cause asthma
- 53 which cause skin rashes, urticaria, eczema
- 36 which cause insomnia
- 52 known as suspect for cancer
- 30 known as suspect for liver and/or kidney disorders

The list does not end there, but if these noxious substances were removed from the taxpayers' food supply, might we all have to pay a great deal less tax? Should we not have some say in the matter? In 2006 the NHS bill for drugs is said to have been £8 billion (National Audit Office). Paid for by us, remember. Why should we be ignored for over 30 years? Well, at the very least get a copy of *FIND OUT* and use it ostentatiously!

Some of these additives are made by the same companies who make a fortune out of Ritalin and many similar medications which must be a very lucrative exercise. This can be confirmed by nosing about on the Web, by spiders with enough curiosity!

People on government committees are usually asked to declare their interests in businesses whose interests might conflict with the matters under discussion, for example, the pharmaceutical industry. Most will declare a number of investments but will continue to be allowed to take part in the proceedings that make the decisions on what is allowed. Are these decisions right?

In 1987, Dr Neil Ward, of the University of Surrey, linked hyperactivity to both nutritional deficiencies and food intolerances. Ward surveyed the parents of 486 hyperactive children and 172 non-hyperactive controls. The parents of the hyperactive children reported that more than 60% exhibited increased behaviour problems when exposed to synthetic colourings and flavourings, preservatives, cow's milk, and certain chemicals. In contrast only 12% of parents of the controls reported a connection between food additives or colourings and worsened behaviour.

Ward identified a subgroup of hyperactive children with known sensitivities to synthetic food colourings and exposed the children to these chemicals. Of 23 exposed to the food colouring tartrazine, 18 responded by becoming overactive, 16 became aggressive, 4 became violent, and several developed eczema, asthma, poor speech, or poor coordination. In contrast, only one control subject showed minor behavioural changes after drinking tartrazine. Two other colourings, 'sunset yellow' and amaranth, also caused significant behavioural effects in hyperactive subjects.

Ward uncovered one possible explanation for the effects of the food colourings. The hyperactive children in the study had statistically lower zinc and iron levels than controls. Therefore, when hyperactive children known to be sensitive to the colourings tartrazine and 'sunset yellow' were exposed to these chemicals, their blood serum zinc dropped markedly. 'Several studies,' Ward notes, 'have shown that zinc-deficient animals are more prone to stress and are aggressive when compared with normal cases.'

Previous research also has strongly linked tartrazine to hyperactivity. I am sure that if the additives can do this to a five-year-old child, it makes us all shudder to think what they may be doing to the unborn.

I would get *FIND OUT* from Foresight and take it shopping with you. I would discuss this with the supermarket staff and suggest that they introduce it to their managers. The more interest we can get at commercial level, the more likely we are to get the additives controlled. A great many of those allowed in the UK are forbidden in other EU countries. **Why can the British government never take on board the useful things the EU does,** and only concur when they make really silly regulations? It is a mystery – except that the establishment is doubtless more sympathetic to big business moguls, with whom they can identify and socialise, than they are to the little children suffering from unnecessary illnesses.

I am sure you have gathered by now that there are many modern causes of ill-health which are interacting. Two issues may need to be addressed:

Firstly, deficiencies can make you more prone to developing allergies. Defences can be weakened if the immune system is undermined by lack of zinc and by other deficiencies. Enzyme systems may be compromised. Vaccinations are, in some cases, causing these deficiencies, or may be polluting in other ways.

Secondly, and directly conversely, the allergies may lead to the deficiencies. Irritation from detergents can make the skin sore, and this will call for zinc, oils and vitamins A, E, and B. Inhaled pesticide, smoke and/or flame retardant can irritate the lungs and create a demand for selenium and vitamins A and E to soothe them. Organophosphate pesticides will also create a shortage of manganese, as they inhibit the uptake from the gut. Calcium and zinc are used up in driving lead out of the body and so on. These minerals are needed to make enzymes work, but being so overworked they are then unavailable to 'do their stuff'.

Do you, or does anyone in your family have asthma, eczema, migraine, epilepsy, insomnia, depression, ME, or irritable bowel syndrome? Try in the first instance using the Foresight booklets

FIND OUT and *WATCH IT* as you shop. The problem could be as simple as a noxious additive! Be sure also to 'eat organic' and you will avoid a lot of pesticides!

If, after a few weeks, you are not clear of the symptoms, try eliminating the food groups we have talked about: milk, gluten-grains, belladonna family, caffeine, citrus. About two out of three times it *is that simple*. Then, if in doubt, check with a nutritionist that your replacement diet is adequate.

Vanessa's story:

For years, Vanessa had many health problems attributed to both candida and endometriosis. The endometriosis needed laser treatment followed by medication. Systemic candidiasis was diagnosed, which also included the ovaries, and this was proving to be obstinate to modem medicine. No medical solutions helped. Lots of antifungal medicines were prescribed but to no effect. For five years Vanessa turned to all sorts of complementary remedies including exclusion diets. With this history, Vanessa and her husband believed that they would need extraordinary preconceptual help if they were to have a baby. They did not want to go down the usual route of IVF, IUI and ICSI. They wanted a natural conception and birth.

Searching for preconceptual care on the internet, they found Foresight, and started on the programme. Vanessa's first hair analysis showed she had high copper levels but all other minerals were next to normal. Her husband's, on the other hand, reflected much lower mineral levels, especially that of zinc. Unfortunately, their mineral levels improved sufficiently to allow an unplanned conception to take place but not enough to carry the pregnancy to full term, and a miscarriage occurred a few weeks later.

Taking care, and after two more cycles of hair analysis and supplements, Vanessa conceived naturally, which led to a healthy baby boy.

'Smiley Miles is in very rude health, chatty, active, very charming, like Daddy,' said Vanessa.

Often people know their allergens, but have not really bothered to acknowledge them! I often hear:

'Really? Yes, I'd always thought oranges gave me a headache, but I thought, no, they can't because they are meant to be good for you, aren't they?'

'I think cheese makes my eczema worse, definitely. Would this mean that milk affects me, too?'

'I always feel a lot better when I'm slimming and I don't eat bread.'

You just need a bit of encouragement to take it the rest of the way! This way, it doesn't cost anything to get it right! If this does not answer your problems, get back to us for the address of a doctor who understands testing for allergies.

To summarise:

Ever-increasing pollution of the biosphere has brought with it an ever-increasing cascade of adverse reactions (allergies, intolerances), especially in the very young and/or the zinc-deficient and the undernourished, whose enzyme systems and immune systems lack the needed support. Babies and small children who fall into both categories are particularly unlucky. Breastfeeding offers the best protection for babies. Making breast milk is much easier if you have everything you need in the way of vitamins and minerals, to do so and to keep yourself going. This avoids post-partum depression (exhaustion and feelings of inadequacy) which appears if you have not enough nutrients for energy, plus enough to supply 'happy-making' milk! When milk is satisfying and abundant, weaning onto 'solid' foods can be done very gradually at the baby's own pace, and this will help to avoid making a whole load of allergies in the next generation! Knowing this, it is surprising that the medics are so willing to inject tiny babies with half-dead bugs, bullock's lymph, mercury and so on. This adds credence to Dr Scheibner's opinion that allergy follows on the backs of the vaccination programmes.

On the following pages there is more help from Gail Bradley:

Allergy

In 1906 Clement von Pirquet, a pioneer in the study of immunisation, defined allergy as *'observable altered reactions to environmental substances'*. Unfortunately, as more research was done on allergy, allergists split into two camps: those who believed the answers lay in closely studying the immune system and those who were more concerned with considering a wider perspective.

Immunologists had discovered that when a foreign body enters the blood, the host body produces special protein substances called antibodies, which circulate in the blood and bind with the foreign body to neutralise it. An allergic person produces more antibodies than is necessary, and these irritate various tissues, causing a range of conditions, including asthma, eczema and hay fever. Immunologists can check for four types of reaction, using blood tests. If one or more is not positive, then allergy is said not to be present.

However, only a minority of people have been found to have symptoms which fit this diagnosis. What about the many others who experience 'observable altered reactions'

Not all doctors trod the immunologists' path. There were still some who continued to follow through the ideas of Francis Hare, a British psychiatrist who wrote a book in 1905 called *The Food Factor in Disease*. But they were few, and they failed to convince the medical establishment of their ideas, so today most of them are in private practice, or in retirement!

Some doctors decided on new approaches and theories on the basis of studies they read in medical journals. Yet even reputable journals sometimes publish very bad research. This has also happened in the field of allergy. Many research projects assume that if there is no quick reaction to a test, allergy is not present. In food allergy this may be quite erroneous. Sometimes a person may not react to a food for many hours, even days.

Jennifer Masefield:

> *Dried encapsulated foods used for double-blind provocation tests may not give accurate results, because the actual state of the food may be the important factor. Some people can*

tolerate cooked cabbage but react to raw cabbage. The preparation of food can alter the allergen.

Often certain food reactions are only caused by food combinations, so testing of foods in isolation will not produce a reaction.

If an allergic person has not been exposed to an allergen for a long period he/she may have lost sensitivity to it. However, reactions may return after repeated exposures. In a multiple allergic patient who is repeatedly changing his/her diet to maintain better health, the sensitivity swing will make food allergy tests give different responses at different phases of the sensitivity level, for each excluded allergen or ingested allergen. This can give very confusing results, leading to an assumption of psychosomatic illness. If an allergen is excluded for only a few days, sensitivity is initially heightened and will show on testing.

At least two states in the USA have passed laws requiring examination for undiagnosed organic conditions either causing or exacerbating psychiatric symptoms. Many studies are now linking allergy with conditions such as migraine, epilepsy and hyperactivity. Self-help groups are increasing in number, and more doctors are becoming interested.

Relevance in preconception care

Foresight clinicians pay special attention to allergy for a number of reasons:

If a prospective parent is suffering from a food allergy, health is impaired, and there may be malabsorption which will generally lead to nutritional deficiencies.

Allergies in either prospective parent seem to lead to allergies in their offspring, which can seriously impair development.

Clearing up allergies may mean that drugs do not need to be taken to alleviate the symptoms caused by the allergens.

Allergies may cause excessive mucus which can lead to blocked fallopian tubes, which cause infertility.

214

If the mother's allergies are not resolved and she is breastfeeding, she may find her baby suffering, eg from colic, because of a masked cow's milk allergy in the mother.

Investigating allergy

There are a number of ways of investigating allergy, with varying degrees of effectiveness. We list below some of the main ones.

1. The clinical history is most important and, ideally, should include reference to the wider family, especially parents. Allergic symptoms may have been present early in life, may alter and not be diagnosed as the cause of later problems found in, for example, the hyperactive, learning-disabled child, the delinquent teenager, and/or the aggressive husband who abuses his wife and children.

2. Questionnaires can be useful in identifying symptoms. The list of symptoms on such questionnaires can be extensive. Indeed, it is this very wide range which makes some doctors so sceptical, and the investigation so difficult.

3. Cytotoxic blood tests, performed by skilled technicians, are approximately 75% reliable for food allergy only, so can give useful guidance.

4. Skin prick tests and sublingual testing, which are sometimes used, are unreliable for food allergy.

5. Miller Provocation testing, a form of skin test, is more reliable and can be used to establish dosage for treatment.

6. Elimination and rotation diets are the most reliable methods. Many doctors specialising in ecological medicine (sometimes called clinical ecology or environmental medicine) put patients on a special diet to check for allergies. Depending on what the clinical history and questionnaires have revealed, it may mean cutting out all dairy produce and cereals, including refined carbohydrates. Basically this means eating meat and vegetables and the more unusual fruits such as pears. But not all meat and vegetables may be allowed. Often a patient will be asked to eat just lamb and game to start with if it is suspected that beef, pork and/or poultry may be allergens.

Easier than this is just eliminating one food group and noting the effects. This is often tried with the major allergens, which tend to be the foods/drinks most commonly ingested in a country, such as wheat, yeast, chocolate, tea, coffee, eggs and milk in the UK.

If this does not improve the situation you may wish to try a rotation diet, designed to give each specific food only one day in, say, five or seven days. The following rotation diet has worked well with many Foresight patients. It should be used in conjunction with a food diary, in which every food and drink taken is noted, with the time. There should be a separate column for comments, which will include any effects felt, either physical or emotional, and the time they were experienced. This is very important, since we have said that the reaction may not be immediate. Remember, you are going to have to play detective, so you want all the evidence you can collect. (You may first wish to try the diary without the rotation diet.)

A word of warning: whatever type of diet you try, be it elimination or rotation, when you come off an allergen you are usually going to suffer some sort of withdrawal symptoms that will make you feel worse. It may be similar to having a hangover, as you are often addicted to the foods to which you are allergic. Persevere, because you are going to feel better than ever once you are over the effects! It is probably wise to start your new diet when the next few days are free of pressure.

If you do find allergies, seek advice from Foresight or one of the self-help organisations, a nutritionist who understands allergy, or a doctor who is experienced in nutritional medicine, to ensure that your diet and nutritional supplements provide all the nutrients you require. This is especially important if you are planning a pregnancy or are pregnant.

A rotation diet for the detection of allergy

Monday	Tuesday	Wednesday	Thursday
Chicken	Pork	Lamb	Turkey
Banana	Sago	Brown rice	Maize
Pineapple	Dates	Rice flour	Cornflour
Beetroot	Apple	Orange	Leeks
Spinach	Pear	Grapefruit	Onions
Swiss chard	Lettuce	Satsuma	Asparagus
Pineapple juice	Endive	Mandarin	Chives
	Chicory	Lime	Grapes
	Artichoke	Carrot	Sultanas
	Sunflower seeds	Celery	Grape juice
	Apple juice	Parsnip	
		Parsley	
		Grapefruit or orange juice	

Friday	Saturday	Sunday
Fish	Rabbit	Beef
Millet	Lentils	Potato
Millet flakes	Green beans	Potato flour
Cabbage	Peas	Tomato
Savoy cabbage	Black-eyed beans	Aubergine
Brussels sprouts	Broad beans	Cucumber
Broccoli	Mung bean shoots	Marrow
Cauliflower	Plums	Melon
Kohlrabi	Peaches	Tomato juice
Swedes	Apricot	
Avocado	Cherry	
Figs	Prunes	
Water	Prune juice	

Do not despair! You will find there are many alternatives to our usual foods, which will add interest and variety to your diet. If you look in your local healthfood or wholefood store you will see many different types of flour, grain and milk. You may also find that your allergies change over time, and if you sort out your nutritional imbalances allergies sometimes become a thing of the past.

Always try to choose an organically grown food, free of additives.

The rotation diet is designed to give each specific food only one day in seven. The diet eliminates the most common allergens, cow's milk, grains and eggs. Also, all stimulants such as coffee, tea, chocolate and the sugars. No drink should be taken except the juice of the day and water. All foods must be boiled in plain water, steamed, plain grilled or cooked in the oven in a covered dish. No fats, oils, gravies are to be used. During the trial period NO FOOD OTHER THAN THOSE LISTED MAY BE TAKEN AT ALL.

During the first week of the diet adverse reactions may take place due to the withdrawal of cow's milk etc., if these are allergenic substances. For a few days the reactions may be quite strong, akin to alcohol withdrawal in the first few days of abstinence.

The participant may be more hungry than usual, however, and it is important to have enough food available.

The diet will have ensured a fast of six days from any offending food, so the reaction to any allergen will probably be fairly immediate and may take the form of a running or stuffed-up nose, headache, stomach pain, feeling of bloatedness, extreme lethargy, irritability etc. The day this occurs can be marked on the diet sheet. It is then possible to test the foods eaten on this day one at a time.

Having thus worked out a basic diet of 'safe' foods, it will then be possible to test common allergens, such as cow's milk, eggs, other fruits, the gluten grains – wheat, oats, barley, rye – etc. After three weeks' abstinence the reaction may be strong, and at first only a small quantity of the substance should be given. If the reaction is very severe, a teaspoonful of bicarbonate of soda in water will help alleviate the symptoms. After an adverse reaction a return to known safe foods for a few days will be necessary before testing for another possible allergen. After a few weeks it should be possible to identify all food allergies in this way.

The treatment of food allergies will depend on a number of factors, including how extensive the allergies are. You may be able to get by with simple elimination, though this is no cure. There are various desensitising methods, ranging from drops to injections. The most practical and successful is probably enzyme potentiated desensitisation, though, as with all methods, it does not work for everyone. Any doctor who is practising as a clinical ecologist, or using a nutritional approach in his work, will be able to diagnose and treat you. You will not be able to get desensitisation done except by a doctor.

Allergies to chemicals, such as food additives, pesticides and chemicals used in the workplace and home, may also be present. These are often difficult to diagnose and eliminate.

Coeliac condition

There is a condition in which the sufferer cannot metabolise gluten, a protein found in wheat, barley, oats and rye. It can cause severe physical and mental symptoms if it is not diagnosed, mainly because of the severe deficiencies arising from the malabsorption. Coeliac condition has been found to exacerbate infertility problems, especially in zinc-deficient women. Treatment is by avoidance of gluten-containing grains.

Parasites

Irritable bowel syndrome is present in about 20% of people (both male and female) who come to Foresight. The term encompasses abdominal pain, inflammation of the gut-wall, bloating, flatulence, diarrhoea and malabsorption of nutrients.

In many cases, if allergies and coeliac condition have been eliminated as possible causes, there can be candida or intestinal and other parasites. Stomach parasites include helicobacter, often responsible for stomach ulcers. Parasites from drinking water include cryptosporidium, about which we are usually warned when there is an outbreak. Intestinal ones we have had detected in Foresight people are blastocystis hominis, giardia lamblia, the homely threadworms and some amoebic-type buglets.

All, or any, of these need to be coped with ahead of the pregnancy, as the diarrhoea and inflammation can cause gross discomfort, and will result in malabsorption of essential nutrients. This could, at best, severely compromise the health of the future baby, and at worst it could precipitate a miscarriage

Foresight can arrange for a stool test and help from a homeopath. This will give you the diagnosis. You can then obtain help from a trained herbalist, a homeopath or from Ainsworths Homeopathic Chemists.

DIY preparations that have been found to be helpful are Paraclear, a herbal preparation, and Citricidal, a preparation made from grapefruit seeds. One of our most experienced doctors suggests 600 mg of garlic every day for three months. After any treatment, or self-treatment, test again to make sure it has been successful.

Be careful to avoid starting a pregnancy until you are certain it has completely cleared up. It can take three to six weeks, as the parasites lay eggs which later hatch out and restart the colony! The treatment is therefore a series of carefully timed doses, and needs to be done accurately.

To summarise:

If allergy doesn't turn out to be the whole answer, seek out a nutritional therapist, get her to arrange a stool test and this will tell you if you have candida albicans (a mouldy infestation of the gut) or some other type of parasite. She can then advise you further on combating these with diet and herbal remedies.

Within a few months there should be a Brand New You, feeling much brighter and stronger — and able to stay that way for the rest of your life. Commensurately, your ova, or sperm, as the case may be, will also be brighter, stronger, better nourished, and more purposeful!

Onwards!

CHAPTER 8
Electromagnetic Pollution
– or 'electrosmog' to you and me

In the excellent *Powerwatch Handbook*, published in 2006, Alasdair and Jean Philips remind us that as early as the 1920s, the Marconi Company began its first speech transmissions from Chelmsford in the United Kingdom. What advances there have been in less than a century! From messages in Morse tapped from headland to headland, to television programmes on a mobile phone to 'our foreign correspondent', now standing amid scenes of devastation and mayhem from every corner of the globe – live.

The point of this chapter is to talk about whether the actual **technology** involved, and the fallout from this, is affecting our health, our fertility and/or our future baby's health. Because sometimes it does.

Foresight started learning about electromagnetism rather late in the day, in the early 1990s. We met Alfred Riggs, possibly the most informed person on the planet on this subject. He told us of the dangers of becoming sensitised to 'electrosmog', which you cannot see, smell, hear or feel in most cases, but which is now all around us as never before. 'Minor' reactions to the bombardment include headaches, dizziness, sleeplessness, fatigue and depression, the ubiquitous 'stress of modern life'. More alarming consequences can include heart disease, leukaemia and other cancers. There are questions over chromosomal damage in babies, cot death, infertility and miscarriage.

In the year 2000 an 'expert group' was set up to study the effects of electromagnetic fields on human health. We are grateful to Alasdair and Jean for letting us know their conclusions:

'...that in making decisions about the siting of base stations, planning authorities should have the power to ensure that the radio frequency fields to which the public will be exposed will be kept to the lowest practical levels that will be commensurate with the telecommunications operating effectively.'

Once again you spot the deliberate mistake, I am sure. The Expert is on the side of the commercial interest. Pollution must be kept as low as possible, but this endeavour must not interfere with the ever-rising need for telecommunication. Therefore the limit set will not in any way be linked to the health implications. It will be linked to the demand for – well, gadgets and wonder-toys that generate electrosmog. As their use proliferates, so this mobile 'limit' will rise in line with commercial interests.

Once again, we do not want to wait for 'the government', 'the medics' or any other august body who rely on 'the Expert' to protect us, or even warn us. We need to be looking out for ourselves, and most particularly for our future children.

There are in this country already in the region of 2½ million people suffering from a new and difficult-to-manage condition called EHS or electro-hypersensitivity. To put it in a nutshell, too much exposure to electromagnetism has heightened their response to this, and each time they are exposed again, they become ill. For example, going near to mobile and cordless phones, to certain types of lighting, or to power lines or electrical appliances of all sorts affects them. People who have the condition very severely, cannot be in a room with a mobile phone that is 'live', for example. They can feel dizzy, sick, headachy or just tired to the point of being completely 'wiped out'. For those who are, or believe they may be suffering from EHS an extremely helpful and informative website now exists: **www.electrosensitivity.org.uk**

To me, because my mind is always veering in one direction, this raises the question, 'what does all this electrosmog do to the sperm, the ova, and the unborn child?'

What do we know so far? We know that carrying a mobile phone in the trouser pocket while it is on means deformity and death to sperm (I have recently heard of someone who did so all the time, who has had a tumour in the upper thigh).

Dr Imre Fejes of Szeged University Hungary is one of the lead researchers in the study of human reproduction and embryology who studied a group of 221 men over a 13 month period. Sperm from very active users of mobile phones was compared with that of non users. The results showed that men who carried a phone with them on stand-by throughout the day had significantly lowered sperm concentration. Their counts averaged at 59.11 million per millilitre of seminal fluid compared with 82.97 million not continually exposed to mobile phone radiation. Men who made lengthy calls had fewer rapidly motile sperm – 36.3 million compared with 51.3 million for men who made no calls. It is believed that mobile phones could be the main contributory factor in the falling rates of male fertility. Sperm counts among British men have fallen by 29 percent over the past decade which has shown the largest increase in the use of mobile phones. More worrying is that I increasingly find that mobile phone microwave energy is now only a small part of a whole orchestration of microwave energy enabled devices that are increasingly finding their way into our households. We know from biology and physics that the human body acts as a half wave dipole antenna. Electromagnetic radiation which includes microwave energy and Earth radiation consist of energy flux and therefore energy is conveyed into the tissues of the body itself. Some of this energy passes straight through (the magnetic field) and some is absorbed depending on the frequency setting up eddy currents as it passes through. This energy will affect people in different ways according to how electro sensitive they are and their differences in height, weight, bone structure, and body fat.

The police in recent years have been using a TETRA mast base station. This sends out a more powerful signal. Since this, they have found that carrying their phone in the trouser pocket caused prostate cancer, wearing it on their belt gave colon cancer, and wearing it in the breast pocket gave breast cancer. This latter is very unusual in men. For further information regarding TETRA and health issues go to: **www.tetrawatch.net**

I think we can conclude that there is enough evidence that too much contact with these gadgets etc. could be more harmful than most people realise, or than the powers-that-be are willing to admit/allow themselves to realise, if intervention would interfere with a multi-million pound enterprise.

Gail's story:

The six years that Gail and her husband had tried for a baby seemed like an eternity. Two years after the wedding there was still no baby. Then in 2001 a referral for Gail and her husband at a hospital for an investigation came up. The examination revealed everything was perfectly fine except for some cysts that were 'too small for removal'. IVF was organised and although there were plenty of embryos, there was no implantation in the first two IVF attempts.

A friend introduced them to Foresight and they started on the programme. They also employed the help of a Foresight practitioner. However, following the lead of medically orientated friends, they felt a need to try for a third IVF attempt with a private fertility specialist, although results of their hair mineral analysis were well below recommended levels for conception. Scans performed by the private clinic indicated three cysts on the left ovary (which previously were too small to remove) and adhesions in the uterus, all of which were then surgically removed. The implant failed. They decided to put the fourth IVF on hold in order to get Gail's body back to full fitness.

Foresight had suggested that perhaps a specialist in electromagnetic pollution, Roy Riggs, could identify a problem. Both were sceptical, but they decided to call him in. Roy found the whole house safe except for their bedroom where there was a problem exactly where their bed was located. They moved their bed into another room, continued with the Foresight programme, and began to experience health. 'Everything felt as if it was coming together. The combination was working well.'

Late in December Gail was four days late. She was keenly aware of her cycle. They were about to attempt the fourth IVF but Gail decided to do a pregnancy test and as usual it proved negative. Two days later, urged by instinct, she did a second pregnancy test which proved positive! 'Ah! I just sat there and couldn't believe it. My husband in surprise asked, "What does positive mean?" "It means we've *done* it!"'

A little boy was conceived on Gail's birthday and was announced on Daddy's. He was born 7lb 8oz by caesarean section. 'He is a fantastic, lovely, laughing little boy and so happy.'

Gail says, 'We changed our food to organic, threw out household chemicals such as air sprays, all our products are now eco-friendly. I have kept up with the Foresight programme all through breastfeeding and found it so helpful.'

So what do we do?

It is possible to hire two instruments from **www.emfields.org** and carry out your own safety check. The first instrument called the Acousticom 2 is easy to use and comes with full instructions. It will accurately measure microwaves and high radio frequencies [RF] such as Wi-Fi, DECT phones, mobile phones and phone masts. It will not measure the electric fields or magnetic fields coming from your mains electricity. You will need to hire the EMFields ELF meter for this, which measures electric, and magnetic fields produced from your home electrics, transformers, power lines and substations. About 90% of microwave and RF measured in an average home is produced by a combination of DECT cordless phones and your own computer Wi-Fi systems. So either dump the DECT telephones and replace them by the older landline phones or if you are addicted to using a cordless phone then buy a low radiation set, called [Eco+ DECT phones] available on line or from www.emfields.org. To rid the house of Wi-Fi create a home network system using an Ethernet connection from your modem to any electric socket which uses your own electric ring circuit to transport the internet connection throughout the house and to any computer in any room. These wired home network systems are available from most computer shops.

Say No to Wireless Smart Meters

The UK government recognizes the non-thermal health problems of gas and electricity wireless smart meters and **allows you to refuse them**. Australia has already reached 10% refusals.

Stop Smart Meters! (UK) is an independent, not-for-profit voice calling for an immediate halt and reversal of the UK's Smart Meter programme. This programme intends to fit smart meters in every home by 2020 – unless we prevent it.

There are many serious problems presented by web-enabling our electricity, gas and water supplies and turning our homes into wireless networks by fitting smart meters that can emit high levels of WI-FI radiation throughout our homes every few minutes. Smart Meters are **NOT** mandatory – you are lawfully entitled to refuse one on whatever grounds you like. And if you would like to help other people do the same, you can download a free leaflet raising awareness about Smart Meters within your own community. See more at: **http://stopsmartmeters.org.uk/**.

International Agency for Research on Cancer (IARC), an agency of the World Health Organisation, recently published a report, reclassifying radiation from mobiles and WI-FI from category 3, with "no conclusive evidence" of causing cancer, to category 2b – a "**possible human carcinogen**" – along with diesel exhaust, chloroform, jet fuel, lead and DDT.

Outside your own house is more difficult. If it is a terraced house, there may be considerable debilitating and cancer-making fields coming through the wall from the back of a neighbour's television or VDU. It is possible to buy wallpaper with a sandwich effect – plain wallpaper on both sides of an aluminium foil lining. The rays cannot pass through aluminium. This can be put up and painted over, or wallpapered over again with one of your choice. There is also a carbon-based paint that is impenetrable. This is black, but can also be painted over. There are silver mesh curtains that look just like ordinary net curtains, I am told, which can go up at the windows and will not let rays through. All/any of these may be helpful if circumstances are really difficult. **www.powerwatch.org.uk** is the relevant website. If the bed is vulnerable then it is important that the bedstead is wooden and the mattress has no metal springs, i.e. it should be wool or latex etc. These beds can be obtained from Greenfibres in Totness, or Healthy House in Ruscombe. See Useful Addresses in the back of the book.

Pylons, base stations, telephone wiring, mobile phone masts (also their boosters, and most especially TETRA masts) and TV broadcasting masts are all giving off electromagnetic signals at their various frequencies. In Germany, builders are not allowed to put up houses within 500m of a mast. Here, we can build right next door to them and furthermore, we plonk masts on the roofs of hospitals and schools.

Again, if you stand around in your house, garden, patio, place of work, wherever, with the Acousticom 2 the flashing coloured lights will give you a reading of the strength of any nearby phone mast or neighbour's Wi-Fi system in an easy to read format. Remember to turn off your mobile phone whilst taking any readings from this instrument, as it will cause interference and give you a higher reading than you are actually measuring.

Do not blame your neighbour, he probably knows nothing about it, but help him to work out what is best for his family too. Maybe have an Acousticom party and see how all of you can best protect your neighbourhood? We are all on the same side, and we all need to help each other as much as possible.

Sadly your local MP is unlikely to be helpful. (Please contact me immediately if you *are* an MP and intend to do something about this! Welcome on board!) The government line has been, *'you can complain on the grounds that they are unsightly, and we will take your complaint seriously, but you cannot complain on health grounds, as nothing is proven in that area.'* This is a crafty angle as it gives the industry the right and the reason to hide the masts – in petrol station signs, in church steeples, in chimney stacks. *'The locals thought it was ugly, so we have to put it out of sight.'* This is typical officialdom. What I call a 'clever-clever' but not intelligent response.

Yes, they are hidden and people do not know they are there, so this solves the problem of coping with the 'fuss'. Their friends in Telecom are happy – even gleeful. Probably punching the air over a glass of beer because the problem has been solved for them. Up go the masts.

The problems of the families where the breadwinner or the young mother is dying of cancer, or where a precious child has been diagnosed with leukaemia, are not solved, however.

Officialdom has yet to arrive at the stage of mental development where avoiding huge numbers of personal tragedies is more important than making huge amounts of money. We all need to come together over this, and push for their enlightenment.

The next problem is the electromagnetism from underground. This is where father and son Alfred and Roy Riggs have done such brilliant work. We will go over here to the chapter written for you by Gail Bradley, with additions to bring it up to date by Roy Riggs.

Physical Hazards

Information you need to check out at work and at home – is it safe for the unborn baby?

Some years ago if you opened a book on occupation health you would rarely find a mention of reproductive hazards. Now, with women of child-bearing age forming a large part of the workforce, and with recognition that occupational hazards can affect the male reproductive system, there are whole books on the subject, as well as large parts of others. The hazards are many, ranging from physical ones, such as radiation, VDUs, noise, light and heat, to chemical ones, such as formaldehyde and benzene. Here we consider radiation, which generates so much damage.

Ionising radiation

Rays of ionising radiation include alpha, beta and gamma rays, neutrons and X-rays. They are so powerful that they shatter atoms they touch, causing them to lose electrons, thereby developing an electric charge. These charged particles are called ions, hence the term 'ionising'. Because of their power these rays are extremely damaging to tissues in the body, and can cause death quickly or slowly. They penetrate the body without a person knowing. They hit atoms and molecules, breaking them up to form free radicals and oxidising agents. These two chemical groups may be quite damaging as they break up proteins, destroy chromosomes and change other chemicals. The results may be death of the cells, immediately or earlier than the usual lifespan, changes in the growth and division of the cell such that there may be no growth or uncontrolled growth (cancer), or prominent changes in the way the cell works.

Man has always been exposed to some ionising radiation. However, Dr Rosalie Bertell has pointed out that 'natural' levels have increased from an exposure of 60 millirems a year in 1940 to 100 in the 1950s to 200 millirems in the 1980s, mainly due to weapons testing. No one disputes that more of us are exposed to more radiation than ever before.

Frequently we are reassured that low doses, such as that received in an X-ray, are safe. But the truth is that no level of radiation has been proved safe and it is likely that any level is potentially harmful. A quick look through, for example, the Bulletin of the Atomic Scientists reveals a number of studies which relate radiation dosages to malformations such as Down's syndrome, Patau syndrome and Edwards syndrome, severe mental retardation, perinatal loss and neurological damage, to mention but a few. Dr Bertell worries that scientists only ask about the risks of cancer from radiation exposure when it has other, more serious effects. She is especially concerned about the genetic pool: 'Children are now being born weakened by radioactivity, prone to enzyme disorders, allergies and asthma directly caused by cell mutations.' She talks of a weakened new generation less able to cope with an ever-increasing dose of radiation in the environment. 'By the fifth generation of children born into the post-nuclear age the damage to the entire gene pool will be very clear indeed.' She denounces the international 'safety' level that power stations work to: '… maximum 500 millirems a year to the public or plant workers, equivalent to 100 chest X-rays'. Other researchers have also indicated that even increases in background radioactivity, within natural levels, may have damaging effects on the foetus and may be a reason for higher malformation rates.

X-rays have been the subject of much research and concern, especially since Dr Alice Stewart shows that they could harm the foetus, causing a high risk of childhood leukaemia. Animal research confirms these adverse effects, in both males and females. When mature eggs of female mice were irradiated the offspring had a high incidence of cancer. Where dominant mutations have been produced in male germ cells by X-rays, low birth weight results.

Radiation Exposure in Hospitals & Clinics

X-rays: 0.6% of all cancers diagnosed in the UK are caused by medical X-rays (700 of the 124,000 a year). (Herzog, P & Rieger, CT, 'Risk of cancer from diagnostic X-rays', *Lancet* 2004 Jan 31: 363(9406):345–51, 2004)

NB: If you have to have an X-ray, consult a homeopath. There are homeopathic nosodes (remedies) to X-rays, which offer some protection from side effects. Alternatively, ring Ainsworths Homeopathic Chemists before you have the X-ray. You can take a nosode before and after.

Mammograms: The dose from a single mammogram is about seven times the dose rate of a single chest X-ray. (There is mixed debate over whether the survival rate among women diagnosed by mammogram is any better than that of those who did not have a mammogram.)

Ultrasound: UK survey showed that, for 1 in 200 babies where the pregnancy was terminated because the ultrasound showed major abnormalities, the diagnosis post-mortem was less severe than predicted and the termination was probably unjustified. Research concluded some adverse effects; a summary of the safety of ultrasound in human studies published in May 2002 concluded that *'there may be a relation between prenatal ultrasound exposure and adverse outcome.'* Some of the reported effects are listed below:

- Growth restriction
- Delayed speech
- Dyslexia
- Non-right-handedness (seen as marker of damage to developing brain)
- Damage to nerve myelin sheath
- Irreversible loss of brain cells

NB: Beverley Beech of the Association for Improvement in Maternity Services (AIMS) and I have both sadly noted a number of occasions in which an early scan was given at 8–9 weeks, where the baby was seen to be kicking about and had a normal heartbeat. However, at the second scan a month or so later, the parents are told, 'We are sorry to tell you, but your baby has died. He did not develop beyond 8–9 weeks. You must just have been lucky enough to catch a glimpse of him just before he died.' It would be hard to expect the scanners to say that what they did may have been responsible, but I think it is time they took stock. This tragically happens far too often to be nothing but a strange coincidence.

For those of you invited to go along for a scan, ask the reason. Is it just 'routine'? Is it to help you 'bond' with your baby? (You will do this anyway.) Is there any really worrying medical reason? What is this?

Obtain all the details and then make your own mind up, in the light of all of the above. Your baby has to rely on you to protect him, when he needs this.

CAT scans: These expose you to between 40 and 100 times the dose of a conventional X-ray examination and represent the largest source of radiation exposure in both the UK and the USA. The Health Protection Agency reported that in 1998, CAT scans constituted 4% of all medical examinations, contributing to 40% of the collective effective dose of X-rays.

MRI scans: These use strong magnetic fields and radio frequency fields to build up a picture. Despite this about a million MRI scans are performed each year in the UK.

Non-ionising radiation

Non-ionising rays, including ultraviolet, infra-red, lasers, microwaves, radar, radio frequency waves and extra low frequency waves, are naturally produced by the sun and also created in the home, in industry and in military activity. Although they are not powerful enough to create ions, no one should be fooled about their safety. The chief of research of non-ionising radiation at the National Institute of Environmental Health Sciences, North Carolina, Donald McCree, has said: '*In animal experiments, [the Russians] have found that this radiation causes changes in almost every system: behaviour, blood chemistry, the endocrine functions, reproductive organs, and the immune system.*

In studies of human workers exposed to microwave equipment for many years, they have reported abnormally slow heart beats, chest pains, and birth defects. And they've found a lot of more subjective effects, things like insomnia, irritability, headaches and loss of memory.'

Of major concern to us here are sunlight, ultraviolet, microwaves, radar and radio frequency waves.

Sunlight

'Light is a primal element of life.' Indeed, without it we would not have life as we know it. We tend to talk about the benefits of 'fresh air' without being aware of the beneficial effects of natural light. Yet research has shown that natural light and artificial light have different physiological effects in animals, including human beings, which show in a variety of physical and mental conditions, such as tumours and hyperactivity.

Clearly, artificial lighting is an essential part of modern lifestyles. But it is possible to buy full-spectrum lighting, which is very similar to natural light and quite different from fluorescent, neon and other artificial forms. Full-spectrum lighting covers more specific wavelengths, especially the blue or ultraviolet ones that are missing from artificial lighting (see below.) If they are blocked out, an endocrine deficiency can arise. Mice kept in artificial light conditions died prematurely or had very small litters, suggesting the need for further research. Full-spectrum lighting has been shown to help alleviate seasonal affective depression. Sunlight has been found to help with the elimination of toxic metals from the body and the metabolism of desirable minerals.

Ultraviolet

Ultraviolet rays can be UV-A or UV-B type. The UV-B are the ones that give you sunburn, but although UV-A is weaker, one expert says it does the same damage, and may even be worse. To get brown, you need the same overall exposure, so with UV-A, it just means that you will have to sunbathe longer. However, UV-A penetrates deeper than UV-B, and may cause damage to collagen, blood vessels and elastic tissues. UV-B may therefore be safer, because the UV-A lulls you into a false sense of security. Also, once exposed to UV-A, the body is more susceptible to the aging and carcinogenic effects of UV-B radiation.

There is now quite a scare about sunbathing and skin cancer. To induce skin cancer in animals, it is necessary to give a larger-than-normal dose of ultraviolet light so that burning occurs. There also seems to be a direct relationship between the number of free radicals formed in the skin when it is exposed to sunlight and the tendency for that skin to burn.

Stop the free radicals forming and you considerably reduce the sun burning. (Free radical formation can be inhibited by certain nutrients in the diet, such as vitamins A, C and E).

Another factor that may be significant is cholesterol, which may be changed into a number of products when the ultraviolet strikes the skin, one of which, cholesterol alphaoxide, can act as a free radical and cause cancer. Oils and fats applied to the skin, or sunbathing creams may also stimulate cancer formation.

So should you avoid ultraviolet light? This is not the good idea that the advertisements would have us believe, since it means avoiding natural sunlight, or at least parts of it, and the ultraviolet portion is the most biologically active. Ultraviolet wavelengths can kill bacteria – and infections are definitely to be avoided in pregnancy! Ultraviolet treatments are provided by law to miners in Russia, as they have been found to help remove dust from the lungs.

Computer monitors

Cathode ray tube (CRT) type monitors were widely used in the workplace and home until a few years ago. There was considerable debate over their safety, especially for the pregnant woman, but few conclusions were drawn. Thankfully, computer technology has now marched ahead, making CRT monitors a thing of the past. These screens have now almost all been replaced by flat colour screens known as TFT-LCD, which are very slim and give off almost zero magnetic fields. Laptop computers also give off very low electromagnetic fields but when run from the mains can radiate very high electric fields. If you use your laptop, make sure it is operated in battery mode. *It is better never to use it on your lap at all.* Be sure your monitor is a modern flat-screen one. This is really important.

Microwaves

Microwaves can penetrate deeply into the body, causing its temperature to rise. High-intensity microwaves can lead to permanent damage. For example, the heat generated can cause the cell lining of the testicles to degenerate, therefore damaging them. It is also suspected of causing breast cancer, especially where a microwave oven is placed at breast height. The problem arises because the breast has poor blood supply so the heat is not dissipated. Microwaves may also cause genetic damage: one study has shown that more Down's syndrome children were fathered by men exposed to microwaves than by fathers not so exposed. The highest concentrations of microwaves in the home are emitted from DECT cordless phones, cordless baby monitors and wireless computer networks (Wi-Fi). To reduce your levels of microwave exposure in the home *replace your DECT cordless phones with landline phones.* Buy baby alarm monitors of the type that route the signal through your household electric circuit. Replace your Wi-Fi systems with a cable or ADSL modem/router.

Digital Cordless Baby Monitors
(by Roy Riggs)

Over the past five years, with the help of parents, I have measured a variety of baby monitors and the DECT pulsing ones seem to be far more disruptive to the infant's sleep and state of contentment (causing restlessness, irritability and crying). Wired ones and the plug-in ones (that use the electricity wiring to communicate between units) do not seem to cause the same problems. The older type of analogue ones, which are still available from a number of brands, seem OK if kept at least one metre from the cot/bed. I have had various reports by parents that their babies did not sleep well and cried a lot when they used DECT monitors but were OK when no baby monitor was used. When they then tried a cheaper analogue monitor, the infant then slept as well as they did with no monitor.

Powerwatch UK strongly recommend that only low-band (35 to 50 MHz) analogue baby monitors are used. These use analogue frequency modulation (FM, like VHP radio stations) that does not pulse at all. The analogue ones are often identifiable by their low number of channels (typically 2–4). You can hire or purchase suitable equipment (i.e. the A-COM and the Electrosmog Detector) from EMFields (www.emfields.org) to check out the microwave environment from all sources that may surround your baby. It is preferable to check the place where the baby will be sleeping **before he is born**.

Most baby monitors are now advertised as using DECT phone technology which runs at 1890 MHz or 2400 MHz, which is 1.89 GHz or 2.4 GHz. 2.4 GHz is the microwave oven frequency. These are identifiable by the large number of claimed channels (usually at least 30 and often up to 120), which DECT automatically switches between. These emit sharply pulsing bursts of microwave radiation 100 times every second all the time they are turned on. **Avoid using these.**

With 'talk back' digital baby monitors, where parents can talk back to the baby, both units continuously emit pulsing radiation (on two different frequency channels – one for each way), not just when the baby is making a noise or the parent is talking to them. There are also some camera-based monitors which run at 2.4 GHz. Since these have to transmit video and sound, it is likely that they would have a higher power output. Also, the manufacturers note that these cannot be used in conjunction with computer wireless networks due to interference. **Avoid these also**.

The baby monitor mats that check temperature, heartbeat, breathing etc. should only be used if you have medical reasons to believe that your baby might be in danger of sudden infant death (SIDS only occurs 1–23 days after vaccination – see Viera Scheibner's work and the Useful Reading List at the end of this book). When used with a wireless baby alarm they carry high levels of microwave radiation (up to 6 volts per metre) right into the cot and we believe that will not do your baby any good at all. **Avoid these also**.

I do not recommend the use of wireless video baby monitors that allow you to see your baby on your TV or a portable TV monitor. If you really need that level of baby watching, then have a proper wired closed-circuit TV (CCTV) system installed – do not put a TV wireless transmitter in your child's bedroom and irradiate them unnecessarily (this can cause cancer).

Electricity

People living near high-voltage power lines have sometimes complained that their health was affected by them, though this has been dismissed as nonsense! However, in March 1988, the chairman of the Central Electricity Generating Board launched a £500,000 study into the effects of high-voltage lines on health. At the launch, officials were still being dismissive of the likelihood of any link, despite the fact that other countries accept the risks that the electromagnetic fields generated by these lines can damage health. Russia limits the time a farm worker can spend near them to three hours, while the USA will not allow houses to be built near them. The New York Power-Lines Project results showed that there was an increase in child cancers and significant behavioural and central nervous system effects associated with proximity to power lines. One group of researchers found an increase in all birth defects from conceptions that occurred during the time the father worked on high-voltage systems. Men working in high-voltage switching yards were found to father more congenitally malformed children than would be expected. A number of animal studies have reported health problems including foetal abnormalities.

Dr Nancy Wertheimer and her colleagues found an association between the use of electric blankets and infertility and birth defects. They hypothesised that strong electromagnetic fields may be generated by electric blankets under certain circumstances. The seasonal variation of rates of birth and birth defects may agree with the time periods of peak electric blanket use. Dr Wertheimer's studies have also indicated a possible link between women living in homes in which electric heating cables have been installed in the ceilings and higher rates of miscarriage.

Heat

Extremes of heat and cold cause stress to the body, which can be disadvantageous in the preconception period. But as well as these general stress effects, there may be specific ones associated with heat.

In the man, heat can interfere with sperm production, since the testicles need to operate at a lower temperature than the rest of the body. Hours of sitting, such as happens with taxi and lorry drivers, travelling salesmen and business executives, may result in excess scrotal heat. Skin-tight underwear or frequent hot baths can have a similar effect.

In women, a high body temperature (hyperthermia) can cause damage to the foetus. Hyperthermia tends to stop the division of cells and very high temperatures may even kill cells. In the foetus cell division is basic to growth so stopping it can have devastating consequences. Both brain size and function have been affected.

High temperatures may occur with infections and people have queried if problems arise as a result of the infection or the high temperature itself. Research suggests the latter alone can cause damage. One study of brain-damaged children revealed that their healthy mothers had taken regular prolonged saunas. The researchers advise that prolonged saunas should be avoided during the first three to five months of pregnancy. Short saunas, six to ten minutes long, such as are taken by the Fins, may be safe. (NB: However, as there is some doubt, I would avoid them.)

EMFs and pregnancy

Two epidemiology studies published in 2000 and 2002 suggest that a substantial proportion of miscarriages might be caused by maternal EMF exposure. They theorised that the added risk of miscarriage for a pregnant women exposed to EMFs may be 5 to 10 per cent. Overall, Dr De-Kun Li and his team for the 2002 study found that **women exposed to peak levels of 1.6 microtesla or greater were nearly twice as likely to miscarry as women not exposed to such strong fields.** (Li, DK et al, 'A population based prospective cohort study of personal exposure to magnetic fields during pregnancy and the risk of miscarriage', Epidemiology, Jan: 13(1):9–20, 2002)

Reducing your EMF and microwave exposure

- Keep at least one metre from the front of televisions.
- If you have an old-type cathode-ray VDU monitor replace it with a TFT or plasma display unit both at work and at home.
- Do not use a laptop on your lap.
- Minimise your use of electric appliances at worktop height in the kitchen.
- Move clock radios at least one metre away from your pillow.
- Reduce your use of electric household appliances such as vacuum cleaners, food mixers and hairdryers.
- If you have power lines over, or a substation next to, your garden, avoid sitting in the vicinity.
- Keep beds away from electric storage heaters, both sides of the wall.
- Don't hold a cordless phone or mobile phone near to your 'bump'. Preferably, don't use one at all.
- **Don't wear support bras that contain metal**. These can act as passive antennas near radio frequency sources such as mobile phones.
- Sprung mattresses should be replaced with one of the many non-sprung mattresses that are now on the market.
- Avoid standing or working near a switched-on microwave oven, electric cooker or washing machine.
- Do not use hairdryers and keep the unit well away from the growing foetus. Hand-held hairdryers use high currents both to drive the motor and to produce heat and are one of the highest sources of EMF exposure.
- Never keep any type of electric blanket turned on when you are in bed.
- Do not use DECT cordless phones or baby alarms.

I am so grateful to Gail and Roy for all of the above.

As you will have gathered, the problems of underground radiation come mainly from either underground rivers, or from cracks in the substrata – especially where the substrata is granite, which is mainly the peninsula, Devon and Cornwall, or the very north of England and Scotland.

If you look at a geophysical map of the United Kingdom showing the areas of granite substrata, and also have a map of deformities in children, you will see they very largely coincide. I have pointed this out to people and the reply is usually, 'Ah yes, but those are also the areas of highest poverty.'

'Poverty' is always some sort of catch-all excuse. However, there may be a connection with a phenomenon that makes people feel ill, dizzy and sick, sleep badly, be increasingly liable to cancer, and be generally under the weather (quite apart from the elderly being more susceptible to mental infirmity and the babies more likely to be born deformed). This phenomenon might, in very many cases, have a direct bearing on their ability to go out to work and earn a decent salary.

If anything is ever going to bring an end to 'poverty' it is getting people well, and therefore better able to use their strength and their brains, and getting their babies born likewise.

So what do we do?

We suggest you call in Roy Riggs who is an expert geopathic and electromagnetic energy surveyor. He will advise you on how to protect your family from the excesses of modern electromagnetic pollution. **www.royriggs.co.uk**

He can then tell you exactly where the lines go. Where, if necessary, you need to move critical bits of furniture like the bed, and/or the favourite chair you sit in to eat, or to relax in the evening. It is also **absolutely vital** to know where to put the cot when the moment comes. Babies are known to be very magnetically sensitive, and to be unable to sleep in an electrosmog position. They are also more liable to cot death, cancer and leukaemia, if exposed to large amounts. Get Roy to check the type and position of the baby monitor.

Roy came to look at the house we are now living in before we bought it. He found a line that goes along inside the wall of two of the bedrooms, about a foot inside the wall. When he told us, the erstwhile owners of the house were very intrigued. He showed them how the line went across the pillow of their bed. The woman told us how she always woke up with a splitting headache and had tried all sorts of solutions from conventional and alternative medicine. The man told us how he woke up with a pain in his neck every morning which he put down to an old rugby injury. In the weeks before the move took place, they moved the bed, and the pains ceased to happen.

It is a great shame that this is not part of the normal house survey when people move house, as so much pain and illness could be eliminated if people knew the best spots to put their furniture.

I am not an expert on this area of Foresight work (but I know a man who is!). I would therefore suggest that:

a) You contact Foresight and borrow our DVD of Alf Riggs (Roy's father, who was arguably the world authority on electromagnetism) giving his talk a few years before his death. In this, he showed exactly what he did, and explained everything in a way that can be easily understood.

b) If you can, I would also try to hear a talk, read a book, or at least have a look at the website of Roger Coghill, MA (Cantab.) C. Biol. MI Biol. MA Environ Mgt, who is another highly intelligent radiesthesist. Roger is very much into the harm being done to the bees, as he is convinced that the stress and confusion electrosmog is causing them lies behind this 'mystery virus'. He is also convinced it is causing sterility in the little songbirds and other small wild animals by zapping their ovaries. If we all become more aware, it may be possible to find ways to minimise the hazards for them. I would look at Roger's website and see if there are things we can do to improve conditions for the wildlife as well as for ourselves. It is only fair. We do not have the right to destroy their environment and their fertility as well as our own.

c) Also, look at Powerwatch UK and read Alasdhair and Jean Philips' excellent book, *The Powerwatch Handbook*, which will give you lots of useful pointers, in enormous detail, on how to keep your house safe. I would also borrow an

Acousticom and nose around with it. There are probably a million things that we do not yet know about electromagnetism because for most of us, we have only just become aware of it. But if we can make every effort to minimise the risks we *are* aware of, we will need to worry a lot less.

d) If you have a fertility problem, have had a miscarriage or a Down's syndrome baby, or suffer from any of the symptoms described above, I would get Roy in and suss out your house, garden and workplace.

e) If you know anybody with cancer, or any of the symptoms described, let them know what can be done.

If you have radio masts on the top of your local school, hospital or nursery, or in the church tower, I would complain about it! For further advice on how to identify and deal with both electromagnetic and geopathic energies in the home and workplace, use Roy Riggs and Powerwatch's websites to gather together the information you need. Good luck!

www.royriggs.co.uk
www.powerwatch.org.uk

Discuss all of it with your neighbours, and help your community as much as you can. You can make a lot of difference to people's lives.

I am so old now I may not be around much longer, so all of you need to take it all on board, and carry the knowledge forward. Do not allow "progress" to destroy our wonderful world!

Onwards!

CHAPTER 9
Chemical Hazards

'Nearly every chemical to which the pregnant woman is exposed will ultimately reach the foetus.' So says Dr Joan Spyker, an eminent toxicologist. In 1984, Gail Bradley commented: 'We must also remember that the foetus does not have a mature system to detoxify all the poisons that may be passed on to it.'

In a study spearheaded by the Environmental Working Group (EWG) in collaboration with Commonweal, researchers at two major laboratories found an average of 200 industrial chemicals and pollutants in umbilical cord blood from 10 babies born in August and September of 2004 in U.S. hospitals. Tests revealed a total of 287 chemicals in the group. The umbilical cord blood of these 10 children, collected by Red Cross after the cord was cut, harbored pesticides, consumer product ingredients, and wastes from burning coal, gasoline, and garbage.

Environmental Working Group, July 14, 2005

Even in the UK, I am afraid we have to conclude that our Hero is up against it!

I think we now have to think on even further than Dr Spyker. The use of powerful medical drugs and hormones has become more and more common. We now know that when chemicals are voided (urinated or defecated) they enter the biosphere and become cumulative until they can be found in measurable quantities in earth, water and so on. Of course these quantities will be small at present, and certainly not all the biosphere pollution has passed through people first! Much has come from smoke, pesticides, fluoride, industrial waste etc. discharged into rivers direct from the factories, incinerators and farmland. Poison such as that used to dip sheep is dumped into rivers etc (illegal, but it happens!).

At the same time we are told of the demise of the bees, butterflies and the small birds, to think of but a few 'bio-tragedies'. We need to become more thoughtful and a lot less gung-ho with every type of chemical. We seem to have been the most destructive generation so far and it has gone on long enough.

One health problem the establishment does seem to be becoming more aware of is obesity. Presumably because it is the most visible! Walking in any town in the United Kingdom now, you can spot the tendency!

The standard answer trotted out by the Establishment is 'too much food/the wrong type of food, and too little exercise'. Yes, well, this has to be factored in. But how much is down to these simplistic answers, and how much is down to exogenous hormones, statins, steroids, insulin, pig's thyroxin, tranquillisers and the like, urinated happily into the biosphere by the pill-taking public and farm animals, and now coming from our tap water? All these drugs are known to have 'weight gain' listed among their side effects.

Then what about the growth promoters, antibiotics etc. given to livestock? Firstly, is meat more fattening to us when the animals are reared on substances meant to be more fattening to them? Secondly, as their excrement seeps from the fields into the water-table, is this too laced with chemical 'growth promoters?

We cannot all be totally neurotic, but I think two at least partial solutions to all today's problems would be:

(a) we do all we can to stay as healthy as possible, so we do not need to take medical drugs; (b) we use as few chemicals as possible, to keep the environment, and our own unborn children, as free from gunk as possible.

My grandmother lived to be 103 years old (compos mentis to the end) and never took a medical pill, even an aspirin, all her life. 'I've watched what happens to my friends,' she used to say; 'when they start going to the doctor they get worse, not better. Your body knows what to do. Leave it alone and let it get on with it.'

Problems and Solutions

We can look at the problems we find commonest in our own lives, and the solutions:

1. We can **eat organic food**, avoiding promoting further use of pesticides such as organophosphates, chemical fertilisers such as potassium, phosphorus and nitrates, and 'growth promoters' in the livestock. We could ask our local supermarket why they do not stock more of it. We could maybe even have a vegetable patch and grow our own, or hire an allotment.

2. We can ask florists for **organic flowers** (essential for maternity greetings and hospital gifts), and so discourage use of chemicals on flowers (using soapy water for greenfly on our own roses).

3. We can **avoid inorganic 'bug killers'** in our own garden and kitchen. Common table salt discourages snails and slugs. So do coffee grounds. Picking things off food plants by hand is the easiest way to get rid of them. Feeding all plants with organic seaweed manure also seems to be a very good way of making plants strong enough to stand up to mould, blight, black spot etc. Pinch the hose into a small jet to knock the blackfly off dahlias etc. A line of flour will deter ants from coming into the house – it sticks to their legs and they don't like it!

4. If you **eat mainly fresh food** you will not come across additives much, but if you buy Foresight's booklet *FIND OUT*, you can avoid any of the really unhelpful ones. It may also help the cause if you flourish it under the noses of the supermarket staff. Better still, give one to the manager! Explain what a lot of harm it is doing to the children.

5. **Avoid toothpaste that contains fluoride.** It is an endemic poison and used as a rat killer in the United States. All other European countries have given up putting it directly into the drinking water because of the health effects and the effects on the environment. Nevertheless, if we and 69 million other people spit it into the waste water twice a day, the cumulative effect must be horrendous. Think of the poor little fish wondering why they feel so queasy – and what the Dickens is happening to their genitalia? Apart from that, we know fluoride affects thyroid function. People keep telling me, 'I'm on thyroxine...' The thyroid is very near the inside of the

mouth, if you think of facial geography. If the lining of the mouth is absorbing fluoride, then it must be reaching the thyroid. And then, how about the baby's thyroid? Remember Dr Spykes saying anything the mother is exposed to reaches the foetus. Don't let's clobber his/her little thyroid. Fluoride-free toothpastes are: Kingfisher, Tom's of Maine, Aloe Vera (I think the nicest) and Euthymol.

6. **We needn't use the contraceptive pill or copper coil.** Nobody needs an extra cancer risk. Wildlife doesn't need these. They have to drink the river water too. We can learn natural family planning – it is more thoughtful for the future fertility of all the species in the world.

7. **Shop wisely:** I intended listing all the noxious materials that are put in a whole range of cosmetics and what are loosely termed 'bathroom products'. However, when I came to consult Foresight's little booklet *WATCH IT*, compiled in 2007 (with Trojan work by Maria Griffiths), I found there were 67 such chemicals – all with chillingly long and complicated names! I realised you would never want to sit and read through them any more than I wanted to copy them out! However, I noted that 39 of them were known to be carcinogenic (cancer-causing) and 12 were listed as causing miscarriage, 41 were skin and/or eye irritants, 16 were said to affect the central nervous system, 11 were said to cause 'mild or serious insanity'(!?), 10 to cause nausea and vomiting, 10 to cause asthma and 9 were said to be teratogenic (baby-damaging).

Reading through the list, I realised we were once again sitting ducks for the pharmaceutical industry. They pop little surprises into our face creams etc that cause eye irritation, asthma etc and then benefit from the expensive little medicaments we use to try to get better.

So, the good news is there is this little booklet, *WATCH IT* which you can take shopping. As with *FIND OUT*, flourish it in the areas where you buy your cosmetics, so that worried staff can let manufacturers know that we are all switched on and nosing around among their products – and not buying them!

The other bit of good news is that there are now 26 different firms making products they claim are free from noxious chemicals! You will have to check them out regarding what is available where and prices etc but they are widely available and also listed in the back of *WATCH IT*.

8. Many **household cleaners** are also pretty suspect! Some are said to contain arsenic.

   EDTA (ethylene-diaminetetraacetic acid) is found in some bleaches, and causes headaches and skin rashes. Once in the river, it kills fish and shellfish.

   Hydrochloric acid is a severe irritant to the eyes and skin, and is found in toilet cleaners.

   Isopropyl is found in liquid cleaners and detergents. It is said to be a central nervous system depressant that can cause vomiting and coma.

   Naphthalene in toilet cleaners etc. and in pesticides is said to be poisonous to human beings, it irritates the skin and eyes, **and** it is carcinogenic.

   Oxalic acid, also found in toilet cleaners, is another hazardous one that is also said to damage the liver and kidneys.

   Paradichlorobenzene, **sodium bisulphate** and two more chemicals in toilet cleaners and disinfectants can trigger allergies. Lots of different products in laundry powders and soaps are said to be carcinogenic.

   So what do we do?
   Use good old hot water, table salt, and bicarbonate of soda. It has the merit of being cheap, baby-friendly and not rough on the biosphere – or on us!.

Furniture and Furnishings

'Hard' furniture, meaning mainly made from wood, is safe so long as it is genuine! It may be best bought second-hand, so that nothing 'modern' has been done to it, like treating it in advance for woodworm etc. Some wood is treated with arsenic to prevent mould and rotting. However, 'old' furniture may also have been treated at some stage.

Always find out exactly what you are buying. If there are woodworm holes, leave it alone!

Beware the fitted kitchen and bedroom furniture that is made from 'chipboard'. This is sawdust stuck together with noxious solvents and resins which can out-gas benzene, nitrophenals, formaldehyde and other volatile compounds which can be allergenic. Maybe stick to old family stuff or buy second-hand and give it a lick and a promise, a coat of beeswax polish or a coat of eco-paint?

The good news is that it is now possible to buy carpets, curtain material and so on, **free from chemicals**. Blendworth, at Horndean, near Petersfield, do this. They ask you if you would like it sprayed with moth proofing, fire retardant or Scotch guard or similar stain proofing? Just say no. If you are not asked this, find out if this has already been done. If so, ask for a length without any of it. This can come straight from the factory without anything added.

To my way of thinking, this should be cheaper as they have not had to do anything with it. However, it will probably not be, but it certainly should not be more expensive!

There are places you can go to get mattresses and bedding that are organic, not treated, and, in the case of mattresses, free from metal springs (which can now be made 'live' by the mobile phone masts – frying tonight!). These splendid suppliers are Green Fibres and Healthy House (see Useful Addresses).

It is enormously important for your baby's cot mattress and bedding to be organic.

Non-organic mattresses can be full of wool from dipped sheep which can give off **organophosphates**. Although there is no 'scientific proof' I have always been concerned that this might be a contributory factor to cot death. In New Zealand all baby mattresses are put in waterproof covers and there is said to be no cot death. (Why has our government not taken this on board?).

There is the London Hazards Centre (www.lhc.org.uk) which can be quite informative on specific issues regarding chemicals.

Issues that are hopefully more under our control include private swimming pools. Avoid the copper-containing **algaecides** and be somewhat sparing with the **chlorine** – consistent with keeping the water bug-free.

I would be wary, for the moment, of **'low energy compact fluorescent' light bulbs (CFLs)**. In 2008 the Health Protection Agency warned that the flickering nature of the light they emit could cause migranes, epilepsy and rashes as well lupus. More recently German scientists have warned that the bulbs should not be left on for extended periods as they emit poisonous materials, including phenol, naphthalene and styrene. It is also well known that they contain mercury. LED light bulbs are a much safer option.

Environmentally friendly household products, using organic ingredients, such as cleaners, washing-up liquid and tablets, washing powders and liquids etc are widely available, for example Ecover, Sonett etc. Other products can cause allergies. This is often skin irritation (hellish, but not life-threatening), but in some cases the products can cause asthma (which can be).

Scraping off old paint – particularly that painted on in the 1960s or earlier – can produce **lead** dust, so it is best to cover up with overalls and wear rubber gloves and a face mask. Otherwise we can breathe in quite a lot of the dust or absorb it through the skin – and it can take us months (working with hair charts and supplements) to get it down again!

If you are an artist and you use lead-based paint, **then do not lick your brushes**. This fills you with lead and can give you cancer of the tongue and throat. It can also cause miscarriage, premature birth, stillbirth and birth defects. If you are pregnant it also causes fetal malformation or death.

Solvents such as **benzaldehyde** can act as central nervous system depressants and cause generalised malaise and allergy as well as allergic irritation. **Butyl cellosolve** can cause headaches, nausea, liver and kidney damage and birth defects. **Ethanol** in other solvents can cause irritation of the eyes, throat and airways, and inhaling it could lead to lack of coordination and stupor. **Ethylene glycol monobutyl ether acetate** can damage internal organs and nerves through the skin, while **hydroxyanisole** is a skin and eye irritant and can cause cancer.

Toluene, used to remove wallpaper, can cause birth defects such as deformed ribs, which can prevent the baby from breathing properly, and cancer as well as the more usual allergic reactions.

From all of this, I am sure you have gathered that the preconceptual period and pregnancy are not very good times for DIY and home decoration! This is very inconvenient, as I know so many of you move house at about this time and set about decorating in a big way. But as you see, you have to pick your way, and be very, very careful what you use, as so much of what is out there can be hazardous.

Safe paints and a good range of colours are available from: Ecos Organic Paints, (www.ecosorganicpaints.co.uk / mail@ecospaints.com / 01524 852371). If you ring them, they will send a colour card straight away. You can also ask for small test pots which is useful to ensure the right colour choice. You will get the paint within two or three days and as far as I know, at the time of going to press, these are the only truly non-toxic paints available.

If you are doing anything other than just painting, check everything you use with Foresight's little booklet *WATCH IT*, and if in doubt, consult the London Hazards Centre.

Water pipes are covered in Chapter 3.

Other Hazards

Nappies: There are substances such as bleach, in the paper of disposable nappies, that can shrink the genitalia of little boys, so our Hero is not going to thank you for using those. Even if the makers managed to get round that one, there would still be the growing problem of mountains of undisposed-of 'disposables'. One toxic problem for future generations to deal with which they will put down to lack of foresight. They say there is **already** a huge floating island of plastic waste out in the Atlantic Ocean. So it looks as though the time has come to go back to good old terry towelling. I used to put it on like a kilt for the first few weeks, while their legs were so very tiny.

I expect I will be executed, hung, drawn and chopped into pieces if I mention the potty? But, I will. In my day we used to sit them on the potty a few minutes after their feed – they do a wee then. Then they are put into a dry nappy that stays dry for a little longer. You do not expect them to be dry in between feeds, of course, or get ambitious about 'potty training'. However, many of them will wee every time they are put on the potty, and some of them, if encouraged, will poo into a potty most of the time, and I don't care what the experts tell you, it saves quite a lot of work and I think the babies are far more comfortable and less likely to get sore. But obviously they wee in between times, and obviously they poo when they want to. I suppose the potty phobia of some 'experts' is due to some baby being maltreated by an idiotic parent who expected too much.

Some **soap products** etc. can give babies rashes. Nappies that are just wet, I would simply wash in very hot water and then hang them outside, location and weather permitting. On the whole, babies do not need lotions and powders etc. – just being washed with clean warm water will do.

If, however, very obvious **nappy rash** appears:

- Use a cream called Morhulin ointment, made with fish oils. It smells a bit fishy, but does the trick. Of course other organic nappy balms are widely available too.

- Think about what you ate if you are breastfeeding eg sugar, citrus, wheat etc? Work out what it is your baby is not tolerating.

- If your baby is also 'eating' by now, what was it he/she ate? Keep a food diary if you need to, and it will soon become clear what is causing the upset.

Very obvious 'people-pollutants' in adults are **mercury dental amalgams** and/or fluoride. Mercury amalgam fillings should now be a thing of the past. See Chapter 3 and the entry on the Association of Mercury Free Dentistry in the Useful Addresses Section.

Some areas are now putting **fluoride** in the water again. This is despite much opposition, since it has been found to cause upset stomachs, headaches and flu-like symptoms, also an increase in ovarian and women's cancers generally. One study in Florida found a fourfold increase in the birth of Down's syndrome babies which reverted to the normal rate per year after the addition of fluoride to the water was discontinued.

If your water board is adding fluoride to your water, I would:

- Discontinue using toothpaste with fluoride in it.
- Drink bottled water.
- Have very quick showers rather than luxuriating in a bathtub, as it can be absorbed through the skin.
- Take plenty of selenium and vitamin E as these fight fluoride.
- Discuss this with your water board. They expect you to pay them money for what they are supplying so you should have your say. Introduce them to the National Pure Water Association and ask them to discuss the issue/arrange a meeting/take them the NPWA literature. Do what you can.

Ask your dentist if the white fillings you are having instead of amalgam ones are free from fluoride? Otherwise you are going 'out of the frying pan into the fire'. Do not have a permanent source of fluoride put into your mouth. Many dentists are a bit in love with fluoride as they get a lot of propaganda directed their way. Take him/her the NPWA literature also. Remember, your mouth is your own.

AIMS, the Association for Improvements in the Maternity Services, has once again done some valuable research and has linked the giving of painkilling drugs in childbirth with the child later going in for street drugs at adolescence. While we are going to all this trouble to smooth the baby's path all through pregnancy, it seems a pity to put a stumbling block in the way the day your baby enters this world. It has been 50 years since I last gave birth, but I still have a pretty clear recollection of the whole event! Well, you lie there thinking, 'Could there not have been another way of doing this?' However, today, there are water births, reflexology, acupuncture and I am sure that homoeopathy has something up its sleeve. People tell me of home births where they were walking about until the last half hour and of warm hot water bottles, fore and aft...Generally, I would say, it all seems to be much more human and friendly than it used to be – and anyway, remember that it only goes on for so long. If you possibly can manage to keep your children drug-free you will probably have a much easier ride when they are teenagers, and believe me, that will be worth it (although I do understand that may not be precisely what is on your mind as you go into the second stage of labour!).

I remember Beverley Beech (director of AIMS) telling us about Queen Victoria being the first person to beg her physician to find something to make childbirth easier. You cannot really blame her as she had to give birth in full view of the Prime Minister of the time, and others, so it was a particularly stressful situation. But it is interesting that Edward VII was so louche and uncontrolled, so unlike his parents in every way. Despite all they did, they could not make any headway with him. Their anguish over his behaviour was probably a factor that contributed to his father's very early death.

See the website for the Independent Midwives (www.sagefemme.co.uk / 7 Lynworth Road, London N2 9LR 02078 732327). I would be sure to contact them for a chat when you are making up your minds what best to do about the birth. We have to factor in the prevalence of MRSA, C. difficile and so on in the hospitals while making the decision. If you decide on a hospital birth however, see Ainsworths the homeopaths for the possible infections. This can be an effective way of coping with the hazards.

The last of the major health hazards, one might say the biggest of the bugbears, is **vaccination and immunisation**. Once again I will refer you on to those who have made a lifetime study of this, and your decisions are your own. However, as it is pushed in some quarters as though the babies' lives depended on it, I will just point out where you can obtain a more balanced perspective:

- There is a very informative website: **vaccineinfo4parents.org.uk** with information from 14 doctors in books and 17 Informative papers.
- Get the book Behavioural Problems in Childhood: The Link to Vaccination by Dr Viera Scheibner and her video and check out her website: www.vierascheibner.com.

- See also The Vaccination Bible by Lynne McTaggart, editor of What Doctors Don't Tell You. The magazine What Doctors Don't Tell You has up to date information
- You can also get in touch with Magda Taylor, of The Informed Parent, PO Box 4481, Worthing, West Sussex, BN11 2WH, Tel: 01903 212969, www.informedparent.co.uk. She is a huge source of relevant information.
- There is also an organisation called JABS, Tel. 01942 713565, www.jabs.org.uk. They have formed to get compensation for victims' families.
- See also the booklist at the back of this book

If you know anybody with an autistic child, I would ask if you can spend a day with them. See at first hand exactly what the issues are. First hand is always the best way to understand any problems. Few of those who wholeheartedly advocate vaccination will have ever spent a day with an autistic child – let alone been in charge of him or her.

I would also contact a good homoeopath. Foresight can help with this. Things that they can do to help:

- Give separate homoeopathic dilutions of measles, mumps and rubella that will prevent the illness from being severe, as the body will have been primed to deal with it.
- Once the child has caught the infection, they can give homoeopathic dilutions which will mean it is not severe and is over quite soon.

Vitamins and minerals will also help.

The Department of Health has assured me that GP practices will be 'disciplined' if they threaten to strike families off their register for not letting their children be given a vaccine. So be sure to tell the DofH if you are threatened. If possible let your husband ring them as officialdom is usually more impressed by a male voice – this is galling but true!

Over 2,000 families know their child became autistic after the MMR jab. This is presumably 4,000 parents and approximately 8,000 grandparents. This makes around 12,000 people. Are they **all** likely to be wrong? In the USA, the connection between the

MMR jab and autism has at last been acknowledged. I expect the UK will be the last to get the message, as always.

As well as behavioural problems, Dr Scheibner has also linked vaccination to cot death. In Japan, they gave up vaccinating children under two years old, and cot deaths virtually disappeared! Why should we ignore all this evidence? How dare the government tell us to do so? There are now 17 papers on the web telling the truth. We all need to read these and take the information in. (vaccineinfo4parents.org.uk)

You get the general gist. We do not wish you to get too neurotic and jump at every shadow, but the modern world is not foeto-friendly or baby-friendly. However, we can make it much more so, without having to go completely bananas or to break the bank. Just concentrate on your own home and make it a place your body can truly relax in and feel safe. Make your own decisions on what goes on – for you and your baby.

Every little you can manage to get sorted out helps your own family, your long-suffering tax-paying country, the local wildlife and the rest of the world. Everything you do makes you and your family that significant little bit fitter. Feel joyful about this. Then what everybody else pollutes you with will not get to you so much!

I hope you have enjoyed reading this and I hope it has inspired you. I hope you and your friends can get together and take it all forward.

Onwards!

Information from the Soil Association

New types of 'Scientific' Pollution!

Genetic Modification

Do not be fooled by government statements. They cannot be trusted to give you the truth!

What is GM?

Genetic modification involves taking a gene from one organism (plant, animal, fungus, micro-organism) and inserting it into the genetic material of another. There are five main types:

1. Plant ↔ plant
2. Plant ↔ animal/micro-organism
3. Animal ↔ animal
4. Micro-organism ↔ animal
5. Micro-organism ↔ micro-organism

GM foods come from plants and animals whose DNA has been altered through the addition of genes from other organisms.

How to protect yourself and your family from GM:

- Grow as much of your own food ORGANICALLY as possible, and buy only organic.
- Write to your MP and MEP if you do not want GM food, particularly UNLABELLED GM food, in this country.
- Support groups fighting GM on your behalf, like ISIS and the Soil Association.
- Look for the Soil Association logo on organic food when you buy it.

The argument and evidence against GM:

It has become increasingly evident that GM technology is inherently hazardous and unreliable both in agriculture and in medicine. Mae Wan Ho on Institute i-sis.org.uk

So claims an eminent scientist, whose career spans over 30 years with many years of research in the field of molecular genetics, as well as biochemistry, evolution and biophysics.

If the kind of detrimental effects seen in animals fed GM food were observed in a clinical setting, the use of the product would have been halted and further research instigated to determine the cause and find possible solutions. However, what we find repeatedly in the case of GM food is that both governments and industry plough on ahead with the development, endorsement, and marketing of GM foods despite the warnings of potential ill health from animal feeding studies, as if nothing has happened. This is to the point where government and industry even seem to ignore the results of their own research! There is clearly a need more than ever before for independent research into the potential ill effects of GM food industry, most importantly with animal and human feeding trials.

Press Release from the Soil Association – 16th November 2007

(We are so grateful for their permission to reproduce this in this book.)

Nearly all the milk, dairy products and pork in UK supermarkets are being produced from animals fed on GM crops, and none of this is labelled, according to a Soil Association investigation. Tests of animal feed and a survey of company policies have revealed that all the supermarkets are widely allowing the use of GM feed. The report found that around 60% of the maize and 30% of the soya fed to dairy cattle and pigs is GM. **[1]** Most consumers are unwittingly eating food produced from GM crops everyday.

Supermarkets have been trumpeting their non-GM food policies, having removed all of their own-label foods made **directly** with GM ingredients by October 2002 in response to consumer concerns. However, unknown to most of the public, supermarkets did **not** prohibit the use of GM animal feed. Because of a legal loophole, there is no requirement to label food produced from GM-fed animals so shoppers will find it hard to avoid food produced from these. **[2]**

Currently, the only food standard that guarantees the non-use of GM feed is organic. The basic food industry mark, the 'Little Red Tractor', allows the use of GM feed. Even ethical labels like

'Freedom foods' allow animals to be fed GM crops. For non-organic food, Marks & Spencer offers the only refuge in offering all its milk and fresh meat from non-GM feed, but it does allow GM feed for its frozen and processed foods. All meat and dairy foods can and should be produced from non-GM feed. Unlike the dairy and pig sectors, the poultry sector has widely adopted non-GM feed policies, though around a third of eggs are from GM-fed hens. **[3]**

This GM stealth invasion of the UK food-chain is denying consumers their right to make fully informed choices. For years, the Food Standards Agency has been assuring consumers they would not be exposed to GM material by eating meat and dairy products from GM-fed animals. Scientific studies **have now found** small amounts of GM DNA in milk and animal tissues from GM-fed livestock. **[4]** And studies on GM-fed livestock are finding horrendous effects, including **lesions on the gut, toxic effects in body organs, unexplained deaths and stunted growth in their offspring. [5]** This raises concerns about the long-term health impacts on humans consuming products from GM-fed animals.

Patrick Holden, Soil Association director said: 'This amounts to deception on a large-scale. This is not just accidental contamination, hundreds of thousands of tonnes of GM grain are being used to produce our food each year. Biotechnology companies have clearly used imported animal feed as a Trojan Horse to introduce GM into the UK food chain, despite the fact that the British public have voted overwhelmingly against GM.

'The research on the presence of GM DNA in food from GM-fed animals and the impacts on animals is alarming. **We urge the public to only buy meat and dairy that are known to be produced from non-GM fed animals, and to write to the supermarkets and ask them to stop allowing the use of GM feed**. While it is excellent that Marks & Spencer and the poultry industry have restricted GM feed already, all retailers and food sectors should follow their lead. We also call on the supermarkets to label these products so they are being honest with their customers.'

A key concern is that future supplies of non-GM feed will be threatened unless there is wide-spread consumer awareness on this issue and pressure on the food industry to ensure that meat and dairy products come from livestock raised on non-GM feed. **[6]**

In the past, supermarkets have resisted direct demands for the use of non-GM feed, citing inadequate supplies of non-GM soya or excessive costs for farmers. **The Soil Association has established that supplies are abundant and can expand to fit demand.** The retail cost is minimal and should be paid for by the retailers, not farmers. The example of the poultry sector shows it can be done. **[7]**

Although food from GM-fed animals does not have to be labelled, animal feed **does** have to be labelled if it contains GM ingredients. Most feed (75%) is now labelled as 'GM', however, our survey found that most farmers (59%) did not know if their feed was GM. Soil Association tests also revealed a high level of breaches of the EU labelling laws – nearly 20% of feed contained GM soya above the 0.9% labelling threshold but bore no GM label. **[8]** The FSA are responsible for enforcing the legislation but are **not conducting any tests to do so.**

References:

[1] Silent Invasion – the hidden use of GM animal feed in the UK, Soil Association, November 2007. Full report available on request from The Soil Association.

The Soil Association tested 37 feed samples from dairy, pig and poultry farmers and surveyed supermarket and feed company sourcing policies. 73% of the feeds tested contained GM soya, with 27% containing soya that was over 70% GM. The company information showed that GM maize (used in the refined form, maize gluten, and so hard to identify in tests) is also widely used. The dairy sector is worst: in the tests, 51% of the soya was GM and it is widely using maize estimated to be around 60% GM. The pig sector is also a concern: the soya was 20% GM and soya makes up a larger proportion of the feed.

Based on our findings, we estimate that around 400,000 tonnes (290,000t of GM maize gluten and 146,000t of GM soya) are imported each year to produce manufactured feed for the dairy, pig and poultry sectors (out of a total of 467,000t of maize gluten and 1,123,000t of soya used in manufactured feed for these sectors). Note, the total amount of imported soya and maize gluten that **contains** GM is far higher. If imported grain used for 'home-mixing' of feed by farmers and the small amounts used for fattening beef and sheep (but not wholly grass-fed animals) are included, the total GM feed used would be higher.

[2] The Soil Association is calling on the Government and European Commission to introduce a legal requirement for GM labelling for foods produced from GM-fed animals. This is supported by the public:

An NOP survey in 2006 found that 87% of the UK public believe food from GM-fed animals should be labelled (up from a finding of 79% by the National Consumer Council in 2001).

A Europe-wide petition for such labelling collected a million signatures by February 2007.

NOP poll of 1000 UK adults carried out 9–11 June 2006 and weighted to be nationally representative.

'One million EU citizens call for labelling of GM foods', by Helena Spongenberg, 5 February 2007, EU Observer.

[3] In 2008, the only general sources of meat and dairy foods from non-GM-fed animals are:

For milk and pork: Marks & Spencer provides the only major source of non-organic milk and fresh pork produced from non-GM fed animals. In all other supermarkets, milk and pork is produced from GM-fed animals, *apart from organic food* and Sainsbury's 'Farm Promise' milk available in some stores.

For chicken: the British poultry industry is the one sector to have mostly excluded GM feed. Apart from Iceland, own-label fresh chicken and turkey in the major supermarkets and Lloyd Maunder poultrymeat is all produced from non-GM feed. However, frozen chicken, processed chicken products (e.g. chicken nuggets), chicken served in restaurants and take-aways are often not British but supplied by importers, and probably from GM fed animals.

For eggs: own-label eggs in the major supermarkets are produced with non-GM feed, except for Iceland. **All organic eggs** and the following egg brands are produced with non-GM feed: 'Woodland', 'Corn Gold', 'Columbus omega-3 rich', and 'Church and Manor' duck eggs. Nearly all 'free range' and 'barn' eggs are produced from GM feed. And there is no requirement for Lion Quality Eggs or 'free range' eggs to be produced from non-GM feed. This means non-organic eggs sold by independent retailers, including some 'free range' eggs, may, unless labelled otherwise, be from GM-fed chickens. About half of caged eggs, including probably most used in processing and catering, are produced with GM feed.

For frozen and processed meat and dairy foods: organic is the only general option for products such as yoghurt, cheese, cream, butter, ice cream, frozen meat, bacon, ham, sausages, meat pies, corned beef and ready meals.

M&S is well ahead of the other supermarkets. However, the Co-op, Sainsbury's and Waitrose offer a few non-organic meat and/or dairy items produced from non-GM feed, besides their own-label fresh chicken, turkey, eggs and farmed fish. Iceland offers no non-organic products from non-GM fed animals.

[4] Until 2005, studies which tried to detect GM DNA in milk, eggs and tissues from GM-fed animals had only detected *non-GM* DNA from the crops, indicating that GM DNA was also probably present in low quantities even if it had not been detected (Chowdhury *et al*, 2004; Phipps *et al*, 2003; Einspanier *et al*, 2001). On this basis, although it was not strictly supported by the science, the FSA and biotechnology industry claimed consumers would not be exposed to GM material by eating food from GM-fed animals. Now, however, TAKE NOTE: **four studies by different scientific teams have detected GM DNA in milk and pig and sheep tissues** from GM-fed animals (Sharma *et al*, 2006; Agodi *et al*, 2006, Mazza *et al*, 2005; reports by Ralf Einspanier, 20 October and 20 December 2000).

[5] The Soil Association report includes a review of GM feeding trials (12 animal and 1 human) that found **negative health effects** (all controlled against non-GM crops). Their report also describes

some of the ways in which these findings were dismissed by the FSA / European Food Safety Authority and the biotechnology companies, and lists eleven scientific reasons why genetic engineering changes the biology of plants, posing risks to health.

1. Russian rat trial of GM soya: very high mortality and stunted growth in the offspring (Ermakova, 2005)

2. Italian mice trial of GM soya: metabolic effects on body organs (Malatesta *et al*, 2002 and 2003; Vecchio *et al*, 2004)

3. FSA-commissioned human trial of GM soya by Newcastle University: GM DNA transfers out of food into the body's gut bacteria (Netherwood *et al*, 2004)

4. Monsanto rat trial of GM maize: changes in body organs indicating toxic effects (report by Monsanto, 2002; review by Dr Pusztai, 2004; Séralini *et al*, 2007)

5. Aventis chicken trial of GM maize: mortality doubled and significant change in composition of meat (reports for the Chardon LL hearing, 2002; review in 'Food safety – contaminants and toxins', CABI publishing, 2003)

6. Aventis rat trial of the novel protein of GM maize: reduced body weight and metabolic effects (same references as for Aventis chicken trial)

7. UK study on sheep: in a few minutes, the genes in the GM maize move into the bacteria in the mouth, changing their characteristics (Duggan *et al*, 2003)

8. Monsanto rat trials of GM oilseed rape: reduction in body weight and increased liver weight (significant as the liver is the organ of detoxification) (US FDA, 2002; Opinion of the Scientific Panel on Genetically Modified Organisms, 2004)

9. Australian mice trial of GM peas: allergic reactions, including inflammation of lungs (Prescott *et al*, 2005)

10. Calgene mice trials of GM tomatoes: gut lesions and 7 of 40 died within two weeks (review in 'Food safety – contaminants and toxins', CABI publishing, 2003)

11. UK Government-commissioned rat trial of GM potatoes by Rowett Research Institute: gut lesions (Ewen and Pusztai, 1999)

NB: These studies were all designed to identify health impacts; the animal trials often referred to by the biotechnology companies are largely **irrelevant** as proof of safety, being mostly studies carried out for commercial purposes on the efficacy of the feed, rather than 'toxicological' studies involving tissue analysis.

[6] Due to promotion by the biotechnology companies, the area of GM soya is rapidly expanding in Brazil, the main global supplier of non-GM soya. GM soya now accounts for 45–50% of the total, up from 20–25% in 2005. The market for certified non-GM feed must be secured to ensure the current non-GM area remains and that the industry segregates the GM and non-GM crops.

[7] **Based on calculations by the Royal College of Agriculture, the increase in costs of using non-GM feed at the retail end would be only 2–4p/kg for pork and bacon, and 0.4p/l for milk, if the non-GM soya premium is 7%.**

[8] Since 18 April 2004, according to EU legislation, feed containing GM material or derivatives of GM crops must be labelled as GM. Unfortunately this had been discontinued. The only exception is if the feed producer uses a non-GM source but some EU approved GM material up to 0.9% is later found to be present due to contamination. 19% of the feed samples we tested (seven of the 37 samples) had no GM label, yet contained GM soya over 0.9% threshold. Remarkably, the soya in five of these samples was over 80% GM. Worse, two were pure soya feeds made of 100% GM soya.

- Plant ↔ plant transfer between plant species
- Transfer between cross-kingdom gene transfer
- Transfer between plant – bacteria

'GM crops scrapped as mice made ill', Selina Mitchell and Leigh Dayton, The Australian, 18 November 2005

'Transgenic Expression of Bean α-Amylase Inhibitor in Peas Results in Altered Structure and Immunogenicity', Vanessa E. Prescott,

Peter M. Campbell, Andrew Moore, Joerg Mattes, Marc E. Rothenberg, Paul S. Foster, T. J. V. Higgins, and Simon P. Hogan

'Identification of a Brazil-Nut Allergen in Transgenic Soybeans', Julie A. Nordlee, MS, Steve L. Taylor, PhD, Jeffrey A. Townsend, BS, Laurie A. Thomas, BS, and Robert K. Bush, MD (http://content.nejm.org/cgi/content/full/334/11/688)

Pesticide Damage

From Occupational and Environmental Medicine, Vol 51, 693–699

Time to pregnancy and occupational exposure to pesticides in fruit growers in The Netherlands

J de Cock, K Westveer, D Heederik, E te Velde and R van Kooij

Department of Epidemiology and Public Health, Wageningen Agricultural University, The Netherlands.

Objectives: Although pesticides are regularly used in agriculture, relatively little is known about possible adverse health effects, especially reproductive effects, due to occupational exposure. This explorative study investigates the relation between exposure of the fruit grower to pesticides and fecundability (probability of pregnancy) in a population of fruit growers.

Methods: The analysis is based on self reported data and includes 91 pregnancies during 1978–1990 of 43 couples. Cox's proportional hazards model was used to analyse time to pregnancy after correction for gravidity and consultation with a physician for fertility problems.

Results and Conclusions: Application of pesticides solely by the owner was associated with a long time to pregnancy, resulting in a fecundability ratio of 0.46 (95% confidence interval (95% CI) 0.28–0.77). Similarly a low spraying velocity (< or = 1.5 hectares/h) resulted in a fecundability ratio of 0.47 (95% CI 0.29–0.76) and is associated with the use of older spraying techniques and tractors without a cabin. These factors were assumed to cause high exposure, which was confirmed by exposure measurements in the field. The effect of high exposure was mainly apparent if the couple had intended to become pregnant in the period from

March–November (fecundability ratio 0.42, 95% CI 0.20–0.92). This is the period in which pesticides are applied. Out of the spraying season the effect of a high exposure was absent (fecundability ratio 0.82, 95% CI 0.33–2.02). In the high exposure group 28% of the pregnancies had been preceded by consulting a physician because of fertility problems, compared with 8% in the low exposure group. **These findings indicate that an adverse effect of exposure to pesticides on fecundability is likely.**

 We are grateful to the Soil Association for allowing us to reproduce part of their recent literature on the whole subject of genetic modification in animal feed.

We need to be aware!

Onward!

CHAPTER 10

Talking to the 'powers-that-be' on what could be done to help

Must the citizen even for a moment, or in the least degree, resign his conscience to the legislation? Why has every man a conscience, then? I think that we should be men first, and subjects afterward. It is not desirable to cultivate a respect for the law, so much as for the right. The only obligation which I have a right to assume is to do at any time what I think right. Law never made men a whit more just; and, by means of their respect for it, even the well-disposed are daily made the agents of injustice.

Henry David Thoreau, 'Civil Disobedience', 1849

In the penultimate chapter I have decided to list all the steps I can think of that the Government could take that would make our lives easier, while we fight to get our country (and our planet) back to health and sanity – and thus back to fertility and normal family happiness.

1. **They could take more interest in promoting organic growing, and thus healthier soil and food:**

    -   By taxing agricultural chemicals such as artificial fertilisers and pesticides more heavily to discourage use.
    -   By giving much bigger subsidies to organic farmers and organic market gardeners.
    -   By seeing that all built-up areas have land set aside for allotments, especially where people are in high-rise apartment blocks.
    -   By encouraging future town planners to give each house enough garden to have a patch for vegetables, possibly a few fruit trees and/or space for a few hens.
    -   By banning outright genetically modified foods or animal feed, as many dangers and no benefits have been identified. The Soil Association will be able to help with

advice on avoiding bringing in GM foods, including animal foodstuffs. Dr Mae-Wan Ho is also a brilliant scientist in this area. This is extremely important. The portents are dire.

- By encouraging the growing of fruit and vegetables on school premises wherever possible. Learning about organic growing should become part of the curriculum.
- By encouraging, and if necessary funding, agricultural colleges to teach organic farming.
- By encouraging the growing of organic flowers for hospital and maternity greetings, as organophosphate contamination is not helpful in these circumstances.
- By presenting a prestigious award for the supermarket providing the highest percentage of organic food.

2. **The Government could promote a 'National Loaf' as in World War II**, with an approximately 85–90% extraction rate, fortified with powdered brewer's yeast. They could juggle with the recipe until they managed to approximate natural, organic whole-wheat.

3. **The Government should ban all the food additives known to cause health problems**, most of which are already banned in other European countries, Canada, Australia and so on. On this issue, they should recognise the fact that the 'research' they are shown is worthless. The way this is conducted, the 'experts' dose small rodents with huge, poisonous doses of a substance until half of them die. They then pronounce that one fiftieth of this dose is safe! **There is no evidence to support this**, and all the more informed health professionals know that with some people (especially children) even a homeopathic dose of a toxic substance can set up a reaction in the body.

Most people know by now that the reason these substances continue to be produced is because the same pharmaceutical companies that make them also make the medications that have to be taken to alleviate the illnesses that they cause. For example, they make tartrazine, known to cause hyperactivity, then they make the Ritalin. This way they manufacture the illness, and then the cure/masking medicine, and get paid handsomely for both! Those doing the suspect 'research' will also be involved in the pharmaceutical industry.

When politicians make decisions on these issues on behalf of the hapless sufferers and sufferers' parents, they need to remember that these parents are both taxpayers and voters. They are becoming more vigilant than they used to be.

It would not be too great a request for all the dangerous additives not to be used in food manufacture in 4 months' time (giving time to reform recipes), and all to be off the shelves in 12 months' time, with leniency over time scale to be withdrawn if there is resistance. The safe list (see *FIND OUT available from Foresight*) has every type of additive they need. Those alone can suffice.

4. **The Government needs to become equally informed regarding pesticides.** The organophosphate pesticides are still present on many of the foods we eat. Christopher Robbins in his book *Poisoned Harvest*, published in 1991, maintained that only 13% of the substances used at the time were really necessary. We gather that since this time pesticide use has dropped to 47%. Good. But there is another 34% to go!

Advice should be taken from the particularly successful organic farmers, from the Soil Association, Friends of the Earth, Garden Organic and the Good Gardeners' Association – and NOT from the manufacturers of the pesticides! The more that poisonous and nerve-damaging pesticides can be eliminated, the less 'mental illness', 'behavioural problems', epilepsy, multiple sclerosis, motor neuron disease, Alzheimer's etc. there will be. (The trace element manganese carries oxygen to the mitochondria of the brain cell. The organophosphate pesticides prevent the uptake of manganese from the gut into the blood, making the blood short of manganese, and so the cells short of oxygen – thus, over time, reducing the ability of the brain cells to function.)

5. **The Government should ensure all carpets, furnishing materials, pillows, duvets, mattresses etc are free from**

pesticides used for moth-proofing, and from fire-retardant and other chemicals. This is particularly important with cot and pram mattresses and bedding, also pen mats, children's car seats and pushchairs.

6. **The Government should prevent veterinary use of 'flea killer' drops** on the necks of cats and dogs. These are organophosphates and can give the pets epilepsy. Also they can affect children who cuddle and stroke them, as they get contaminated. The same applies with 'flea collars'. (A bath was how we used to get rid of fleas.)

   Reducing the use of pesticides should be discussed with PAN (Pesticides Action Network), the Soil Association, Friends of the Earth and Garden Organic, with a view to withdrawing time scale lenience unless cooperation from the manufacturers is forthcoming, in the same way as with additives.

7. **Cigarettes** should be labelled 'Smoking can reduce fertility and cause miscarriage, premature birth and malformation.' The ban on smoking in public places is excellent and should be retained despite opposition from tobacco addicts!

8. **Alcohol** should not be sold to pregnant women, as well as children. There should be notices in pubs, and in the liquor aisles in supermarkets, saying 'Alcohol can reduce fertility, cause miscarriage and damage the unborn child.' School children should be taught that alcohol causes depression, impedes mental functioning and can cause mental illness and violence. They need to know this.

9. **Pubs should close** at 11pm as formerly. Drinks such as alcopops should be made significantly more expensive. If they have been made containing colourings etc that are known to be addictive, these should be removed.
   Teenagers should be taught about alcoholism and foetal alcohol syndrome in school.

10. **Coffee** should be labelled: Research has revealed that drinking coffee can contribute to miscarriage. Pregnant

women are advised to avoid it. It will also cause crying and sleeplessness in the breastfeeding baby.

11. **Education on the effects of street drugs** on mental health, fertility and on the unborn child should be given in all secondary schools (www.talkingaboutcannabis.com).

12. **The use of medical drugs Seroxat and Prozac** should be reviewed in the light of the increase in deeper depression and suicide amongst users.

13. **The Department of Health should acknowledge the harmful effects of exogenous hormones**, both psychologically and physically – the contraceptive pill, stilbestrol, fertility drugs such as Clomid, and HRT. More publicity should be given to psychological consequences, and to thrombosis, heart disease, cancer risks etc, so women will be able to take control of their own destinies and not be used as money spinners for the drug companies. The pill should not be available on the internet.

14. **Natural family planning** (NFP) should be promoted as the method of choice at all schools and family planning centres and on the internet. It can be used with barriers in the fertile phase if preferred. All FPCs should publicise health problems associated with pill use, including later fertility problems directly due to the pill. Natural family planning (fertility awareness) should also be taught as part of biology in all secondary schools. Advice should be sought from Mrs Colleen Norman (www.fertilityet.org.uk).

15. **Genitourinary medicine needs to be given more publicity.** Clinics should be advertised widely. Notices, with easily remembered helpline phone numbers/website addresses should be put up in prominent places. The websites should list all the symptoms as well as effects on future fertility for both men and women, and the links to problems in pregnancy.

16. **Medical schools should be asked to give more attention to nutrition and illness caused by deficiencies, and to allergic illnesses, candida and intestinal parasites.** All these areas are

germane to most modern illnesses, but appear to be largely missing from basic medical training, and too few doctors specialise in them. The Government should set up a think tank composed of people from alternative medicine to advise them. They should **not** be intimidated by the outdated prejudices of the medics, which are largely fuelled by ignorance of the methods and the achievements of those working in the alternative field.

The antagonism is keeping a lot of very useful work from helping the large majority of the general public whose illnesses are caused by contemporary environmental hazards, not to mention by the side effects of the medical drugs themselves. Cooperation and exchange of information between the two groups should be encouraged.

17. **The NHS should set up its own laboratories for hair mineral analysis**, and to analyse water, dust and other environmental factors relevant to the intake of trace minerals and heavy metals. Training for health professionals in interpretation should be given!

18. **The Government should ban adding fluoride** to the water supplies. This has been discontinued all over Europe after the experiment failed. The contribution to stomach problems, depression, thyroid problems, osteoporosis, women's cancers and the increase in Down's syndrome babies should be recognised. Efforts should be made to find ways of chelating it out of people/children who start to show signs of dental fluorosis and other adverse reactions.

19. **Fluoride in toothpastes should be discontinued**, owing to the link to thyroid dysfunction.

20. **Fluoride being added to white filling material for teeth should be discontinued**, as it will be slowly released into the saliva for many years, and this could also affect thyroid function.

Massive amounts of research on the harm done by fluoride can be obtained from NPWA, the National Pure Water Association, and from the internet. It should be forbidden outright that any more of this endemic poison is put into our water supplies. (It is a waste product of the pesticide industry; once we reduce our use of pesticides, disposing of it will not be such a problem!) See also *The Case Against Fluoride* by Paul Connett, James Beck and HS Micklem.

21. **The Government should ban the use of mercury dental repair amalgams**, as they have been found to cause mental problems and infertility especially in dentists and dental nurses, their spouses and their children. This will also be the case with some patients. By now there are plenty of alternatives available. (More attention paid to diet will greatly reduce the number of cavities in any case!)

The Association for Mercury Free Dentistry should be the body to give official advice and should replace the BDA, who are stuck in a time warp. There are plenty of types of white filling available. However, these should be fluoride-free!

22. **Tuna fish should be tested for mercury contamination** before being tinned, or sold fresh.

23. **The Government should become aware of the contribution made by electromagnetic pollution to cancer, infertility and the malformation of babies** – also sleeplessness, leading to depression and mental illness. In Germany, mobile phone masts are sited away from dwellings, as are pylons. The UK should study the findings from other countries, and apply them, as soon as possible.

24. **DECT (cordless) telephones** need to be discontinued.

25. **Switching off street lighting at night** should be extended as widely as possible. Having no glaring street lights in the middle of the night would make urban dwellers' sleep patterns much more normal. Probably millions of prescriptions for sleeping pills could be saved. This would also help the environment, and save taxpayers' money.

It should be introduced thoughtfully, with people told well in advance, explaining all the advantages, but suggesting that people review their home lighting and security.

26. **The Government should upgrade the role of the surveyors' house surveys to include a geopathic survey.** This would involve Acousticom and other scanning for electromagnetic pollution from cracks in granite substrata and from underground rivers, as well as man-made hazards, such as pylons, mobile phone masts, electrical substations etc. Experts should be called in to give extra training in the use of the instruments.

27. **In semi-detached or terraced housing or blocks of flats, the intrusion of electromagnetism from adjoining dwellings should be investigated.** Instructions/grants for reinforcing the defence of a property with insulated wallpaper, carbon paints, silver mesh curtains etc. should be mandatory.

28. **Surveyors should also be required to test the water supply** of the house for lead and copper contamination, also aluminium. The two former are present in excess in the hair of approximately 10% of the couples who we see. This is usually from the tap water due to a corroding joint, where either a lead connecting pipe is joined to a copper one, or two copper pipes have been joined with a lead-containing solder. This will cause corrosion and contamination of the water, so it needs to be removed.

    Lead over 0.01 ppm or copper over 0.2 ppm should not be allowed. Corroding pipes should be replaced, possibly with ABS plastic (kite mark BS7291) if the water is acidic.

29. **The Government should make sure all water connecting pipes** from the mains to the boundary stopcocks of private properties **are no longer lead**. In some areas where the water is acidic, ABS plastic may be the material of choice for piping, rather than copper.

30. **Algaecide for swimming pools** should not be allowed to contain copper.

31. **The aluminium contamination of water** can be from aluminium gel used in the reservoir for collecting peaty particles. The effluent from this needs to be monitored more efficiently.

32. **The Government needs to ban the addition of aluminium** to deodorants. It can be absorbed into the body, and will ultimately affect brain function and be a contributory cause of Alzheimer's. We regularly find high levels of it in the head hair of those who use the deodorants, showing it is circulating in the blood. It will therefore reach the brain.

33. **The Government should forbid the use of aluminium in antacids.** It is a stomach irritant and is present to increase sales.

34. **The Government should ensure that if artists' paints contain lead, they should be labelled** as such. Alternatively, this could be banned.

35. **The Government should make a study of permanent hair dyes** regarding substances that have been found to cause bladder cancer in hairdressers. Hair dyes, which contain lead should be banned. Braids for use in making plaits in African hair need to be made free from lead and cadmium.

36. **The Government should forbid the addition of copper or aluminium to epilepsy medication** as it will increase the likelihood of fits. A biochemically trained body needs to be set up to monitor the formulae for medicaments to be sure they do not contain substances designed to perpetuate the condition they are prescribed for, and thus increase the sales of the drug. The NHS drug bill is said to be costing the taxpayers over £8 billion a year, so it is time all of this was investigated, and controlled.

37. **The giving of aspirin in pregnancy should be urgently reviewed** by an independent body. The links with maternal post-partum haemorrhage, HDNB (haemorrhagic disease of the newborn), and bleeding into the eyes and sub-dermal bleeding in the babies need studying, as do strokes in young mothers following labour. All of these problems seem to have come to light comparatively recently, and are receiving insufficient attention.

38. **The Vaccination Question needs to be studied again.** WDDTY (What Doctors Don't Tell You) have written *The Vaccination*

273

Bible. Dr Viera Scheibner has written *Behavioural Problems in Childhood: The Link to Vaccination.* There is a magazine, *The Informed Parent* that comes out monthly. There is also an organisation called JABS (Justice, Awareness and Basic Support for vaccine-damaged children). See also the website vaccineinfo4parents.

It is believed that in this country, 2,000 children every year become autistic after the MMR vaccine. This means that over 70 years, 140,000 children would be so afflicted. How would the country cope with this huge population needing constant care? How many of the so-called disaffected or difficult teenagers we have are 'sub-clinically autistic' but never diagnosed – although possibly sectioned or imprisoned at a later date? Dr Scheibner also believes the cascade of allergic illness – irritable bowel syndrome, eczema, asthma and epilepsy – followed the cascade of immunisations that started in the 1950s. Certainly, the timings are coincidental, and **no other explanation is so convincing**. If so, we are losing 2,000 children to autism, 2,000 children to asthma and approximately 400 to cot death every year. 2,000 lose their sanity, and 2,400 lose their lives, to save about seven deaths a year from measles? Is this intelligent? Deaths from measles would be much less likely, possibly non-existent, if treatment with nutrients and homeopathy were used.

Every MP making a decision on this should spend a day with an autistic child, and a day with a little mite screaming with itching eczema, and time with a tiny child fighting an asthma attack – made worse by the crying with terror that makes it even more severe. **Nobody should ever legislate about things they have never seen or experienced**, or even talked about with someone who has. Please see the list of suggested reading.

39. **The Government should be less dismissive of people running the voluntary organisations** and **charities for health problems**. We have our fingers on the pulse of the nation. We are in touch with all the groups who are suffering from

any number of disadvantages. We know the day-to-day problems and in many cases we know the causes.

Much of the suffering (which, quite apart from the personal angle, is disabling and very expensive to the nation) could be avoided altogether if we were listened to, and our recommendations acted upon. We are in many ways far more representative of the nation than are 'scientists' or other so-called 'experts', who are not necessarily honest, disinterested, experienced in the practical aspects of a problem, or well informed.

Most 'experts' are paid to have a certain point of view. 'Qualifications' do not necessarily mean that people are intelligent, independent or right. They are just powerful. Common sense coupled to years of experience of coping with the problem in 'real life' situations will provide more practical and effective solutions in most cases, and it would be a better idea to embrace these than the view of an 'expert' totally divorced from his subject. Please consider this viewpoint.

If government **cooperated** with the relevant voluntary organisations, they could tap into a wealth of concentrated, 'hands-on' experience for each particular problem. They have a huge untapped resource to draw upon. If they took advantage of this, **so much** could be achieved so quickly.

The volunteers have no axe to grind. They have a much more in-depth grasp of the problems in their specialised area than any other body.

The Government is using too much 'paper knowledge' and 'think-tank' reports – and having too little **conversation** with the experienced people on the ground.

If the Government seeks advice from the people who do research, the only answer they will ever get is: '**It needs more research**.' This is how these people make their livelihood. There will **never** be a conclusion as this would inhibit their income. Surely this is self-explanatory?

In many areas where the Government needs to take action, the problems are not hard to grasp. The research is all done and all out there, including on the internet. The Government needs to be more easy to communicate with and more executive. Please consider this and consult with us.

Thank you.

CHAPTER 11
Onwards!

So we are nearing the end of what has been quite a marathon for all of us – but I hope a joyful one. Let's just recap exactly what there is to do:

1. Optimise the diet

Build up the sperm and the ova with living nutrients so they are healthy and energetic in their union to create a new life! Eat fresh, raw, organic natural food, as near to straight out of the ground as you can manage! The old McCarrison Society mantra of 'Nothing added, nothing taken away' is a good rough guide. No GM. Avoid as many additives as you can manage. Use and flourish *FIND OUT* as you shop!

If, for example, in the supermarket, you find a product that could cause asthma, eczema, epilepsy or cancer, just have a conversation and **tell them so**! If several thousand of you introduce them to this book, who knows what we might achieve? **'The customers are saying…'** can be a powerful phrase to the hard-pressed rep whose mortgage depends on his commission. There are safe alternatives to all the unsafe additives. Change is possible – tell him this is just a wake-up call, not a death knell to his producers.

Anyway, most of what *you* choose will not have had any additives near it and if you are growing your own, a lot of it will have never seen a supermarket!

Leave the dead stuff in the tins and the packets on the shelves and bring home real food and cook it yourselves, with élan!

2. Hair mineral analysis

If you have not done so already, I would get this done ASAP. The benefits are twofold:

If the beneficial minerals are all well up where they are meant to be i.e. into the recommended range on your chart, then this eliminates a whole tranche of hazards – from physical and mental problems in the future baby, to exhaustion and depression in the mother, to lactation failure and early weaning, with all the misery of a screaming baby with colic and diarrhoea... The mother's body working as it should, will safeguard against it.

The other side of the coin is the elimination of the destructive substances aluminium, cadmium, mercury and lead, and the reduction of over-high copper. Getting rid of the body-burden of unwanted metals can similarly guard against disaster with the foetus and depression for the mother. The details about the problems caused by low trace minerals and high toxic metals are given in Chapter 3.

The better we can get the hair levels, and thus the levels throughout the body, the easier it will be to conceive, the smoother the course of the pregnancy and the breastfeeding and the healthier and more intelligent the future child will be. It is worth sticking with it.

3. Common social poisons

These include alcohol, tobacco, cannabis etc, caffeine, tranquillisers, anti-depressants, sleeping pills, over-the-counter medical drugs. Well, the more we get rid of the first four poisons, the less we need the rest of them! So it is more or less a puzzle with the solution built in.

Alcohol in relatively small quantities can enhance the fun of a social gathering, but an excess inevitably means for the next few days you are less organised, less even-tempered, and much less efficient! You will feel more put upon, and find other people more exasperating than at other times. Observe yourself more closely, and see if I am right! For these reasons alone it does not enhance job satisfaction or family life!

Tobacco is a similar story. Any substance that changes mood, either dramatically or marginally, will kick back proportionally in the opposite direction when the immediate effect wears off.

So, if something appears to 'relax' or 'enliven' you, you can be sure that the directly converse mood will appear in due course! This means you will crave the substance yet again, and the very worst scenario is that addiction can set in. Then gradually you could become a less worthwhile person at home and at work! Avoid it, or you could be an excellent money spinner for the alcohol or tobacco industry!

The tranquillisers, the sleeping pills, the anti-depressants (please put me into a better mood – please help me to find oblivion) are the inevitable follow-on to the 'social drugs' that produced the agitation, sleeplessness, misery and gloom in the first place.

It has to be said, however, that the person seeking the medication may not always be the one using the suspect substances! They may just be on the receiving end of the petulance, gloom and paranoia from a spouse, a relative, a colleague or an employer. Whatever the case, factor these issues into your decisions/reactions, and don't be the one driven to medication!

The effects of street drugs are more easily recognised, so they are more universally condemned. See Mary Brett's chapter regarding street drugs, and her report on the Foresight website. She is on our side!

Chocolate, coffee and tea all contain caffeine, but in small quantities these are not a major problem for most 'non-baby-making' people. However, caffeine, even in quite reasonable amounts, has been linked to miscarriage, so under present circumstances we suggest giving these things a miss in favour of drinks such as organic smoothies, fruit juices and water, and the occasional herb tea, Marmite, Bovril (beef or chicken – not too strong), milkshakes, vegetable juices (carrot or beetroot etc.), Rice Dream, Oatly, Provamel, Horlicks etc. Anything that is known to cause miscarriage will inevitably take its toll on the developing sperm and ova. You know what to do!

4. Contraception

Whatever happens, we want to get away from the pill, which has proved such a disaster for women's health, both physically (thrombosis, cancer, PMT) and mentally (masculinisation, lack of natural maternal instinct, lack of libido, frank mental illness, violence and suicides). It has also been linked to lowered zinc, and thus caused many malformations and hyperactivity, dyslexia, asthma, eczema and so on in the children. Time to throw it away!

So, in the interim, whilst you take time for all the health benefits to kick in (and for your organic vegetables to grow!), we suggest natural family planning (NFP). Find out exactly when you ovulate so that this knowledge can be harnessed. While you are cosseting and feeding up the relevant little ova and sperm, you can avoid unprotected intercourse for the crucial few days coming up to ovulation itself, and thus avoid a conception before you want it, or before your body is quite ready.

If, during the fertile stage, you decide to use barrier methods, I would use liquid honey rather than a spermicidal gel. It seems to work as well, is less likely to set up a reaction, it also has an anti-candida action which is always useful, and I do feel it must be nicer for the sperm! (By this stage we are all feeling quite maternal towards them, even the hundreds of millions who are just the supporting cast!). The easiest form of barrier, if you don't like condoms, is the diaphragm. They can provide and fit these at your local family planning clinic.

Once the mineral levels are optimised and, as far as we can manage, all traces of poisons gone from the body etc, then, as you will know the most propitious date to try, it will be all the easier, and hopefully quicker, to conceive once you are ready to do so!

Colleen Norman at the Fertility Trust, whom I have known for about 40 years, is absolutely ace at teaching NFP, so I suggest that your first point of contact is to visit her website: www.fertilityet.org.uk. Having learned the technique it will be useful for the rest of your life. It will mean you never have to go back to hazardous pills and devices. This will lessen your risk of cancer, depression, thrombosis, migraine, and also of any more infertility in the future.

5. Genitourinary infections

Get these checked out and sorted. If any are on board, these can cause a miscarriage or can prevent conception in the first place. No point in keeping them, as this will stimulate the immune system, and this will use up zinc, which is often in short supply. No problems, as the check-up can be obtained on the NHS, **free!**

To find out where your local GUM clinic is, you only have to ring your nearest big hospital and ask if they have a GUM clinic and, if so, to put you through to them. If not, ask where the nearest one is. They are also very easy to find using the internet.

The doctors in the GUM clinics are some of the nicest people I know, and are surprised by nothing!

If you have a positive result, one option is to take the antibiotic they give you (plus extra B-complex vitamins, an extra probiotic capsule and lots of yoghurt).

Alternatively, the homeopathic chemist Ainsworths at 36 New Cavendish Street, London, W1G 8UF will be able to let you have a remedy for almost any of them. Just ring them up on 020 7935 5330, tell them what you have, and you can pay by card and they will send it to you. All homeopathic remedies are very reasonably priced and completely safe. However, most homeopaths would say that you would be better off consulting one of them on your 'whole body state of health' – and having a 'constitutional remedy' also. Most homeopaths are very knowledgeable and careful and this is likely to be helpful in re-establishing your general health.

Recheck at the GUM clinic afterwards to make sure you are clear of the specific infection, before trying for a baby.

6. Allergies, malabsorption and parasites

Allergies are very common, and very easily solved in most cases, by manipulating the diet or making adjustments to the environment. It may just be as simple as some noxious food additive (study *FIND OUT*) or it may be very commonly eaten foods like grains or milk. Whatever the problem, see if you can puzzle it out and avoid it. Then, not only are you more likely to conceive, but also the baby will be much less likely to be born with allergies of his or her own. It will also usually mean a much pleasanter pregnancy with less sickness and fatigue.

Parasites are a major source of tummy cramps, itching anus, malabsorption, diarrhoea, bloating – all the things you really DO NOT WANT in pregnancy. If in doubt, find a local homeopath – Foresight can find you one – and check it out with a stool sample. He or she will arrange for this to be sent to a laboratory and they will be able to put a name to your problem. Again, as with GUI, your homeopath can give you a remedy, or Ainsworths may turn up trumps again, or a herbalist will know of some useful herbal products. Always recheck a few weeks after the treatment to make sure all is now sorted. Sometimes parasitic infestations appear to die down, and then a few weeks later the survivors have reproduced again. Seek advice on timing of medication, if so. Don't be embarrassed, lots of people have them! All parasites *can* be got rid of, and you will be amazed how much better and more energetic you feel once they are dealt with.

7. Electromagnetism

Again, this can be a vital element in success, although one where it is harder to judge what needs to be done, when and where. The hazards are growing – TETRA masts, mobile phones, DECT phones – and microwave ovens, we are told, can leak. Even vacuum cleaners, hairdryers and VDUs, although innocuous to the average adult, can become hazardous to the unborn and tiny babies.

There are ancient hazards known about in the Middle Ages, but comparatively recently brought to our attention again, such as underground rivers and cracks in the substrata – particularly granite substrata, that sends up rogue electricity... I am told that in the old days, people used to build their cottage 'where the cows lie down', as there 'the ground is peaceful'. Experience and research has taught us that where these hazards are found, they can have a bearing on miscarriage, malformations and illnesses such as leukaemia and other cancers. I therefore asked some very informed people to write some of the chapter on this subject for us. Study these, and if in doubt, I would call in one of Foresight's experts. If you have suffered more than one miscarriage, or if you have had the sadness of a damaged baby – especially if it was due to a chromosomal break (such as Down's, Edwards or Patau syndrome) – I would enlist this particular area of help without delay. You would be amazed at how much difference it can make.

Rob's story:

One of our North Country couples had been struggling for over a year, but the husband had a sperm count of only 15m. He was, however, resistant to the idea of a house check, until Roy was going up North anyway and so the rate would be cheaper! After the visit I heard from the wife that the chair her husband constantly sat on was directly over the edge of an underground river – the friction of the water against the rock always sends up an electrical charge in these cases. Roy can always pick this up – both by dowsing (at which he is brilliant) and with his instruments, which are very expensive and accurate!

After a few months the wife rang me: *'Guess what, Nim, Val (our redoubtable Branch Secretary) came over a few months ago. She asked Robert if he had moved his chair yet. "No," he replied. He doesn't go much for that sort of thing. "Well, come on now," she said, and caught hold of the chair. Rob had to go and help her, she's only a little bit of a thing. "Where will we put it, then?" asked Rob. "Over here," said Val. "There's a table there," Rob said. "Yes, well, we'll move the table, then; it's not going to cost you anything, Robert, you know," replied Val. So they moved the whole room around. A couple of months later he went for another sperm count, and would you believe it, there were 63m! It's like a miracle, isn't it? A mercifully cheap miracle, for once! God bless Val.*

Anovulation, as well as low sperm counts, can be due to electromagnetism. Sometimes just moving the bed or a much-used chair can work wonders with a woman's cycle or with the husband's sperm count. If you wake up in the mornings with a particular ache or pain always in the same place, this can be a reason.

For this reason also, remember to ask Roy to check the place where you are planning to put the cot. Babies are very sensitive to electromagnetism and it may be one of several contributing causes of cot death.

If you have seen Roy and had a positive finding, then you need to move the furniture as he suggested, and possibly replace a metal-sprung mattress. There are many well thought through solutions now available. You may or may not need (according to the findings) silver mesh net curtains, foil sandwich wallpaper, carbon-containing paint, metal-free mattresses, and so on. But it is all there for you if you do.

Remember not to carry a mobile phone while it is 'live' and not to have a cordless (DECT) phone at home. A mobile in the trouser pocket microwaves the testicles. Be aware!

8. New hazards, and new solutions

The answer is to keep one jump ahead of the game!

Hair dyes: Hair dyes turn out to be hazardous. They are absorbed through the scalp into the bloodstream, and have been linked to kidney damage and bladder cancer. The wash-in, wash-out ones, however, are said to be OK. These are obtainable from chemists/health stores/websites etc. Seek them out 'because you're worth it'!

Dental amalgams: Avoid any more mercury fillings, even if you are sticking with the ones you already have, for the time being. It appears that the jury is still out on whether removing the existing fillings – which can create a lot of mercury dust etc. – is the best thing to do. My feelings are that it is probably dependent on how much mercury is leaking from the existing filling and how experienced/conscientious the dentist who is removing them is!

We are lucky that an Association for Mercury Free Dentistry has been formed (www.mercuryfreedentistry.org.uk, The British Society for Mercury Free Dentistry, The Weathervane, 22a Moorend Park Road, Cheltenham, Glos, GL5 0JY, Tel: 01242 226918). These are the people to contact, for an expert opinion.

Cosmetics: Buy Foresight's little booklet *WATCH IT* and see what can lurk in cosmetics, household cleaners, furnishings, decorator's materials, and the like. It is a minefield but navigable and a little extra awareness pays off.

So, when we've made all this amazing effort – what are we going to see in the way of tangible results?

Well, hopefully, first and foremost a conception – the conception of a really beautiful baby with everything he/she needs to be perfectly formed, equipped with a good working brain and a strong immune system. We hope he/she will be conceived in most cases with a surge of living love (not a clattering of test-tubes) and the springing up of a happy and lively little soul!

Hopefully also his/her mum and dad will feel strong and blissfully happy and well able to cope. Above all, they will have a sense of humour about the ups and downs, something that seems abysmally lacking in the 'experts'! This will mean the baby will be reared by maternal instinct – demanding feeding and lots of lovely milk – and Mum will be well able to stand up to any officious advice that would have them separated, harassed by conflicting theories, or put on schedules that are not their own!

Mothers who have plenty of the particularly helpful nutrients (vitamins, omega-3s, zinc and manganese) bond well and lactate abundantly! Plenty of breast milk given when wanted, and no unnecessary crying, will mean much joy, and much less chance of eczema, asthma, hyperactivity etc. Good breast milk is made by good food, plenty of fresh water, and the sheer joy of love between mother and baby. It is not a medical matter – it is a natural happening. Every mouse in the skirting board, every fox in its lair, every rabbit in the burrow, every sow in the stye knows what to do, and (as long as hazards from their environment are not running them ragged) so do women.

If babies are left with their mothers and the mothers are allowed to handle them as they wish (and as the babies wish!), this will hugely reduce the amount of crying which will be a great relief to both mother and baby.

The baby will grow into a much calmer and happier child, which will make learning an easier process. It will make such a happy mother–baby relationship that leaving the baby to 'go out to work' would be an agonising choice, and perhaps fewer mothers would do so. This would make for a generation of much happier babies and children – and parents!

285

Although I worked in one, and adored the babies, my personal feeling is that nurseries are not natural places. Homes are. For life in general, it seems to me, the money angle has got blown out of all proportion. Higher house prices and rents means that 'a roof over our heads' is beginning to use up half our lives and all our family intimacy, fun and happiness.

Women were not meant to be computer-fodder. We are a different sex. A survey by the National Council of Women in 1994 found that 94% of working women with children felt 'stressed' and exhausted. Most would have preferred not to go out to work. It does not seem sensible or kind to ignore these findings. If you are one of the 94% you do not have to be browbeaten! Our babies need us. In many cases we don't have to leave them with strangers. Most of the strangers do not love them. There could never be enough extra-loving, extra-maternal strangers to go round, so that all children could be removed from their own mothers (who love them) and given to another woman who is not capable of replacing that love.

At best, the children will be occupied and amused with affection and without cruelty. At worst, if the staff are unsuitable, as is often the case, they will be lonely and bored and feeling rejected while miserably waiting for Mummy's return. Occasionally, we hear of abuse. What is the point of all this? Who gains in the long term? Not the mothers and not the babies.

Does it mean we are better off financially? As taxpayers, we have to pay for all the very expensive nurseries, nurses and supporting staff. We could do with this money to help us run our own homes. Why is it taken in ever-increasing taxes from the pockets of women to make them do something that 94% of them do not want to do?

Some august 'think tank' has just come up with the fact that the 'Sure Start' programme has cost billions and benefitted nobody. Whoever thought it would do otherwise?

Do not ever be bullied. Do your own thinking, your own nurturing and your own loving. It is **your** life and **your** child.

OK, I hear you say, it would be lovely to stay with the baby all day, but we need the money. Well, I do know the feeling, but there are possible nice little earners that can be done from home, in little snippets of flexitime, maybe while he/she has a nap?

Do you sew? Dressmaking, soft furnishings (but mind the pins) embroidery, knitting, crochet, lampshades?

Do you type? Could you take in typing, website design, and transcribing books? Better still, write your own stories? Think of JK Rowling! Cookbooks – think of Jamie or Nigella. Simpler stuff? Help hard pressed offices with mail outs?

Are you an outdoor type? How about growing organic fruit or veg, or flowers? Keeping hens if circumstances permit? Keeping bees? Thoughts of *River Cottage for Ever* and The *Good Life* seep into the mind...?

Are you artistic? Painting pictures, taking photos, making designs for book covers, greeting cards, wall papers, table mats, paper napkins? Dream it up!

Are you musical? Could you write music, pop songs, ballads, opera!?! I am told this is very difficult to break into, but, hey – who knows?

Have more innovative ideas for flexi-time home-working and send them into us for our website? We could start a page for it in the newsletter? You could lead the way! (It does not mean you have to be alone all day, you can form little groups, and the children will also make little friends...)

I have often wondered whether, when the children go to school, there could be flexible job sharing arrangements, such as a young-at-heart retiree working to fill in the school holidays? Possibly, in an ideal world, the one who had just retired from the job in question. Would she like to come back for about 14 weeks each year to augment her pension, while you take unpaid leave? Alternatively, could you find a student who would like to work off a bit of the student debt problem by working Monday to Friday through the school holidays at your job? Have a bit of 'work experience'? It all depends on the type of work, the expertise necessary, and the whole situation, but these are just ideas to toss around. An advert in the local paper might bring amazing results!

I know Foresight mums do wonderfully well and we get such heartening feedback about our Foresight children. As with plants that are properly fed, they blossom! We hear of their success-getting scholarships, playing in orchestras, playing in chess tournaments, being in teams, getting into their choice of university and so on... We can all do the world a very good turn, producing some outstanding people – we can also save the taxpayer (us) a vast fortune in SCBU time, special needs schools, hospital time, and later mental hospital time and prison time!

I suspect that as our glorious undamaged children grow to maturity, they will produce better music, poetry, fiction writing, plays, TV programmes, dancing, singing, furniture, clothes – whatever! – than we have at present, and some will be playing in orchestras (some are already). They will go in for beautiful architecture, gardens, parks and open spaces, maybe just window boxes, hanging baskets, courtyard allotments. Who knows, they may make Britain a flowering paradise!

Contact with the earth brings tremendous rewards. Tiny children are thrilled as 'their' seeds come up out of the soil and organic gardening makes it possible for them to get involved as they can handle the soil without fear of damage from chemicals.

Children also love pets and benefit from animals in the house where this is possible. With a mother based at home, a much more expanded home environment is possible. Domestic animals will also benefit from an organic environment with much less illness.

As human contamination of earth and water lessens, wildlife will also benefit. This is really important. At the moment sparrows and other little songbirds are disappearing rapidly. This may be partly because of pesticides and voided medicines, but it is also likely to be due to radiation from TETRA masts etc. The poisons and the electromagnetic pollution may be making the birds' eggs, if any, sterile. It may compromise the immune system in the bees.

We cannot do without bees. They pollinate everything. There will be no fruit, only some vegetables, no flowers. If we have no bees, *we* may also disappear, as food production will be very, very difficult. Any protest will be greeted with screams of 'You cannot stop progress!' followed a decade later with 'If only we had realised at the time.'

It has been said that the homing pigeons can no longer navigate by instinct, picking up on vibrations. It has been noticed that they are using sight and going by the road systems. This is a drastic adaptation they have had to make. Other birds may not be so resourceful or adaptable.

Maybe the birds can't manage this, or are finding it totally exhausting/depressing/terrifying. Is this progress? We need to reduce the use of pesticides to nil, and reduce our dependency on mobile phones etc. We also need to reduce the amount of medical drugs, exogenous hormones, alcohol, tobacco, effluent etc that we are urinating into the biosphere!

We do need to follow through on this one. If the songbirds all die, they will **never** come back. Apart from their beauty, we need them desperately to control the insect population. We could lose all our butterflies. How will future populations feel about us? They will say: 'They had a world full of beautiful birds, butterflies and flowers but they created mobile phones so they could chat to one another from the train!'

I remember in the 1970s when the pill first came out, all the men in London started growing huge bosoms. It was from the extra female hormones in the pill finding their way into the women's urine, and hence into the sewage and down to the water tables. This was a somewhat dramatic demonstration that, in the end, a whole population drinks what is in the rest of the population's urine! More and more people are being put on to medical substances. I read the other day that in studies of the cord blood of a sample of American babies, **287 different toxic chemicals were identified**. This means at least this number were in the mother's body. We need to wonder where they came from. Was it food additives, pesticides, medicines, fluoride, lead, mercury, aluminium, tobacco, alcohol, street drugs, disinfectants, hormones, insulin, thyroxin, statins, steroids, hormones, benzodiazepine, Prozac, Seroxat? How much is in the water now? Have we a right to inflict this on our own and each other's babies? On wildlife? On each other?

We need to take stock very quickly as we haven't got much time left to get it right! We need to love money a lot less, and people and animals a whole lot more.

It is becoming clear that we need to breed a generation very much brighter than the one we have at present! Foresight is working on that one, but we cannot leave it all to our babies alone – even if they are little geniuses! We/you, the Foresight parents, need to lead the way.

I am sure that when you have read all of this, you will have seen how limited and inadequate the 'Establishment's' approach to health matters is. They do not look at the whole jigsaw puzzle of life, and see how it all fits together. My MP cries out, 'No, no, I can only talk about one thing, we only have 15 minutes.' The doctor says, 'We cannot look at anything unless there has been a double-blind, randomised, controlled, cross-over trial.' This, of course, could not be done with babies (nor could trials with a lot of other conditions) and it means that only one factor could be isolated and studied – the results would therefore be 'inconclusive' as the problem stems from a series of interacting factors so nothing would be done.

Reforms such as the banning of noxious food additives, pesticides, fluoride, the pill, GM foods, vaccines and so on will probably not take place in the foreseeable future. To understand why, you have to look at the mindsets. The present-day MPs are very wedded to the 'bottom line'. Their background is mainly from small businesses – their own, or a friend's or relative's. They are imbued with the feelings of having to scoop up enough profit to stay in business, pay the mortgage, feed the family, and so on. They find it hard to take a view beyond this. Instinctively, they identify with manufacturers.

Britain needs more women who have brought up a family, more farming people, more organic growers, more alternative practitioners, going into Parliament – people with a wider perspective. If you are in a position of selecting a candidate for election, study their background very carefully. Habitual patterns of thought die hard. Meanwhile, we can all take charge of our own lives – eat good organic food, drink pure water, avoid all the drugs, bugs, plugs and fugs that we can, and do our bit for our own families. All the modern agonies – the alcoholism, the drug taking – are the result of brain malformation from the outset and lead people down the wrong path.

If preconceptual care were there for every baby, so that they did not suffer with foetal alcohol syndrome or foetal tobacco syndrome, that they were not zinc-deficient, nor gender-confused by extraneous hormones, nor polluted by heavy metals, nor ill with chlamydia, nor kept awake all night by electrosmog, and if they were then breastfed, and not vaccinated – well, we might have normal brain power all round and a virtually crime-free world! My late husband, who was the Deputy Director of Public Prosecutions at one time, used to say that the prison population was made up of 92% inadequates and perverts and about 8% master criminals who manipulated them.

If this is so, attention to preconceptual health could maybe rescue the 92%, and there might only be 8% of criminal masterminds to put behind bars! What a saving that would be! It would certainly more than cover the cost of free preconceptual care for everyone!

Talking of covering costs, I read in June 2008 that the numbers of drug addicts and alcoholics on benefits in the UK was 17,000 and that ex-cannabis smokers suffering from psychosis had topped 148,000. (Many of these could respond to Foresight's stop-alcohol programme – supplements, oils, homeopathy and allergy workouts).

The number of claimants with back pain is said to be 123,000. People suffering from back pain usually need osteopathy, along with zinc and manganese to prevent the cartilage in the discs from swelling, and magnesium and selenium to strengthen the muscles.

The number of children born deaf has trebled in the last ten years. This is tragic, and is almost certainly due to lack of vitamin A before birth – due to the mistake by the Department of Health in advising mothers not to take any.

Learning difficulties are due to all the factors we have mentioned elsewhere, and these also have risen in the last ten years from 182,000 sufferers to 282,000. We were not told how many are disabled by epilepsy, MS, ME, arthritis etc but it rises yearly.

Many more people struggle to work with diabetes, migraine, asthma, skin problems, IBS, etc. There are nutritional solutions but most of this could have been fully pre-empted by a pristine pregnancy and a good beginning.

So let's turn things around for the next generation and let's get all the information on the web, so that even those who have these problems but are *not* planning a pregnancy can also have a crack at getting well again.

In this book I have tried to tell you all, after a lifetime of working on all of this, how I think and feel, and what I know. I want you all to take up the baton and run – you and your children are the Custodians of the Future. It is all quite simple, really: let your body be healthy, let your God-given instincts guide you. Have a welcoming womb inside a healthy body, inside a happy home, within a wonderful world.

Much happiness, love and courage to you all. May your God go with you, and may you go with your God.

Onwards!

Love

Nim

APPENDIX 1
Useful Addresses

Active Birth Movement, The Active Birth Centre, 25 Bickerton Road, London, N19 5JT. Telephone: 0207 281 6760 www.activebirthcentre.com

AIMS, Association for the Improvement of Maternity Services, 5 Anne's Court, Grove Road, Surbiton, Surrey, KT6 4BE. Telephone: 08707 651453 www.aims.co.uk

Ainsworths Homeopathic Chemists, 36 New Cavendish Street, London, W1M 7LH. Telephone: 0207 935 5330 www.ainsworths.com

Angus Horticultural (Rock Dust), Polmood, Guthrie, By Forfar, DD8 2TW. Telephone: 01241 829049 www.angus-horticulture.co.uk

ARM, Association of Radical Midwives, 16 Wytham Street, Oxford, Oxon, OX1 4SU. Telephone: 01865 248159 www.midwifery.org.uk

Association for Breastfeeding Mothers, PO Box 207, Bridgwater, Somerset, TA6 7YT. Telephone: 08444 122949. www.abm.me.uk

Biodynamic Agricultural Association, Painswick Inn Project, Gloucester Street, Stroud, Gloucestershire, GL5 1QG. Telephone: 01453 759501 www.biodynamic.org.uk

Biolab Medical Unit, The Stone House, 9 Weymouth Street, London, W1W 6DB. Telephone: 0207 636 5959 www.biolab.co.uk

Breastfeeding Helpline, National, The Breastfeeding Network, PO Box 11126, Paisley, PA2 8YB, Telephone: 0300 100 0212, www.nationalbreastfeedinghelpline.org.uk

Brett, Mary, 6 Pines close, Amersham, Bucks, HP6 5QW. Telephone: 01494 726958

British College of Osteopathy and Naturopathy, 6 Nethershall Gardens, London, SW3 5RP, Telephone: 0207 435 7830 www.bcom.ac.uk

British Homeopathic Association, Hahnemann House, 29 Park Street West, Luton, Bedfordshire, LU1 3BE, Telephone: 08704 443950 www.trusthomeopathy.org

British Society of Dowsers 4–5 Cygnet Centre, Worcester Road, Honley Swan, Worcester, WR8 0EA, Telephone: 0684 576969 www.britishdowsers.org.uk

Penny Brohn Cancer Help Centre, Chapel Pill Lane, Pill, Bristol, BS20 0HH. Telephone: 01275 370100 www.pennybrohncancercare.org

Cerebra Centre for Brain Injured Children, Second floor Offices, The Lyric building, King Street, Carmarthen, Dyfed. Telephone: 01267 244200 www.cerebra.org.uk

Coeliac Society, 3rd Floor, Apollo Centre, Desborough Road, High Wycombe, Bucks, HP11 2QW, Telephone: 0845 305 2060 www.coeliac.org.uk

Compassion in World Farming, River Court, Mill Lane, Godalming, Surrey, GU7 1EZ. Telephone: 01483 521950 www.ciwf.org

Compost, The Compost Centre, Organic compost delivered in SE England. Priest Lane, West End, Woking, Surrey, GU24 9NA. Telephone: 01483 472423 www.thecompostcentre.co.uk

Cryshame (Vaccine damage), Wilton House, Southbank Road, Kenilworth, Warwickshire, CV8 1LA. www.cryshame.co.uk

Dental Nurses with Mercury Damage, Mrs Rebecca Dutton, Mistletoe Barn, Smithfield Road, Bearley, Stratford-on-Avon, CV37 0EX. Telephone: 01789 730330 www.mercurymadness.org

Down's Syndrome Association, The Langdon Down's Centre, 2a Langdon Park, Toddington, Middlesex, TW11 9PS, Telephone: 08452 300362 www.downs-syndrome.org.uk

Eco Paints, Unit 34, Heysham Business Park, Middleton Road, Heysham, Lancs, LA3 3PP. Telephone: 01524 852371 www.ecospaints.com

Ecover, 154 Main Street, New Greenham Park, Newbury, Berks, RG19 6HM, Telephone: 0845 130 2230 www.ecover.com

Endometriosis Society, (Dian Shepperson Mills, MA), 56 London Road, Hailsham, East Sussex, BN27 3DD, Telephone: 01323 846888 www.endometriosis.co.uk

Ecology Building Society, 7 Belton Road, Silsden, Keighley, West Yorkshire, BD20 0EE, Telephone: 0845 674 5566 www.ecology.co.uk

Electro Sensitivity. UK, BM Box ES-UK, London, WC1N 3XX, Telephone: 0845 643 9748 www.es-uk.info

Ewe-too Spinners, Organic Wool, Silver Street, Hordle, Hants, SO41 0FN, Telephone: 01425 616203

Fertility Thermometers, Burkton-Dickenson, Omiss, Ontario, L5J 2M8, Canada.

Flint, Professor Caroline, Midwifery Services, 34 Elm Quay Court, Nine Elms Lane, London, SW8 5DE, Telephone, 0207 498 2322 caroline@birthcentre.com

Foresight, The Association for the Promotion of Preconceptual Care, 3 Lower Queen's Road, Clevedon, N. Somerset, BS21 6LX, Telephone: 01275 878955 www.foresight-preconception.org.uk

Foresight Resource Centre, Telephone: 01483 869944

Freshwater Filters, Unit 3, Old Winery Business Park, Chapel Street, Norwich, Norfolk, NR10 4SE www.freshwaterfilters.com

Friends of the Earth, 137–143 Clapham Road, London, SW9 0HP, Telephone: 0207 490 1555 www.for.co.uk

G and G, Vitality House, 2–3 Imberhorne Way, East Grinstead, East Sussex, RH19 1RL, Telephone: 01342 312811 www.gandgvitamins.com www.gandginfo.com

Garden Organic, Wolston Lane, Ryton-on-Dunsmore, Coventry, Warwickshire, CV8 3LG, Telephone: 02476 30311111517 www.gardenorganic.org.uk

Garthenor Organic Wool, Llanlo Road, Tregaron, Ceredigion, SY25 6UR, Telephone: 01570 493347 www.organicpurewool.co.uk

Green People Ltd, Pondtail Farm, Coolham Road, West Grinstead, West Sussex, RH13 8LN, Telephone: 01403 740350 www.greenpeople.co.uk

Green Party Headquarters, The, 1a Waterloo Road, London, N19 5NJ, Telephone: 0207 549 0310 www.greenparty.org.uk

Greenpeace, Canonbury Villas, London, N1 2PN, Telephone: 0207 865 8100 www.greenpeace,org,uk

Healthy House Ltd, The old Co-op, Lower Street, Ruscombe, Stroud, Glos, GL6 6BU, Telephone: 01453 752216 www.healthy-house.co.uk

Harrison, Donald, Homeopathic Remedies, Telephone: 01974 241376

High Barn Oils, Nunthan House Farm, Barns Green, Horsham, Sussex, RH13 0NH, Telephone: 01403 730326 www.highbarnoils.co.uk

Holland and Barrett Headquarters, Samuel Ryder House, Townsend Drive, Nuneaton, Warwickshire, CV11 6XW, www.hollandandbarrett.com

Hyperactive Children's Support Group, Mrs Sally Bunday, 71 Whyke Lane, Chichester, West Sussex, PO19 7PD, Telephone: 01243 539966 www.hacsg.org.uk

Informed Parent, The, (Vaccination information), Mrs Magda Taylor, PO Box 4481, Worthing, West Sussex, BN11 2WH, Telephone: 01903 212969 www.informedparent.co.uk

Institute of Optimum Nutrition, Avalon House, 72 Lower Mortlake Road, Richmond, Surrey, TW9 2JY, Telephone: 0870 979 1122 www.ion.ac.uk

International Federation of Reflexologists, 8–9 Talbot Court, London, EC3V 0BP, Telephone: 0870 879 3562 www.intfedreflexologists.org

JABS (information on vaccine damage and compensation), 1 Gawswoth Road, Golborne, Wellington, Cheshire, WA3 3RF, Telephone: 01942 713565, www.jabs.org.uk

Just Organic Box Scheme, Freepost, Just Organic. www.justorganic.org.uk

Katzen, Jan, (Foresight American Branch Secretary), 31–51 North 18th Street, Phoenix, Arizona, 5016, USA, Telephone: (Mobile) 602 370 4036, Home 602 954 9540

La Leche League GB (breastfeeding support), PO Box 29, West Bridgford, Nottingham, NG2 7NP, Helpline: 0845 120 2918 www.laleche.org.uk

London Hazards Centre, 213 Haverstock Hill, London NW3 4QP, Telephone: 0207 794 5999 www.lhc.org.uk

MacManaway, Dr Patrick, (Electromagnetism Surveyor), Westbank Natural Health Centre, Strathmilgo, Fife, KY14 7QP, Telephone: 01233 750253 www.geomancy.org.uk

National Childbirth Trust, The (NCT), Alexandra House, Oldham Terrace, Acton, London, W3 6NH, Telephone: 0300 330 0771 www.nct.org.uk

Natural Family Planning (Fertility Education Trust), Mrs Colleen Norman, 218 Heathwood Road, Heath, Cardiff, Telephone: 02920 754628 www.fertilityet.org.uk

Nutri-Link Ltd, Unit 24, Milber Trading Estate, Newton Abbot, Devon, TW12 4SG, Telephone: 08450 760 402 www.nutri-linkltd.co.uk

Organic Meat, Carole Hockley, Newton Farm, Fordingbridge, Near Ringwood, Hampshire, Telephone: 01425 652542 www.hockleysfarm.co.uk

Organic Farmers and Growers Association, The Old Estate Yard, Albrighton, Shrewsbury, Shropshire SY4 AG, Telephone: 0845 330 5122/ 01939 291800 www.organicfarmers.org.uk

Organic Flower Company, The, 28 Mount Street, Shrewsbury, Shropshire, SY3 8QH, Telephone: 01691 683866 www.theorganicflowertcompany.co.uk

Passion for The Planet Radio, Zeal House, Deer Park Road, Wimbledon, London, SW19 3GY, www.passionfortheplanet.com

Pesticide Action Network, The Brighthelm Centre, North Road, Brighton, BN1 1YD, Telephone: 01273 964230 www.pan-uk.org

Plastic Pipes, British Plastics Association, Chestwood, 3 Kneeton Park, Middleton Tyas, Richmond, DL10 6SB, Telephone: 01325 339184 www.plasticpipesgroup.com

Powerwatch, 2 Tower Road, Sutton, Ely, Cambridgeshire, CB6 2QA, Telephone: 01353 778814 www.powerwatch.co.uk www.enfields.org

Price Pottenger Foundation. Le Mesa, 4200 Wisconsin Avenue, NW380, Washington DC, 20016, USA, Telephone: 619 462 7600 www.westonaprice.org

Reeves, John (Mycorrhiza), Eastleigh, Greenfield close, Joys Green, Lydbrook, Gloucestershire, GL17 2QU, Telephone: 01594 861196

Reflexologists, The International Federation of, 76–78 Edridge Road, Croydon, Surrey, CR0 1EF, Telephone: 0870 879 3562 www.intfedreflexologists.org

Riggs, Roy, (Electromagnetic Stress and Geopathic Energy Surveyor), 25 Coleridge Street, Poets Corner, Hove, Sussex, BN3 5AB, Telephone: 01273 732523 www.royriggs.com

Right From the Start, Sarah Woodhouse, Chief Executive, Welcome Cottage, Weveton, Nr Holt, Norfolk, NR25 7TH Telephone: 01263 740935 Email: sarah@rightfromthestart.fsnet.co.uk

Riverford Organic Vegetables, Wash Barn, Buckfastleigh, Devon. TQ11 0LD Telephone: 0845 600 2311 www.riverford.co.uk

Royal College of Midwives, 15 Mansfield Street, London, W1, Telephone: 0207 580 3535 www.rcm.org.uk

Scheibner, Dr Viera, 178 Govett's Leap Road, Blackheath, New South Wales. Australia, Telephone: 0061 24787 8203 www.veirascheibner.org

Scottish Institute of Reflexology, The, www.scottishreflexology.org

Soil Association, The, South Plaza, Marlborough Street, Bristol, BS1 3NX Telephone: 0117 314 500. (information) 0117 914 24444 www.soilassociation.org

Ultrasound Unsound, Shane Ridley, Manor Barn, Thurloxton, Taunton, Somerset, TA2 8RH,

University of Surrey, The Department of Chemistry, Guildford, Surrey, GU2 7HX, Telephone: 01483 300800 www.surrey.ac.uk

Vegetarian Society, The, Parkdale Dunham Road, Altringham, Cheshire, WA14 4QG, Telephone: 0161 925 2000 www.vegsoc.org

Vitacare Limited (Dried Goat's Milk), Utopia Village Unit 1, 7 Shalcot Road, Primrose Hill, London, NW1 8LH, Telephone: 0800 328 5826 www.vitacare.co.uk

What Doctors Don't Tell You, Satellite House, 2 Salisbury Road, London, SW19 4EZ, Telephone: 0870 444 9886, 0208 944 9555 www.wddty.co.uk

Wholistic Research Company, Unit Fiver House Farm, Sandon Road, Therfield, Royston, Hertfordshire, SG8 9RE, Telephone: 0845 430 3100 www.wholisticresearch.com

WISH, Westminster City Council Drug and Alcohol Foundation, 18 Dartmouth Street, London, SW1H 9BL, Telephone: 0207 233 0400 www.daf-london.org.uk

Women's Environmental Network (WEN), Ground Floor, 20 Club Row, Shoreditch, London, E2 7EY, Telephone: 0207 481 9004 www.wen.org.uk

World Federation of Doctors who Respect Human Life. The, PO Box 17317, London, SW3 4WJ, Telephone: 0207 7303059 www.doctorsfed.org.uk

Zed Books (Environment), 7 Cynthia Street, London, N1 9JF, Telephone: 0207 837 4014 www.zedbooks.co.uk

Zinc Bangles, Perfect Pillow, Unit A, Lantsbury Drive, Liverton North industrial Estate, Liverton Mines, Nr Loftus, Clevedon, TS13 4QZ, Telephone: 01287 643333 www.aromrelief.co.uk

APPENDIX 2
Recommended reading and references

Chapter 2: Nutrition

Alice Higgins Foundation – 'Birth outcomes before and after a nutritional programme', Montreal.

Anon. 'Tie Deficiency in Vitamin B6 to Low Agpar', *Medical Tribune,* 2 April 1980, 27

Antonov A.N., 'Children born during the siege of Leningrad in 1952', J Pediatr, 1947, 30, 250–259

Arawaka, T. et al., 'Dilation of cerebral ventricles of rat offspring induced by 6 mercapto purine administration to dams', Tohoku J Exp Med, 1967, 91 143

Baird Cousins, 'Effects of Undernutrition on Central Nervous System Function', Nutr Reviews, 1965, 23, 65–68

Barbara Griggs *The Food Factor – Why we are what we eat,* ISBN 0-670-80201-8

Barnes, B. *Male Infertility – Fighting Back* (2003) Foresight

Bryce-Smith, D (1979) Environmental trace elements and their role in disorders of personality, intellect, behaviour and learning ability in children. Proceedings of the second new Zealand Seminar on Trace Elements and Health. University of Auckland, 22–26 January.

Bryce-Smith, D and Hodgkinson, L (1986) *The Zinc Solution,* London, Century Arrow.

Caldwell D F Oberleas, D (1969) Effects of Protein and Zinc Nutrition on Behaviour in the Rat Perinatal Factors Affecting Human Development 85:2–8

Cannon, Geoffrey, 'Why Hampstead babies are 2lbs heavier', *The Sunday Times,* 28 March 1983

Chaitnow, Leon, 'Candida Albicans. Could Yeast be Your Problem?', Thorsons, 198, 48

Churchill, John A., et al. 'Birth Weight and Intelligence'. Obstet Gynecol, 1966, 28, 425–429

Colquhoun, Irene, Barnes, Belinda, *The Hyperactive Child. What the Family Can Do*, Wellingborough Thorsons, 1984

Davis, A (1954) *Let's Eat Right to Keep Fit*, New York, New American Library

Davis, A (1974) *Let's Have Healthy children*, Unwin paperbacks

Department of Health. 'Folic acid and the prevention of neural tube defects: report from an expert advisory group', Heywood: DoH Health Publication Unit, 1992, 21

DHSS-COMA. 'Diet and cardiovascular disease', London, HMSO, 1984

Doyle, W., Crawford, M.A. et al., 'The association of maternal diet and birth dimensions', J Nut Med, 1990, 1, 7–9

Ebrahim, G.J., 'The Problems of Undernutrition', in: Nutrition and Disease, ed: Jarrett, R.J., Baltimore, University Park Press, 1979, 29

Erdmann, Robert, Meiron Jones, *The Amino Revolution*, London Century paperbacks, 1987, 82

Eric R Braverman, MD with Carl C Pfeiffer, MD, PhD, *The Healing Nutrients Within, Facts, Findings and New Research on Amino Acids,* ISBN 0-87983-384-X

Fletcher, David, 'Cake recipe may prevent spina bifida', *The Daily Telegraph*, 13 January, 1994

Francesca Naish & Janette Roberts, *A Couples Guide to Natural Preconception and Health Care*

Gal, Isobel, et al., *Vitamin A in relation to Human Congenital Malformation*, 149

Graham, Judy, *Evening Primrose Oil*, Wellingborough, Thorsons 1984, 34

Hale, F., *Pigs born without eyeballs*, J Hered, 1935, 24, 105–106

Harrell, Ruth F. et al., 'The Influence of Vitamin Supplementation of the Diets of Pregnant and Lactating Women on the Intelligence of Their Offspring', Metabolism, 1956, 5, 555–562

Hawkins, David, Pauling, Linus, *Orthomolecular Psychiatry, Treatment of Schizophrenia*, San Francisco, CA, W.H. Freeman and Company, 1973

Health Education Council. A discussion paper on proposals for nutritional guidelines for health education in Britain. Prepared for the National Advisory Committee on Nutrition Education by an ad hoc working party under the Chairmanship of Professor V.P.T. James. NACNE, September 1983.

Healthy Parents, Better Babies, Francesca Naish and Janine Roberts, ISBN 0-7171-3007-X

Henry Schroeder, MD, *The Trace Elements and Man* ISBN 0-8159-6907-4

Hodges, Robert E., Adelman, Raymond D., *Nutrition in Medical Practice*, Philadelphia, W. B. Saunders, 1980, 43

Hoffer, A. 'Orthomolecular Nutrition at the Zoo'. Orthomolecular Psychiatry 1983, 12(2). 116–128

Holiverda-Kuipers, J., 'The cognitive development of low birthweight children', J Child psychology and Psychiat, 1987, 28, 321–328

Horrobin, D F (1981) 'The Importance of Gamma-Linolenic Acid and Prostaglandin E1 in Human Nutrition and Medicine', J Holistic Med 3(2): 118–139

Hurley, L (1969) *Zinc Deficiency in the Developing Rat*, Am J Clin Nut 22: 1332–1339

Hurley, L (1980) 'Developmental Nutrition', Englewood Cliffs, New Jersey

Hurley, L et al (1976) 'Teratogenic effects of magnesium deficiency', J Nut 106: 1254–1260

Hurley, Lucille, 'Developmental Nutrition', Englewood Cliffs, NJ, Prentice-Hall, 1980

Jameson, S (1984) Zinc Status and Human Reproduction in: Zinc in Human Medicine proceedings of a Symposium on the role of zinc in health and disease, Isleworth

Jennings, I W, *Vitamins in Endocrine Metabolism*, ISBN 0-433-17320-3, William Heinemann Medical Press (1972), pp.130–131

Jervis, R and N (1984) *The Foresight Wholefood Cookbook*, London, Roberts Publications

Johnson, M K (1975) The Delayed Neuropathy Caused by Some Organophosphorous Esters: mechanism and challenge, *Critical Reviews in Toxicology*, June 289:313

Kamen, B and S (1981) *The Kamen Plan for Total Nutrition During Pregnancy*, New York, Appleton-Century-Crofts 1981, 21–30. This gives a good overview of weight gain during pregnancy.

Kesserm Nucgaekm (1980) *Nutrition and Vitamin Therapy*, New York, Bantam, 1980

Laurence, K.M. et al., 'Increased risk of recurrence of neural tube defects to mother on poor diets and the possible benefits of dietary counselling', Br Med J, 1980, 281, 1509–1511

Lesser, Michael, (1980) *Nutrition and Vitamin Therapy*

Lodge-Rees, E (1983) Prevention versus problems in pediatric science In: *The Next Generation*, Foresight

Lodge-Rees, E (1983) Trace elements in pregnancy In: J Rose (Ed) *Trace elements in health*, London, Butterworths

Marks, John, *A Guide to the Vitamins*, Lancaster Medical and Technical Publishing Co. Ltd, 1979, 46

Mc Carrison, Sir R (1984) *Nutrition and Health,* London, McCarrison Society

Mental and Elemental Nutrients, ISBN 0-87983-114-6 Dr Carl C Pfeiffer, PhD, MD

Mercier, Chas., 'Diet as a Factor in the Causation of Mental Disease', *Lancet*, 1916, i, 561

Montagu, Ashley, 'Life Before Birth', New York, New American Library 1961, 23

Moore Lappe, Francis, *Diet for a Small Planet*, New York, Ballentine, 1975

Mortimer, G. Rosen, 'In The Beginning: Your Baby's Brain Before Birth', New York, New American Library, 1975, 25

MRC Vitamin Study Group. 'Prevention of neural tube defects: results of the Medical Research Council vitamin study', *Lancet*, 1991, 338, 131–7

Naish, F, and J Roberts, *Better Babies*, Random House, Australia (1996), p.57

National Pure Water Association, York.

Nutrition Against Disease, No ISBN Roger J Williams

Nutrition Search Inc. *Nutrition Almanac*, New York, McGraw-Hill Book Company, 1979, 94

Oberleas, D et al 91972) Trace Elements and Behaviour, Int Review Neurobiology Sup

Passwater, R and Cranton, E (1983) *Trace Elements, Hair Analysis and Nutrition*, ISBN 0-87983-265-7

Peer, L.A,. et al., 'Effect of vitamins on human teratology', Plast Reconst Surg, 1964, 34,358

Pfeiffer, Carl C (1975) *Mental and Elemental Nutrients*, New Canaan, Keats

Pfeiffer, Dr Carl C, PhD, MD, *Zinc and Other Micro-Nutrients*, (1978), New Canaan, Keats

Picciano, Mary Frances, 'Nutrient Needs of Infants', *Nut Today*, 1987, Feb, 8–13

Pottenger, F M (1983) *Pottenger's Cats*, La Mesa, Price Pottenger Foundation

Prescription for Nutritional Healing, ISBN 1-58333-077-1, Phyllis A Balch & James F Balch, MD

Price, Weston A, *Nutrition and Physical Degeneration*, The Price Pottenger Nutrition Foundation, La Mesa, California, USA (1945)

Board of Science and Education Report, 'Diet, Nutrition and Health', British Medical Association, March 1986

Reusens, B, et al.,'Controlling Factors of Foetal Nutrition', In: Carbohydrate Metabolism in Pregnancy, eds: Sutherland H.V., Stower, J.M., New York, Springer-Verlag, 1979, 209

Robertson, W.F., 'Thalidomide (Distaval) and vitamin B deficiency', BMJ, 1962, 1, 792

Robson, John R.K., *Malnutrition: its causation and control*, New York, Gordon and Breach, 1972, 401

Rush, David, et al., 'Diet in Pregnancy: A Randomised Control Trial of Nutritional Supplements', Birth Defects Original Article Series, Vol 16, No 3, New York, Alan R. Liss Inc, 1980, 114

Schroeder, H A (1973) *The Trace Elements and Man*, Old Greenwich, Devin-Adair

Seidmann, Daniel S., Laor, Arie, et al. 'Birth weight and intellectual performance in late adolescence.' Obstet and Gynecol. 1992, 79: 545–6

Smith, G.A., 'Effects of maternal undernutrition upon the newborn infant in Holland (1944–1945)', J Pediatr, 1947, 30, 250–259

Smith, J.C. et al., 'Alterations in vitamin A metabolism during zinc deficiency and food and growth restriction', J Nut, 1976, 106, 569–574

Smith, J.C. et al., 'Zinc: a trace element essential in vitamin A metabolism', *Science*, 1973, 181, 954–955

Smithells, R.W. et al., 'Further experience of vitamin supplementation for the prevention of neural tube defect recurrences', *Lancet*, 1983, i, 1027–1031

Smithells, R.W. et al., 'Possible prevention of neural tube defects by preconceptual vitamin supplementation', *Lancet*, 1980, i, 339–340

Sohler, A et al (1977) Blood lead levels in Psychiatric Outpatients Reduced by Zinc and Vitamin C, J orthomolecular Psychiat 6(3): 272–76

Stempak, J.G., 'Etiology of antenatal hydrocephalus induced by folic acid deficiency in the albino rat', Anat Rec, 1965, 151, 287

Suharno, Djoko, West, Clive, E. et al., 'Improvement in the vitamin A status may contribute to the control of anaemic pregnant women', *Lancet*, 1993, 342, 1325

Sutcliffe, Margaret, Schorah, Christopher J. et al., 'Prevention of neural tube defects', *Lancet*, 1993, 342, 1174

The Denner Report, London, HMSO (1990)

The Health Education Council (now the Health Education Authority) has issued many booklets, as well as the NACNE report

Tomorrow's World, BBC 1, 12 November 1987

Trace Element Metabolism in Animals, ISBN 0-443-00713-6 General Editor C F Mills

Tuormaa, T. *The Adverse Effects of Zinc Deficiency*, Foresight

Underwood, E J (1977) *Trace Elements in Human and Animal Nutrition, New York*, Academic Press, ISBN 0-12-709065-7

Vallee, B (1965) Zinc In: Comar, C L and Bronner, E S (eds) Mineral Metabolism, Vol II B, London, Academic Press

Ward, N et al (1987) Placental element levels in relation to foetal development for obstetrically "normal" births: A study of 37 elements, evidence for effects of cadmium, lead, and zinc on foetal growth and smoking as a source of cadmium. Int J Biosocial Res 9(1):63

Ward, N I (1995) Preconceptual Care and Pregnancy Outcome, *Journal of Nutritional and Environmental Medicine*, 5, 205–8

Ward, N. Durrant, S. Sankey, R J. Bound, J P. And Bryce-Smith, D.(1990) Elemental Factors in Human Foetal Development, J of Nutritional Medicine 1, 19–26

Werbach, M, *Nutritional Influences on Illness*, Third Line Press, California, USA (1988)

Williams, R J (1956) *Biochemical Individuality: the basis for the genetotrophic concept*, New York.

Williams, R J (1973) *Nutrition Against Disease*, London, Bantam, page 51.

Wynn, Arthur and Margaret, 'Prevention of Handicap of Early Pregnancy Origin'. Today – Building Tomorrow: International Conference on Physical Disabilities, Montreal June 4–6, 1986, First Session

Chapter 3: Hair Analysis

Abel, Ernest L (1982) Marihuana, Tobacco, Alcohol and Reproduction, Boca Raton, CRC Press

Alary, Michael et al (1993) Strategy for screening pregnant women for chlamydial infection in a low prevalence area, Obst Gynecol 82: 399–404

Anderson R A (1980) Chromium as a naturally occurring chemical in humans. Proceedings of Chromate Symposium, Industrial Health Foundation, Inc, Pittsburg, pp 332–345

Anderson R A and Polansky M M (1981) Dietary chromium sperm count and fertility in rats. Biol Trace Element Res, 3:1–5

Andrews, S H (1981) Abnormal reactions and their frequency in cattle following the use of organophosphorous warble fly dressing, The Veterinary Record 109: 171–175

Anke M et al (undated) Nutritional Requirements of Nickel. Offprint available through Foresight.

Anon (1985) Microwaves The Invisible Danger to Expectant Mums, *Healthy Living*, 2 March

ASH, Oldfield J E, Shull L R, Cheeke P R (1979) Specific effect of selenium deficiency on rat sperm. Biol Reprod, 20:793

Ashton B (1980) Manganese and Man. J Orthomol Psychiatry, 9(4):237–249

Balch J & Balch P, (2000) *Prescription for Nutritional Healing*, Penguin, Putnam Inc., New York.

Ballentine, R (1978) *Diet and Nutrition*, Honesdale, The Himalayan International Institute

Bellinger, D et al (1978) Low level lead exposure and infant development in the first year, Neurobehavioural Toxic and Terat 8: 151–161

Bellinger, D et al (1987) Longitudinal analyses of prenatal and postnatal lead exposure and infant development in the first year, New Eng J Med 17: 1037–1043

Bingol, N et al (1987) Teratogenicy of cocaine in humans, J Pediatr 10(1): 93–96

Bithell, F J and Stewart, A M (1975) Prenatal irridation and childhood malignancy: a review of British data from the Oxford Survey, Br J Cancer 31: 271–287

Blair, J H et al (1962) MAO inhibitors and sperm production, JAMA 181:192–193

Blumer, W R T (1980) Leaded gasoline – a cause of cancer, Envir Int 3: 465–471

Borel J S, Anderson R A (1984) Chromium. in: *Biochemistry of the Essential Ultratrace Elements* (Ed: E Frieden) Plenum Publishing Co.

Brazelton, T B (1970) Effect of Prenatal Drugs in the Behaviour of the Neonate, Am J Psychiat 126: 1296–1303

Bremmer I, Young B W, Mills C F (1976) Protective effects of zinc supplementation against copper toxicity in sheep. Br J Nutr, 36:551

Briggs, M H (1973) Cigarette Smoking and infertility in men, Med J Aust 1:616

Brostoff, J and Gamlin, L (1989) *The Complete guide to Food Allergy and Intolerance*, New York Crown Publisher Inc

Bryce-Smith, D (1977) Lead and cadmium levels in stillbirths, *Lancet* i: 1159

Bryce-Smith, D (1979) Environmental trace elements and their role in disorders of personality, intellect, behaviour and learning in children. Proceedings of the second New Zealand Seminar on Trace Elements and Health, University of Auckland, 22–26 January

Bryce-Smith, D (1981) Environmental Influences on Prenatal Development Thesssaloniki Conference, September

Bryce-Smith, D and Simpson, R I D (1984) Anorexia, Depression and Zinc Deficiency, *Lancet*, ii: 1162

Brzek, A (1987) Alcohol and male fertility (preliminary report), Andrologia 19: 32–36

Bushnell, P J and Bowman, R E (1977) Reversal deficits in young monkeys exposed to lead, Pharm Biochem and behaviour 10: 733–747

Buttram, H (1994) Controversal issues – 1 Candidiasis – The Phantom Illness, Unpublished paper

Caldwell D F, Oberleas, D (1969) Effects of protein and zinc nutrition on behaviour in the rat. Perinatal factors affecting human development, 85: 2–8

Campbell, J M and Harrison, K L (1979) Smoking and Infertility, Med J Aust 1; 342–343

Carruthers M E (1966) Hobbs C B, Warren R L: Raised serum copper and ceruloplasmin levels in subjects taking oral contraceptives. J Clin Pathol, 19:498–450

Catterall, R D (1981) Biological effects of sexual freedom, Lancet i: 315–319

Chaitow, L (1984) Candida Albicans Could Yeast Be Your Problem? Wellingborough, Thorsons

Chavez, G F et al (1989) Maternal cocaine use during pregnancy as a risk factor for congenital urogenital anomalies JAMA 262: 795–8

Clark L C (1996) et al: Effects of selenium supplementation for cancer prevention in patients with carcinoma of the skin. JAMA, 276:1957–1963

Clark L C (1997) Recent developments in the prevention of human cancer with selenium. Selenium-Tellurium Development Assoc Bulletin, November

Clausen, J and Rastogi, S C (1977) Heavy metal pollution among autoworkers in Lead, Br J Ind Med 34: 208–215

Colgan, M (1982) Your Personal Vitamin Profile, London, Blond and Briggs

Consumers Association (1985) Drug and Therapeutics Bulletin, July 23:15

Cowdry, Q and Stokes, P (1989) Aluminium causes senility, The Daily Telegraph, 13 January

Crawford, I Land Connor, J D (1975) Zinc and Hippocampal Function, J Orthomol Psych 4(1): 39–52

Crews M G (1980) Taper U, Ritchey S I: Effects of oral contraceptive agents on copper and zinc balance in young women. Am J Clin Nutr, 33:1940

Crook, W G (1983) *The Yeast Connection*, Professional Books

Crosby, W M et al (1977) Foetal Malnutrition: An Appraisal of Correlated Factors, Am J Obstet Gynaecol 128: 26

David, O J et al (1976) Lead and hyperactivity Behavioural response to chelation: a pilot study, Am J Psychiat 133(10): 1155–1158

Davies, S (1981) Lead, Beyond Nutrition, Summer 12–13

Davies, S and Stewart, A (1987) *Nutritional Medicine*, London, Pan

Davis, A (1954) *Let's Eat Right to Keep Fit*, New York, New American Library

Davis, A (1974) *Let's have healthy children*, Unwin Paperbacks

Doisy EA (1973) In: Proceedings of the University of Missouri's 6th Annual Conference on Trace Substances in Environmental Health, p. 193, Ed: DD Hemphill, Columbia, MO. University of Missouri Press

Doisy EA (1974) Trace Substances in Environmental health. Proceedings of the University of Missouri's 6th Annual Conference, p.193, 1972. In: Trace Element metabolism in Animals. Eds: WG Hoekstra, et al, Vol:2,p,664, Univer Park Press, Baltimore, Maryland

Doisy R J, Streeten DHP, Freiberg JM et al: chromium metabolism in man and biochemical effects. In: Trace Elements in Human Health and Disease (Ed:AS Prasad), Vol II, pp 79–104, New York Academy Press.

Duffy, F H and Burchfield, J L (1980) Long Term Effects of the Organophosphate Sarin in EEGs in Monkeys and Humans, Neurotoxicology 1: 667–689

Duffy, F H et al (1979) Long-Term Effects of an Organophosphate upon the Human Electroencephalogram, Toxicology and Applied Pharmacology 47; 161–176

Eagle, R (1986) *Eating and Allergy*, Wellingborough, Thorsons

Ebrahim, O J (1979) The Problems of Undernutrition In: Ed: R J Jarrett *Nutrition and Disease*, Baltimore, University Park Press

Editorial (1964) The Drugged Sperm BMJ 1: 1063–1064

Eilard, T et al (1976) Isolation of chlamydia in acute salpingitis, Scand J Infectious Dis (Suppl 9), 82–84

Elam, D (1980) Building Better Babies Preconception Planning for Healthier Children, Milibare, Celestial Arts

El-Dakhakny, A and El-sadik, Y M (1972) Lead in hair among exposed workers, Am Ind Hygiene Assoc Journal 33

Elkington, J (1985) *The Poisoned Womb*, Harmondsworth, Viking

Erlichman, J (1993) Sheep dip alarm likely to force ban, *The Guardian* 26 October

Erway L, Fraser AS, Hurley LS (1971) Prevention of congenital otolith defects in pallid mutant mice by manganese supplementation. Genetics, 67:97–108

Erway L, Hurley LS and Fraser A (1966) Neurological defect: Manganese in penocopy and prevention of a genetic abnormality of inner ear. *Science* 152:1766–68

Erway L, Hurley LS and Fraser AS 1970 Congenital ataxia and otolith defects due to manganese deficiency in mice. *J Nutr*, 100:643–654

Evans, H J et al, (1981) Sperm abnormalities and cigarette smoking, *Lancet*, i: 627–629

Everson GJ and Shrader RE: J.Nutr, 94:89, 1968 and Shrader RE and Everson GJ, p 296

Fantel, A G and Macphail, B J (1982) The teratogenicity of cocaine, Teratology 26: 17–19

Freundlich, M et al (1985) Infant Formula as a Cause of Aluminium Toxicity in Neonatal Ureamia, *Lancet* ii: 527–529

Friberg, J and Gnarpe, H (1973) Mycoplasma and human reproductive failure, Am I Obstet Gynecol, 116: 23–26

Fromell, G T et al (1979) Chlamydial infections of mothers and their infants, J Pod 95(1):28–32

Garnys, V et al (1979) Lead Burden of Sydney Schoolchildren, University of New South Wales

Gibbs, C E and Seitchik, J (1980) Nutrition in Pregnancy In: R S Goodhart and M Shils (eds) Modern Nutrition in Health and Disease, Philadephia, Lea and Febiger

Gittelman, R and Eskenazi, B (1983) Lead and hyperactivity revisited, Arch Gen Psychiat 40: 827–833

Gordon, G F (1980) Hair Analysis: Its Current Use and Limitations Part II, *Let's Live*, October: 89–94

Grant, E (1985) The Bitter Pill, London, Corgi

Grant, E (1994) Sexual Chemistry: Understanding our Hormones, the Pill and HRT, London, Cedar

Gruden N (1979) Dietary variations and manganese transduodenal transport in rats. Periodicum Biologorum, 81:567–70

Hall A C, Young B W, Bremmer I (1979) Intestinal metallothionin and the mutual antagonism between copper and zinc in the rat. J Inorg Biochem, 11:57

Hambidge, K M et al (1972) Low Levels of Zinc in Hair, Anorexia, Poor Growth, and Hypogeusia in Children, Pediat Res, 6: 868–874

Hambridge K M (1971) Newer Trace Elements in Nutrition. Eds: W Metrz and WE Cornatzer p.169, Dekker, New York

Hambridge K M (1974) Chromium nutrition in man. Am J Clin Nutr, 27:505–51

Hambridge K M. Rodgerson D O, O'Brien D O (1968) The concentration of chromium in the hair of normal and children with diabetes mellitus. Diabetes. 17:517–519

Hansen, J C et al (1980) Children with minimal brain dysfunction, Danish Bull 27(6): 259–262

Himmelberger, DU et al (1978) Cigarette smoking during pregnancy and occurrence of spontaneous abortion and congenital abnormality, A. Epid 108: 470–479

Hodges, R E and Adelman, R D (1980) Nutrition in Medical Practice, Philadelphia, W B Saunders

Hornsby, M (1993) Insecticide might be "mad cow" link, The Times, 21st August

Hurley, L (1969) Zinc Deficiency in the Developing Rat, Am J Clin Nut 22: 1332–1339

Hurley, L S et al (1976) Teratogenic effects of magnesium deficiency, J Nut 106: 1254–1260

Ip C and Ganther HE (1993) Novel strategies in selenium chemoprevention research. In: Selenium in Biology and Human Health. (Ed RF Burk), pp 169 Springer Verlag, NY, US

Jameson, S (1984) Zinc Status and Human Reproduction In; Zinc in Human Medicine Proceedings of a Symposium on the role of Zinc in Health and Disease, Isleworth, TIL Publications Ltd

Johnson, M K (1975) The Delayed Neuropathy Caused by Some Organophosphorus Esters: Mechanism and Challenge, Critical Reviews in Toxicology, June 289: 313

Kamen, B and S (1981)*The Kamen Plan for Total Nutrition During Pregnancy*, New York, Appleton-Century-Croft (This is an excellent book)

Kaufman, M In: Neville Hodgkinson, Alcohol Threat to Babies, *The Sunday Times*, 31 January 1988

Kime, Z R (1980) Sunlight, Penryn, World Health Publications

Klevay, L M (1978) Hair as a Biopsy Material Progress and Prospects, A Intern Med 138: 1127–1128

Kostial, K and Kello, D (1979) Bioavailability of lead in rats fed "human diets", Bull Environ Contam Toxic 21: 312–314

Kucheria, K et al (1985) Semen analysis in alcohol dependence syndrome Andrologia 17: 558–563

Kunin RA (1976) Manganese and niacin in the treatment of drug-induced dyskinesias. J Orthomol. Psychiatry, 5(1):4–27

Kupsinel, R Mercury Amalgam Toxicity A Major Common Denominato Degenerative Disease, J Orthomolecular Psychiat 13(4): 240–257

Lacranjan, 1(1975) Reproductive ability of workmen occupationally exr lead, Arch Envir Health 20: 396–401

Laker, M (1982) On determining trace element levels in man: the uses of blood and hair *Lancet* ii: 260–262

Lazebik, N et al (1988) Zinc Status, Pregnancy Complications and labor Abnormalities, Am J Obstet Gynecol, 158: 161–166

Leach RM (1976) Metabolism and function of manganese. In: *Trace Elements in Human Health and Disease*. Vol:II, pp 235–47, Eds: Prasad AS and Oberleas DY, NY Academic Press, New York

Lesser, M (1980) *Nutrition and Vitamin Therapy*, New York, Bantam

Lester, M Let al (1986) Protective Effects of Zinc and Calcium Against Metal Impairment of Children's Cognitive Function, 145–161

Levander, O A (1982) Selenium: Biochemical Actions, Interactions, and some human health implications. In: Clinical, Biochemical, and Nutritional Aspects of Trace Elements (Ed: AS Prasad) pp 345–368, Alan Liss Inc. New York, US

Lin-Fu, J S (1973) Vulnerability of children to lead exposure and toxicity Eng J Med 289: 129–1233

Lodge Rees, E (1979) Aluminium Toxicity as Indicated by Hair Analysis, I Orthomol Psychiat 8(1): 137–143

Lodge Rees, E (1981) The concept of preconceptual care, Intern J Envir Studies 17: 37–42

Lodge Rees, E (1983) Prevention versus problems in pediatric science In: The Next Generation, Foresight

Lodge Rees, E (1983) Trace elements in pregnancy In: J Rose (Ed) Trace Elements in Health, London, Butterworths

Mann, P (1985) *Marijuana Alert*, New York, McGraw-Hill

Mardh, P H (1981a) Medical chlamydiology: A position paper, Scan J Infect Dis (Supp 32):3–8

Mardh, P H et al (1981b) Endometriosis caused by chlamydia trachomatis, Br J Vene Dis, 57–91

Masefield, J (1988) Psychiatric illness caused or exacerbated by Food Allergies (Unpublished article)

Maugh, T H (1978) Hair: A Diagnostic Tool to Complement Blood Serum and Urine, Science 202: 1271–1273

McConnell K P, Burton R M (1981) Selenium in spermatogenesis. In: second International Symposium on Selenium in Biology and Medicine (Eds: JL Martin and JE Spallholz), Westport, Connecticut: AVI Publishing

Mervyn L (1985) *The Dictionary of Minerals*. Thorson Publishing Group

Merz W: Clinical and Public Health Significance of Chromium In: Clinical, Biochemical, and Nurtritional Aspects of Trace Elements (Ed: AS Prasad) 315–323, Alan R Liss, Inc., New York, USA, 1982

Millstone, E & Abraham, I (1988) *Additives A Guide for Everyone*, Penguin

Moore, L S and Fleischman, A (1975) Subclinical Lead Toxicity, Orthomol Psychiatry 4(1): 6 1–70

Morgan J M (1972) Hepatic chromium content in diabetic subjects. Metabolism 21:313–316

Mortimer, G R (1975) *In the Beginning: Your Baby's Brain Before Birth*, New York, New American Library

Nath R, Minocha J, Lyall V et al (1979) Assessment of chromium metabolism in maturity onset and juvenile diabetes using chromium 51 and therapeutic response of chromium administration on plasma lipids, glucose tolerance and insulin levels. In: Chromium in Nutrition and Metabolism (Eds: D Shapcott and J Hubert) pp 213–222, Elsevier/North Holland

National Research Council Committee on medical and Biological Effects of Environmental Pollutants. Manganese. Washington (1973) National Academy of Sciences, pp 1–191

Needleman, H L et al (1979) Deficits in psychologic and classroom performance of children with elevated dentine lead levels, New Eng J Med 300: 689–696

Needleman, H L et al (1984) JAMA 25 1(22): 2956–9

Needleman, H L et al (1990) New Eng J Med 332: 83–88

Nielson, F H (1984a) Nickel In: Earl Frieden, (Ed) *Biochemistry of the Essential Ultratrace Elements*, Plenum Publishing

Nielson, F H (1984b) Fluoride, Vanadium, Nickel, Arsenic, and Silicon in Total Parental Nutrition, Bull of the New York Academy of Med, 60(2), 177–195

Norwood, C (1980) *At Highest Risk*, New York, McGraw-Hill

Nutrition Search Inc (1979) Nutrition Almanac, New York, McGraw-Hill

Oberleas, D et al (1972) Trace Elements and Behaviour, Int Review Neurobiology Sup

Passwater, R (1980) *Selenium as a Food Medicine*, New Canaan, Keats Publishing Co

Passwater, R and Cranton, E (1983) *Trace Elements, Hair Analysis and Nutrition*, New Canaan, Keats Publishing Co

Pfeiffer C and laMola S (1985) Zinc and manganese in the schizophrenias. J Otrhomol Psychiartry, 12(3)215–234

Pfeiffer CC and Bacchi D (1975) Copper, zinc and manganese, niacin and pyridoxine in the schizophrenias. *J Appl Nutr*, 27:9–39

Pfeiffer, C (1975) *Mental and Elemental Nutrients*, New Canaan, Keats Publishing Co

Pfeiffer, C C (1978) *Zinc and Other Micronutrients*, New Canaan, Keats Publishing Co

Pharoach, P 0 D Ct al (1971) Neurological damage to the foetus resulting from severe iodine deficiency during pregnancy, *Lancet* i: 308–3 10

Phil, R O and Parkes, M (1977) Hair element content in learning disabled children, *Science* 198: 4214

Pitkin, R M et al (1972) Maternal Nutrition, A Selective Review of Clinical Topics Obstet Gynaecol 40: 775

Rayman MP (1997) Dietary selenium: time to act. *Br Med J*, 314: 387–388

Rhodes, A J (1961) Virus and Congenital Malformations: Papers and Discussions presented at the First International Conference on Congenital Malformations, Philadelphia-Lippincott

Riopelle AJ and Hubbard DG: Prenatal manganese deprivation and early behaviour of primates. J Orthomol Psychiatry, 6(4)

Roberts, D (Undated) Pharmacology and toxicology of organophosphorus pesticides, Offprint available from Foresight

Robertson, W F (1962) Thalidomide (Distival) and vitamin B deficiency BMJ1: 792

Robinson, M F (1982) Clinical effects of selenium deficiency and excess. In: Clinical, Biochemical, and Nutritional Aspects of Trace Elements (Ed: AS Prasad) pp 325–343, Alan Liss Inc, New York, New York, US

Rodriguez, A F et al (1986) Relationship between benzodiazepine ingestion during pregnancy and oral clefts in the newborn, a case-control study, Med Clin 87/18: 741–743

Rose, J Ed: (1983) *Trace Elements in Health*, London, Butterworths (and Samarawickrama, G)

Rosett H,et al (1983) Patterns of Alcohol Consumption and Foetal Development, Obstet Gynecol, 61: 539–546

Sandstead, H H (1984) Zinc: Essentiality for Brain Development and Function, *Nut Today*, November, December 26–30

Saner, G et al (1985) Hair manganese concentrations in newborns and their mothers, Am J Clin Nut 41: 1042–1044

Sassenath, E N et al (1979) Reproduction in Rhesus Monkeys Chronically Exposed to Delta-9-THC Adv in the Biosciences, 22–23: 50 1–522

Schelling, J L (1987) Which Drugs should not be Prescribed during Pregnancy, Ther Umsch Rev Ther 441: 48–53

Schofield, C B S (1972) *Sexually Transmitted Diseases*, London, Churchill – Livingstone

Schrauzer G N (1977) White DA, Schneider CJ: Cancer mortality correlation studies, III, Statistical associations with dietary selenium intakes. Bioinorg Chem, 7:23

Schroeder H A (1965) Serum cholesterol levels in rats fed thirteen trace elements. J Nutr, 94:475–480

Schroeder H A (1966) Chromium deficiency in rats: A syndrome simulating diabetes mellitus with retarded growth. J Nutr, 88:439–445

Schroeder H A (1970) Nason AP, Tipton IH: Chromium deficiency as a factor in atherosclerosis. J Chronic Dis, 23:123–142

Schroeder, H A (1973) The Trace Elements and Man, Old Greenwich, Devin-Adair

Schroeder, H and Mitchener, M (1971) Toxic Effects of Trace Elements on the Reproduction on Mice and Rats, Arch Envir Health 23; 102

Schwartz, J et al. (1986) Relationship between childhood blood lead levels and stature, Pediatrics 77(3): 281–283

Shamberger and Frost, D V (1969) Possible protective effect of selenium against human cancer. Can Med Assoc J, 100:682

Simpson, J (1957) A preliminary report on cigarette smoking and the incidence of prematurity, Am J Obstet Gynaecol, 73: 800–815

Singh, N et al (1978) Neonatal lead intoxification in a prenatally exposed infant, J Paediat 93(6): 1019–1021

Smith, C G and Gilbean, PM (1985) Drug Abuse Effects on Reproductive Hormones In: J Thomas et al (eds) Endocrine Toxicology, New York, Raven Press

Smith, I C et al (1973) Zinc: a trace element essential in vitamin A metabolism, Science, 181: 954–955

Smith, J C et al (1976) Alterations in vitamin A metabolism during zinc deficiency and food and growth restriction, J Nut 106: 569–574

Sohler A and Pfeiffer C C (1979) Direct method for the determination of manganese in whole blood, patients with seizure activity have low blood levels. J orthomol. Psychiatry, 8(4):275–80

Sohler, A et al (1977) Blood Lead Levels in Psychiatric Outpatients Reduced by Zinc and Vitamin C, J Orthomolecular Psychiat 6(3): 272–276

Spatling, L and G (1988) Magnesium supplementation in pregnancy: a double-blind study, Br J Obstet Gynaecol 95: 111–116

Spears, J W S (1984) Effect of Dietary Nickel on Growth, Urease Activity, Blood Parameters and Tissue Mineral Concentrations in the Neonatal Pig, J Nut 114: 845–853

Spivey, Fox M R (1975) New York Acad Science 258: 144

Spyker, J M Occupational Hazards and the Pregnant Worker, Behavioural Toxicology Overview, 470

Stenchever, M A et al (1974) Chromosome Breakages in Users of Marijuana, AmlObstetGynaecol, 118: 106–113

Streissguth, A P (1991) What every community should know about drinking during pregnancy and the lifelong consequences for society, Substance Abuse, 12(3): 114–127

Tanaka Y (1977) Low manganese level may trigger epilepsy. JAMA, 258: 1805

Thatcher, R et al (1982) Effects of low levels of cadmium and lead on cognitive functioning in children Arch Envir Health 37(3): 159–166

Tolonen M (1990) Vitamins and Minerals in Health and Nutrition, Ellis Horwood Series in *Food Science and Technology*

Tuormaa, T (1994) The Adverse Effects of Alcohol on Reproduction, A Review from the Literature, Foresight

Tuormaa, T (1994a) The Adverse Effects of Tobacco Smoking on Reproduction, A Review from the Literature, Foresight (Also reprinted in Int J Biosocial Med Res, 14:2)

Underwood, E J (1977) Trace Elements in Human and Animal Nutrition, New York, Academic Press

US Surgeon General's Advisory on Alcohol and Pregnancy (1981) FDA-Drug Bulletin 11(12) July

Vallee, B (1965) Zinc In: Comar, C Land Bronner, C S (eds) Mineral Metabolism, Vol II B, London, Academic Press

Vitale, L F et al (1975) Blood lead – an inadequate measure of occupational exposure, J Occ Med 17: 102–3

Ward, N I (1992) Environmental Aspects of Heavy Metals and Aluminium and the Effect on Human Health, Foresight Mid-Summer Newsletter, 26–38

Ward, N I (1993) Preconceptual care questionnaire research project, In press Details from Foresight

Ward, N I (1995) Preconceptual care and pregnancy outcome, *J of Nutritional & Environmental Medicine 5*, 205–8

Ward, N I et al (1987) Placental element levels in relation to foetal development for obstetrically "normal" births: A study of 37 elements, evidence for effects of cadmium, lead and zinc on foetal growth and smoking as a source of cadmium, Biosocial Res 9(1): 63

Weber, LW D (1985) Benzodiazepines in pregnancy — academic debate or teratogenic risk? Biol Res in Preg, 64: 15 1–167

Wertheimer, N and Leeper, E (1984) Adverse effects on foetal development associated with sources of exposure to 60 hz electric and magnetic fields (Abstract), 23rd Hanford Life Sciences Symposium Interaction of Biological Systems with Static and ELF Electric and Magnetic Fields, Richland, WA

Westrom L (1975) Affect of acute pelvic infectious disease on fertility, Am J Obstet Gynecol, 121: 707–713

Whorton, M D et al(1977) Infertility in male pesticide workers, Lancet:1259–61

Wibblerley, D G et al (1977) Lead levels in human placentas from normal and malformed births, I Med Gen 14(5): 339–345

Williams, R J (1973) Nutrition Against Disease, London, Bantam

Woffinden, B (1994) Cows: mad or poisoned? Living Earth and The Food Magazine, 184:10

Wolff, H et al (1991) Chlamydia trachomatis induces an inflammatory response in the male genital tract and is associated with altered semen quality, Fert Ster 55(5): 1017–1019

Wright, P (1988) Claims that power cables cause Cancer to be investigated, The Times, 18 March

Wynn A and M (1986) Prevention of Handicap of Early Pregnancy Origin Today – Building Tomorrow International Conference on Physical Disabilities, Montreal, 4–6 June

Wynn A and M (Undated) Should Men and Women Limit Alcohol Consumption when Hoping to have a Baby? London, The Maternity Alliance

Wynn M and Wynn A (1981) The Prevention of Handicap of Early Pregnancy Origin, London Foundation for Education and Research in Childbearing

Yale, W et al (1985) Teachers' ratings of children's behaviour in relation to blood lead levels, Br J Dev Psych 2: 285–306

Ziff, S (1985) The Toxic Time-Bomb, Wellingborough, Thorsons

Chapter 4: Voluntary Social Poisons

SMOKING

Abel, Ernest L., Marijuana, Tobacco, Alcohol and Reproduction, Boca Raton, F1, CRC Press, 1983, 31–33

Albernathy JR, Greenberg BG, Wells HB et al.: Smoking as independent variable in a multiple regression analysis upon birth weight and gestation. Am J Public Health, 56:626–633, 1966

Andrews Z and McGarry JM: A community study in smoking in pregnancy. J Obstet Gynaecol Br Commonw, 79:1057–1073, 1972

Bailey RR: The effect of maternal smoking on the infant birth weight. NZ M J, 71:293–294, 1970

Barnes B & Bradley SG: *Planning for a Healthy Baby*, pp 96–97, Ebury Press, London, 1990

Bernard P: Die Workung desRauchens auf Frau and Mutter. Munch Med Wochenschr, 104: 1826, 1962

Bridges BA, Clemmensen J, Sugimura T: Cigarette smoking does it carry genetic risk? Mutat Res, 65: 71–81, 1970

Briggs MH (1973) Cigarette smoking and infertility in men. Med J Austr, 1:616

Butler NR and Alberman ED (1969) Perinatal Problems: The Second Report of the 1958 British Perinatal Mortality Survey. Edinburgh, Livingstone

Butler NR and Goldstein M (1973) Smoking during pregnancy and subsequent child development. Br Med J, 4:573–575

Cadmium in the environment and its significance to man. U.K. Department of the Environment, Pollution Paper No:17, Her Majesty's Stationery Office, London 1980

Campbell AM: Excessive cigarette smoking in women and its effect upon their reproductive efficiency. J Mich Med Soc, 34: 146–151, 1935

Campbell JM and Harisson KL: Smoking and infertility. Med J Austr, 1: 342–343, 1979

Carmichael NG, Backhouse BL, Winder C, Lewis PD (1982) Teratogenicity, toxicity, and perinatal effects of cadmium. Human Toxicol, 1:159–186

Chamberlain G, Philipp E, Howlett B, Masters K: British Births 1970, Vol:2, Obstetric Care, Heineman, London, 1978

Chow, W (1988) Maternal cigarette smoking and tubal pregnancy. Obstet Gynecol 71: 167–174

Clemetson CAB and Anderson L: ascorbic acid metabolism in preeclampsia. Obstet Gynecol, 24: 774–782, 1964

Comstock GW and Lundin FE (1967) Parental smoking and perinatal mortality. Am J Obstet Gynecol, 98:708–718

Crawford MA: Maternal nutrition before conception and the prevention of neurodevelopmental disorders. The McCarrison Society Newsletter, Winter, 1992

Crosby, W.M. et al., 'Foetal malnutrition: an appraisal of correlated factors', Am J Obstet Gynacol, 1977, 128, 22

Davidoff GN, Votaw ML, Coon WW, Hultquist FA, Filter EE, Wexlar BJ: Elevations on serum copper, erythrocyte copper and ceruloplasmin concentrations in smokers. Am J Clin Path, 75:790 1978

Davies, Stephen, Nutritional Medicine. (1987) Pan, London

Denson R, Nanson JL, McWatters MA: Hyperkinesis and maternal smoking. Can Psychiatr Assoc J, 20: 183, 1975

Esber HJ, Menninger FF, Bogden AE, Mason MM: Immunological deficiency associated with cigarette smoke inhalation by mice. Arch Environ Health, 27:99 1973

Evans HJ, Fletcher J, Torrance M, Hardgreave TB (1981) Sperm abnormalities and cigarette smoking. The Lancet, 1:627–629

Fedrick J, Alberman E, Goldstein H (1971) Possible teratogenic effect of cigarette smoking. Nature, 231:529–530

Fedrick, J., Anderson, A., 'Factors associated with spontaneous pre-term birth', Br J Obstet Gynaecol, 1976, 83, 342

Fergusson DM, Horwood U, Shannon FT (1979) Smoking during pregnancy. N.Z. Med J, 89:41–43

Fielding JE and Rosso PK (1978) Smoking during pregnancy. N Engi J Med, 298:337–339

Frazier TM, Davis GH, Goldstein H et al. (1961) Cigarette smoking and prematurity: A predictive study. Am J Obstet Gynecol, 81:988–996

Friberg L, Nystrom A, Swanberg H: Transplacental diffusion of carbon monoxide in human subjects. Acta Physiol Scand, 45:363–368, 1959

Golding J: The Consequences of smoking in Pregnancy. Talk given to a conference on smoking in Pregnancy commissioned by the Health Education Authority, 2 February, 1994

Goujard S. Rumeau C, Schwartz N (1965) Smoking during pregnancy, stillbirth and abruptio placentae. Biomedicine, 23:20–22

Goujard, J., Kaminiski, C, et al., 'Maternal Smoking, Alcohol Consumption and Abruptio Placentae', Am J Obstet Gynacol, 1978, 130, 738

Grant E: Sexual Chemistry. P.135, Cedar Publications, 1994

Grant ECG: Allergies, smoking and the contraceptive pill. In: *Biological Aspects of Schizophrenia*, Ed: G Hemmings, John Wiley & Sons Ltd, 1982

Grant, Ellen, 'The Effect of Smoking on Pregnancy and Children.', In: Guidelines for Future Parents, Witley, Surrey, 1986, 85–86

Gulsvic A and Fagerhol MK: Smoking and immune-globulin levels. The *Lancet*, 1: 449, 1979

Gustavson KH, Hagberg B, Hagberg G, Sars K (1977) Severe mental retardation in a Swedish country. Neuropadiatrie, 8:293–304

Haddon W, Nesbitt REL, Garcia R: Smoking and pregnancy: carbon monoxide in blood during gestation and at term. Obstet Gynaecol 18:262–267, 1961

Halliwell B: Cigarette smoking and health: a radical view, J Roy Soc Health, April, 91–96, 1993

Halliwell B: Free radicals and vascular disease: how much do we know? Br Med J, 307:885 1993

Hammer DI, Calocci AV, Hasseiblad V. Williams ME, Pinkerton C (1973) Cadmium and lead in autopsy tissue. J Occup Med, 15:956

Handelsman DJ, Conway AJ, Boylan LM, Turtle JR:

Haworth JC and Ford JD: Comparison of the effects of maternal under nutrition and exposure to cigarette smoke on the cellular growth of the rat fetus. AM J Obstet Gynaecol, 112:653, 1972

Hellman LM, Jonson HL, Tolles WE et al, Some factors affecting fetal heart rate. Am J Obstet Gynaecol, 82: 1055–1063, 1961

Hemsworth BN: Deformation of the mouse foetus after ingestion of nicotine by the male. IRCS Medical Science, 9: 728–729, 1981

Herriot A, Billewics WZ, Hytten FE (1962) Cigarette smoking in pregnancy. *The Lancet*, 1:771–773

Himmelberger DV, Brown BW, Cohen EN (1978) Cigarette smoking during pregnancy and the occurrence of spontaneous abortion and congenital malformation. Am J Epidemiol, 108:470–479

Holt PG, Keast D, Mackenzie JS: Immunosuppression in the mouse induced by long-term exposure to cigarette smoke. Am J Pathol, 90: 281–284, 1978

Hypoglycaemia and Personality. Br Med J, p 134, April, 20 1974

Jansson I: Aetiological factors in prematurity. Acta Obstet Gynecol Scand, 45:279–300, 1966

Jick H, Porter J, Morrison AS: Relation between smoking and age of natural menopause. The Lancet, 1: 1354–1355, 1977

Jones MS: Hypoglycaemia in the neuroses. Br Med J, 945–946, November 16, 1935

Kallerup HE, Kierkegord-Hansen G, Hansen JC (1976) Exposure to cadmium as a possible precipitating factor in connective tissue disease. Ugerskr Laeger, 138:1396

Kelly J, Mathews KA, O'Conor M (1984) Smoking during pregnancy: effects on mother and the foetus. Br J Obstet Gynaecol, 91:111–117

Kelsey JL, Theodore RH, Bracken MB (1978) Maternal smoking and congenital malformations: An epidemiological study. J Epidem Community Health, 32:103–107

Kjeldsen K: Smoking and atherosclerosis. Munksgaard, Copenhagen, 1969

Kline JO, Stein ZA, Susser M, Warburton D (1977) Smoking: a risk factor for spontaneous abortion. N Engl J Med, 297:793–796

Kraal JH: Immunoglobulin levels in relation to smoking and coffee consumption. Am J Clin Nutr, 31: 198–200, 1978

Kulikauskas V. Blaustein D, Ablin RJ (1985) Cigarette smoking and its possible effect on sperm. Fertil Steril, 44:526–528

Kullander S and Kallen B (1971) A prospective study of smoking in pregnancy. Acta Obstet Gynecol Scand, 50:83–94

Landesman-Dwyer S and Emanuel I: Smoking during pregnancy. Teratology, 19:119–126, 1978

Landmann HR and Sutherland RL: Incidence and significance of hypoglycaemia in unselected admissions to a psychosomatic service. Am J Digest Dis, 105–108, April, 1950

Lehtovirta P and Forss M (1978) The acute effects of smoking on intravillous blood flow of the placenta. Br J Obstet Gynaecol, 85:729–731

Lener J and Bibr B (1971) Cadmium and hypertension. The Lancet, 1:970

Lewis GP, Coughlin LL, Jusko JW, Hartz S (1972) Contribution of cigarette smoking to cadmium accumulation in man. *The Lancet*, 1:291

Lewis GP, Jusko WJ, Coughlin L (1972) Cadmium accumulation in man: influence of smoking, occupation, alcohol habit and disease. J Chronic Dis, 25:717

Linquist O, and Bengtsson C: Menopausal age in relation to smoking. Acta Med Scand, 205: 73–77, 1979

Longo LD (1970) Carbon monoxide in pregnant mother and foetus and its exchange across the placenta. Ann NY Acad Sci, 174:313–341

Longo LD (1977) The biological effects of carbon monoxide on the pregnant woman foetus and newborn infant. Am J Obstet Gynecol, 129:69–103

Lowe CR (1959) Effect of mothers' smoking habits on birth weight of their children. Br Med J, 2:673–676

Mackaness R: *A Little of What You Fancy.* pp 94–95 Fontana Paperbacks, 1985

MacMahon B, Alpert M, Salber EJ: Infant weight and parental smoking habits. AM J Epidemiol, 82:247–261, 1965

Maxwell C and Berry MD (1959) Tobacco hypoglycaemia Ann In Med, 50:1149–1157

McKean HE (1978) Smoking and abortion. N Engl J Med, 298:113–114

Menden EE, Ella VJ, Michael LW, Petering HG (1972) Distribution of cadmium and nickel of tobacco during cigarette smoking. Environ Sci Technol, 6:830

Meyer MB, Jonas BS, Tonascia JA (1976) Perinatal events associated with maternal smoking in pregnancy. Am J Epidemiol, 103:464–476

Meyer MB, Tonascia JA, Buck C (1974) The interrelationship of maternal smoking and increased perinatal mortality with other risk factors. Further analysis of the Ontario Perinatal Mortality Study. Am J Epidemiol, 100:443–452

Meyer MB: How does maternal smoking affect birth weight and maternal weight gain? AM J Obstet, Gyanecol, 131:88–893, 1978

Moiers RL (1973) Relative hypoglycaemia in schizophrenia. pp 452–462, Orthomolecular Psychiatry, Eds: D Hawkins, L Pauling, W.H. Freeman & Co

Moynihan EJ: Trace elements in man. Phil Trans R Soc, London, 288:65 1979

Mulcahy R (1968) Effect of age, parity, and cigarette smoking on outcome of pregnancy. Am J Obstet Gynecol, 101:844–849

Naeye R: The duration of maternal cigarette smoking and placental disorders. Early Hum Dev, 3: 229–237, 1979

Naeye RL (1978) Effects of maternal cigarette smoking on the foetus and placenta. Br J Obstet Gynaecol, 85:732–737

Naeye RL (1981) Influence of maternal cigarette smoking during pregnancy on foetal and childhood growth. Obstet Gynecol, 57:18

Naeye RL and Peters EC (1984) Mental development of children whose mothers smoked during pregnancy. Obstet Gynecol, 64(5):601–607

Naeye RL and Tafari N: Risk factors in Pregnancy, Diseases of the Fetus and Newborn. Baltimore, MD, Williams & Wilkins Co, 1983

Nandi M, Slone D, Jick H, Shapiro S, Lewis GP (1969) Cadmium content of cigarettes. *The Lancet*, 2:1329

Nieburg, P. et al., 'The Foetal Tobacco Syndrome', JAMA, 1985, 253, 2998–2999

O'Lane JM (1963) Some foetal effects of maternal cigarette smoking. Am J Obstet Gynecol, 22:181–184

Ostergaard K (1977) The concentration of cadmium in renal tissue from smokers and non-smokers. Acta Med Scand, 202:193–195

Palmgren B and Wallander B: Cigarettesokning ochabort: kondervativ prospective undersokning av 4312 graviditeter. Lakartidningen, 68: 2611–2616, 1971

Pelkonen O, Karki NT, Koivisto M, Tuimala R, Kauppila A: Maternal cigarette smoking, placental aryl hydrocarbon hydroxylase and neonatal size. Toxicology Letters, 3:331–335, 1979

Pelletier O: Vitamin C and tobacco. In: Hanck A and Ritzel G: Revaluation of Vitamin C. Int J Vit Nutr Res, Suppl:16, 1977

Perinatal Mortality Study, Ten University Teaching Hospitals, Ontario, Canada, Publ: The Ontario Department of Health, Toronto, p 173, 1967

Persson PH, Grennert L, Gensser G, Kullander S: A study of smoking during pregnancy with special reference to fetal growth. Acta Obstet Gynaecol Scand, Suppl. 78:33–39, 1978

Peterson WF, Morense KN, Kaltreider DF (1965) Smoking and prematurity: A preliminary report based on study of 7740 Caucasians. Obstet Gynecol, 26:775–779

Rantakallio P (1978) Relationship of maternal smoking to morbidity and mortality of the child up to age of five. Acta Paediatr Scand, 67:621–631

Rantakallio P (1979) Social background of mothers who smoked during pregnancy and the influence of these factors on the offspring. Soc Sci Med, 13A:423–429

Rantakallio P (1983) A follow-up study up to the age of 14 of children whose mothers smoked during pregnancy. Acta PediatrScand, 72:747

Rantakallio P, Laara E, Isohanni M, Moilanen I: Maternal smoking during pregnancy and delinquency of the offspring an association without causation? Int J Epidemiol, 21: 1106–1113, 1992

Rantakallio P: Groups at risk in low birth weight infants and perinatal mortality. Acta Paediatr Scand, 193 (Suppl): 1–71, 1969

Rantakallio P: The effect of maternal smoking on birth weight and the subsequent health of the child. Early Hum Dev, 2: 371–382, 1978

Rantala ML and Koskimies Am (1986) Semen quality of infertile couples – comparison between smokers and non-smokers. Andrologia, 19:42–46

Ravenholt RT, and Levinski MJ (1965) Smoking during pregnancy. *The Lancet*, 1:961

Ravenholt RT, Levinski MJ, Nellist DJ et al. (1966) Effects of smoking upon reproduction. Am J Obstet Gynecol, 96:267–281

Reinke WA and Henderson M (1966) Smoking and prematurity in the presence of other variables. Arch Environ Health (Chicago) 12:313–316

Roszman TL and Roger AS: The immunosuppressive potential of products derived from cigarette smoke. Am Rev Resp Dis, 108: 1158–1163, 1973

Rush D and Cassano P: Relationship of cigarette smoking and social class to birth weight and perinatal mortality among all births in Britain, 5–10 April, 1970 J Epidemiol Community Health, 37(4): 249–255, 1983

Rush D and Kass EH: Maternal smoking: A reassessment of the association with perinatal mortality. AM J Epidemiol, 96(3): 183–196, 1972

Russell C, Scott TR, Maddison RN (1966) Some effects of smoking in pregnancy. J Obstet Gynaecol Br Commonw, 73:742–746

Rynaerson EH and Moersch FP: Neurologic manifestations of hyperinsulinism and other hypoglycaemic states. J AM Med Assoc, 1196–1199, October 20, 1934

Salzer HM: Relative hypoglycaemia as a cause of neuropsychiatric illness. J Nat Med Assoc, 12–17, January, 1966

Savel LE and Roth E: Effects of smoking in pregnancy: A continuing retrospective study. Obstet Gynaecol, 20: 313–316, 1962

Saxton DW: The behaviour of infants whose mother's smoke in pregnancy. Early Hum Dev, 2: 363 1978

Schroeder HA and Winton WH (1962) Hypertension induced in rats by small doses of cadmium. Am J Physiol, 202:515

Siegers CP, Jungblut JR, Klink F, Oberhauser F (1983) Effects of smoking on cadmium and lead concentrations in human amniotic fluid. Toxicol Letters, 19(3):327–331

Silvette H, Larson PS, Haag HB: Immunological aspects of tobacco smoke. AM J Med Sci, 234: 561–589, 1967

Simpson, W.J., 'A preliminary report on cigarette smoking and the incidence of prematurity', Am J Obstet Gynacol, 1957, 73, 800–815

Sontag LW and Wallace RF: The effects of cigarette smoking during pregnancy upon the fetal heart rate. AM J Obstet Gynaecol, 29:77–83, 1985

Sterling, H.F. et al., 'Passive smoking in utero: its effects on neonatal appearance', British Medical Journal, 1987, 295, 627–628

The Health Consequences of Smoking: A Report of the Surgeon General: U.S. Department of Health Education and Welfare, 1039(1 0):1 23–137, 1973

Thomas W, Holt PG, Keast D: Effect of cigarette smoking on primary and secondary humoral response of mice. Nature, 234: 240–241, 1973

Thomas WR, Holt PG, Keast D: Humoral immune response of mice chronically exposed to cigarette smoke. Arch Environ Health, 30:78–80, 1975

Underwood P, Hester LL. Latiffe T et al: The relationship of smoking to the outcome of pregnancy. Am J Obstet Gynaecol, 91:270–276, 1965

Underwood PB, Kesler KF, O'Lane JM et al. (1967) Parental smoking empirically related to pregnancy outcome. Obestet Gynecol, 29:1–8

US Public Health Service, 'The Health Consequences of Smoking for Women'. A Report of the US Surgeon-General, Office on Smoking and Health, US Dept of Health and Human Services, Rockville Mid, 1980

Viczian M: Ergebnisse von Spermautersuchungen bei Zigarettenrauchen. Z Haut Geschlectskr, 44: 183–187, 1969

Virkkunen M (1984) Reactive hypoglycemic tendency among arsonists. Acta Psychiatr Scand, 69:445–452

Virkkunen M: Reactive hypoglycemic tendency among habitually violent offenders. Nutr Rev, Suppl, 94–103, May, 1986

Ward N.I.(1994) The effect of cadmium from smoking activity (non, active and passive) on the outcome of pregnancy. Foresight Spring Newsletter, pp 0–13,

Ward NI, Watson R, Bryce-Smith D (1987) Placental element levels in relation to foetal development for obstetrically normal births: A study of 37 elements. Evidence for effects of cadmium, lead and zinc on foetal growth, and smoking as a cause of cadmium. Int J Biosocial Res, 9(1):63–81

Wichmann L: The value of semen analysis in predicting pregnancy. Act Universitatis Tamperensis, ser A, vol 346, 1992

Wideman GL, Baird GH, Bolding OT: Ascorbic acid deficiency and premature rupture of membranes. Am J Obstet Gynecol, 88: 592–595, 1964

Wilder J (1943) Psychological problems in hypoglycaemia. Am J Digest Dis, 10, 11:428–435

Wynn M and Wynn A (1981) The Prevention of Handicap of Early Pregnancy Origin, pp 28–33, Foundation for Education and Research in Childbearing, 27 Walpole Street, London SW3

Yager H: Alveolar Cells: depressant effect of cigarette smoke on protein synthesis. Proc Soc Exp Biol Med, 131, 147–150, 1969

Yerusnaimy (1964) Mothers' cigarette smoking and survival of infant. Am J Obstet Gynecol, 88:505–518

Zabriskie JR: Effect of cigarette smoking during pregnancy: Study of 2000 cases. Obsted Gynecol, 21:405–411, 19634039.

ALCOHOL

Abel EL, Sokol RJ: Incidence of Fetal Alcohol Syndrome and economic impact of FAS-related anomalies. Drug Alcohol Depend, 19: 52–70, 1987

Abel EL: Fetal alcohol syndrome and fetal alcohol effects. New York, Plenum Press, 1983

Alcohol and Brain Development. West JR, Ed. New York, Oxford University Press, 1986

Alcohol and Pregnancy Outcome: D D Lewis, Director ALFAWAP Trust Fund Ltd. December 1983. Midwives Chronicle and Nursing Notes.

Alcohol and the Safety of the Unborn Child Woollam *The Journal of the Royal Society for the Promotion of Health.*1981; 101: 241–244

Alcohol and the Unborn Child – The Fetal Alcohol syndrome The National Council of Women Working Party on Alcohol Problems, 36 Lower Sloane Street, London SW1D 8BP, 1980

Alcohol Misconceptions: Lindsay Reid. From Nursing Times, October 14, Volume 88, No. 42, 1992.

Alcoholism: Clinical and Experimental Research, Vol 14, No 5, September/October 1990. Moderate Prenatal Alcohol Exposure: Effects on Child IQ and Learning Problems at Age 7. Years. Ann P Streissguth, Helen M Barr, and Paul D Sampson.

Barnes DE and Walker DW: Prenatal ethanol exposure permanently reduces the number of pyramidal neurons in right hippocampus. Dev Brain Res, 1: 333–340, 1981

Barr HM, Streissguth AP, Darby BL, Sampson PD: Prenatal exposure to alcohol, caffeine, tobacco and aspirin: effects on fine and gross motor performance in 4 year old children. Develop Psychol, 26: 339–348, 1990

Beattie J: fetal Alcohol Syndrome – The incurable hangover. Health Visitor, 54: 468–469, November 1981

Bennet HS, Baggenstgors AH, Butt HR: The testes, breast and prostate in men who die of cirrhosis of liver. Am J Clin Pathol, 20: 814–828, 1950

Blanchard BA, Riley EP, Hannigan JH: Deficits on a spatial navigation task following prenatal exposure to ethanol. Neurotoxiol Teratol. 9: 253–258, 1987

Branchley L and Friedhoff AJ: Biochemical and behavioural changes in rats exposed to alcohol in utero. Ann NY Acad Sci. 273: 328–330, 1976

Brzek A (1987) Alcohol and male fertility (Preliminary report) Andrologia, 19:32–36

Carlsen, H., Guverman, A et al. 'Evidence for decreasing quality of semen during past 50 years.' BMJ 305: 609–13

Chernick V, Childiaeva R, Ioffe S: Maternal alcohol intake and smoking on neonatal electroencephalogram and anthropometric measurements. Am J Obstet Gynecol, 146(1): 41–47, 1983

Chernoff G: A mouse model of the Fetal Alcohol syndrome. Teratology, 11: 14A, 1975

Chernoff GF: The Fetal Alcohol Syndrome in mice: An animal model. Teratology, 15: 223, 1977

Clarren SK and Smith DW: The Fetal Alcohol Syndrome. New England J Med, 298: 1063–1067, 1978

Clarren SK, Avord EC, Sumi SM, Streissguth AP, Smith DW: Brain malformations related to prenatal exposure to ethanol. J Pediatr, 92(1): 64, 1978

Clarren SK: Neuropathology in the Fetal Alcohol Syndrome, In: Alcohol and brain development. Ed: JR West, pp 158–166, New York, Oxford University Press, 1986

Clarren, S K, and Smith, D W (1978) The Foetal Alcohol Syndrome. New England Journal of Medicine 298, 1063–1068

Coles CD, Smith MPH, Fernoff PM, Falek A: Neonatal ethanol withdrawal: characteristics in clinically normal, nondysmorphic neonates. J Pediatr, 105(3): 445–451, 1984

Davies : Zinc, nutrition and health. 1984–85 Yearbook of Nutritional Medicine, pp113–152, Keats Publishing, New Canaan, Connecticut

Dehaene F, Samaille-Villette P, Crepin G, et al: Le syndrome d'alcoolisme fetal dans le nord de la France. Rev L'alcoolisme, 145–148, 1977

Dixit VP, Agarwal M, Lohiya NK (1983) Effects of a single ethanol injection into the vas deferens on the testicular function in rats. Endokrinologie, 67:8–13

Dr Ernest Nobel, Director of the National Institute on Alcohol Abuse and Alcoholism 1976–1978.

Ellis FW and Pick JR: Beagle model of Fetal Alcohol Syndrome. Pharmalogist, 18: 190, 1976

Ferrier PE, Nicod I, Ferrier S: Fetal Alcohol Syndrome. The Lancet, 2: 1496 1973

Flynn A, Miller SI, Mather SS, Golden NL, Sokol RJ, Del Villano BC: Zinc status of pregnant alcoholic women: A determination of fetal outcome. The Lancet, 572–575, March 14, 1981

Forbes R: Alcohol-related birth defects. Publ Health, London, 98: 238–241, 1984

G F Chernoff (1977) The Foetal Alcohol Syndrome in Mice: An Animal Model. Teratology 15: 223–230

Goodlett CR, Kelly SJ, West JR: Early postnatal alcohol exposure that produces high blood alcohol levels impairs development of spatial navigation learning. Psychobiology, 15: 64–74, 1987

Gray JK, Streissguth AP: Memory deficits and life adjustment in adults with Fetal Alcohol Syndrome: a case study. Alc Clin Exp Res, 14: 294 1990

Gusella JL, Fied PA: Effects of maternal social drinking and smoking on offspring at 13 months. Neurobehav Toxicol Teratol, 6: 13–17, 1984

Hanson JW, Jones KL, Smith DW,: Fetal alcohol syndrome: Experience with 41 patients. JAMA, 235: 1458–1460, 1976

Hanson JW, Streissguth AP, Smith DW: The effects of moderate alcohol consumption during pregnancy on fetal growth and morphogenesis. J Pediatr, 92:457–460, 1978

Havlicek V, Childiaeva R, Chernick V: EEC frequency spectrum characteristics of sleep states in infants of alcoholic mothers. Neuropadiatrie, 8: 360–373, 1977

Helwig HI, Hoffer EM, Thulen WC et al: Urinary excretion of zinc in chronic alcoholism. Am J Clin Pathol, 45: 156–159, 1966

Immune Deficiency and Apparently Increased Susceptibility to Infection in the Foetal Alcohol Syndrome. Nutrition Reviews 40: 45–47, 1981.

Ioffe S, Childiaeva R, Chernick V: Prolonged effects of maternal alcohol ingestion on the neonatal electroence-phalogram. Pediatrics, 74: 330–335, 1984

Jameson S: Effects of Zinc deficiency in human reproduction. Acta Med Scand, 593 (suppl); 1–89, 1976

Jones KL and Smith DW: Recognition of Fetal Alcohol Syndrome in early infancy. *The Lancet* 2: 999–1001, 1973

Jones KL and Smith DW: The Fetal Alcohol Syndrome Teratology, 12:1 1975

Jones KL, Smith DW, Hanson JW: The Fetal Alcohol Syndrome: Clinical delineation. Ann N.Y. Acad Sci, 272: 130 1976

Jones KL, Smith DW, Streissguth AP et al: incidence of Fetal Alcohol Syndrome in offspring of chronically alcoholic women. Pediatr Res, 8: 440–466, 1974

Jones KL, Smith DW, Streissguth AP, Myrianthoupolis NC: Outcome in offspring of chronic alcoholic women. *The Lancet*, 1076–1078, 1974

Judges 13: 7

K L Jones, D W Smith, C N Ulleland and A P Streissguth (1973) Pattern of Malformation in Offspring of Alcoholic Mothers. Lancet 1: 1267–1271

Kaufmann, Matthew. In: Hodgkinson, Neville, 'Alcohol Threat to Babies', *Sunday Times*, 31 January 1988

Kelly SJ, Black AC, West JR: Changes in the muscarininc: Cholinergic receptors in the hippocampus of rats exposed to ethyl alcohol during the brain spurt. J Pharm Exp Ther, 249: 798–04, 1989

Kronick JB: Teratogenic effects of ethyl alcohol administered to pregnant mice. Am J Obstet Gynecol, 124:676–680, 1976

Kucheria K, Saxena R, Mohan D (1985) Semen analysis in alcohol dependence syndrome. Andrologia, 17:558–563

Landesman-Dwyer S, Keller L, Streissguth AP: Naturalistic observations of newborns; effects of maternal alcohol intake. Alc Clin Exp Res, 2: 171–177, 1978

Landesman-Dwyer S, Ragozin AS. Little RE: Behavioural correlates of prenatal alcohol exposure; A four-year follow-up study. Neurobehav Toxicol Teratol, 3: 187–193, 1981

Landesman-Dwyer S, Sackett GP, Metzoff A: Prenatal nicotine and alcohol exposure and sleep-wake patterns in infants. Paper presented at Society Research in Child Development, Detroit, MI, April 1983

Laurence KM, James N, Miller MH, Tennant HB, Campbell H: Double-blind randomized controlled trial of folate treatment before conception to prevent recurrence of neural-tube defects. Brit Med J, 282:1509–1511, 1981

Lemoine P, Harousseau H, Borteyru J-P, Menuet J-C: Les enfants de parents alcoholiques: anomalies observes a propos de 127 cas. Quest Medical, 25: 476–482, 1968

Lewis DD: Alcohol & Pregnancy outcome. Midwives Chronicle & Nursing Notes, 420–423, Dec. 1983

Library, The Royal College of Physicians, 1725

Lipsett MB: Physiology and pathology of the Leydig cell. In: MC Bleich, MJN Moore, Eds. Seminars in Medicine, Engl J Med, 85: 682–688, 1980

Little RE: Moderate alcohol use during pregnancy and decreased infant birth weight. Am J Publ Health, 67(12): 1154–1156, 1977

Little, B B, Snell, L M, Rosenfield, C R, Gilstrapp, L C, and Gant, N F (1990) Failure to Recognize Foetal Alcohol Syndrome in Newborn Infants. American Journal of Diseases in Children 144, 1142–1146

Majewski F, Bierich JR, Loser H, Michaelis R, et al: Zur Klinik und Pathogenese der Alkoholemybryopathie uber 68 Falle. Munch Med Wochensch. 118:1635–1642, 1976

Martin DC, Martin JC, Streissguth AP, Lund CA: Sucking frequency and amplitude in newborns as a function of maternal drinking and smoking. In: Currents in Alcoholism, Vols,5. Ed: M Galanter pp359–366, New York, Grune & Stratton, 1979

Martin JC, Martin DC, Lund CA, Streissguth AP: Maternal alcohol ingestion and cigarette smoking and their effects on newborn conditioning. Alc Clin Exp Res, 1: 234–247, 1977

Martin JM: The Fetal Alcohol Syndrome: Recent findings, Alc Health And Res World, 1(3): 8 1977

Masters WH and Johnson VE: Human Sexual Inadequacy. Boston, Little, Brown and Company, 1970

Mendelson JM, Ellingboe J, Mello NK, Kuehnli J (1978) Effects of alcohol on plasma testosterone and luteinizing hormone levels. Alc Clin Exp Res, 2:255–258

Mulvihill JJ and Yeager AM: Fetal Alcohol Syndrome. Teratology, 13: 345 1976

Mulvihill JJ, Klimas JT, Stokes DC, Risemberg HM: Fetal Alcohol Syndrome: seven new cases. AM J Obstet Gynecol, 125(7): 937 1976

National Institute of Alcohol Abuse and Alcoholism (1977) Critical Review of the Foetal Alcohol Syndrome. Rockville MD, Alcohol, Drug Abuse and Mental Health Administration

Neurotoxicology and Teratology: Vol 11 pp 493–507. Neurobehavioral Effects of Prenatal Alcohol: Part III. PLS Analyses of Neuropsychological Tests. Ann P Streissguth, Fred L Bookstein, Paul D Sampson and Helen M Barr.

Noble EF: Fetal Alcohol syndrome. Drug Survival News, 6: 3, Nov–Dec, 1977

Noonan JA: Congenital heart disease in Fetal Alcohol Syndrome. Am J Cardiol, 37:160 1976

O'Connor MJ, Brill NJ, Sigman M: alcohol use in primiparous women older than 30 years of age; Relation to infant development. Pediatrics, 78(3): 444–450, 1986

Olegard R, Sabel KG, Aronsen M, Sandin B, et al.: Effects on the child of alcohol abuse during pregnancy. Acta Paediatr Scand Suppl, 275: 112–121, 1979

Papara-Nicholson D, Telford IR: Effects of alcohol in reproduction and fetal development in guinea pig. anat Rec, 127: 438–439, 1957

Pettigrew AG, Hutchinson I: Effects of alcohol on functional development of the auditory pathway in the brainstem of infants and chick embryos. In: Mechanism of alcohol damage in utero. Eds: M O'Connor and J Whelan, pp 26–46, Ciba Foundation Symposium 105, London, Pitman Publishing, 1984

Pieroq S, Chandauasu O, Wexler I: Withdrawal symptoms in infants with Fetal Alcohol Syndrome. J Pediatr, 90(4): 630 1977

Plant, Moira, Reported in: Gill, Kerry, 'Alcohol "safe in pregnancy"' The Times, 4 Nov 1987

Prof David W Smith, University of Washington in Seattle with references from Hanson et al, J Amer Med Assn, 1976, 235, 1458.

Publ. Hlth, Lond (1984) 98, 238–241. Alcohol Related Birth Defects. Ronald Forbes, Hon. Executive Director, Alfawap Trust Fund Ltd. From The Society of Community Medicine

Quelette EM, Rosett HL, Rosman NP, Weiner L: Adverse effects on offspring of maternal alcohol abuse during pregnancy. N Eng J Med, 297(10): 528–530, 1977

Quelette EM, Rosett HL: A pilot prospective study of the Fetal Alcohol Syndrome at the Boston City Hospital: Part II, The Infants. Ann N.Y. Acad Sci, 273: 123–129, 1976

R V Patwardhan, S Schenker, G I Henderson, N N Abou-Mourad and A M Hoyumpa Jr (1981) Short Term and Long Term Ethanol Administration Inhibits the Placental Uptake and Transport of Valine in Rats. J. Lab. Clin. Med 98: 251–262

Randall CM, Taylor WJ, Walker DW: Ethanol-induced malformations in mice. Alc Clin Exp Res, 1: 219–223, 1977

Randall CM, Taylor WJ, Walker DW: Teratogenic effects of in utero ethanol exposure, Alcohol and Opiates; In: Neurochemical and Behavioural Mechanisms K Blum, Bard DL, MG Hamilton, Eds, New York Academy Press, pp. 91–017, 1977

Report from the Select Committee on 'Inquiry into Drunkenness', House of Commons Library, 5 August, 1834

Riley EP, Barron S, Hannigan JP: Response inhibition deficits following prenatal alcohol exposure: A comparison to the effects of hippocampal lesion in rats. In; Alcohol and Brain Development, J.R. West, Ed., London, Oxford University Press, 1986

Rosett HL, Snyder P, Sander LW et al.: Effects of maternal drinking on neonate state regulation. Dev Med Child Neurol, 21(4): 464–473, 1979

Rosett HL, Snyder P, Sander LW, Lee A et al.: Effects of maternal drinking on neonatal state regulation. Dev Med Child Neurol, 21(4): 464–473, 1979

Sampson PD, Streissguth AP, Barr HM, Bookstein FL: Neurobehavioural effects of prenatal alcohol; Part II, Partial least squares analysis. Neurotoxicology and Teratology, 11: 477–491, 1987

Sander LW, Snyder P, Rosett HL et al.: Effects of alcohol intake during pregnancy on newborn stat regulation; A progress report. Alc Clin Exp Res, 1(3): 233–241, 1977

Sandor GCS, Smith DF, MacLeod PM: Cardiac malformations in the Fetal Alcohol Syndrome. J Pediatr, 98(5): 771–773, 1981

Sandor S, Elias S: The influence of acetyl-alcohol on the development of the chick embryo. Rev Roum Embryol Cytol (Ser Embryol) 5: 51–76, 1968

Schenker S, Becker HC, Randall CL, Henderson GI: Fetal Alcohol Syndrome; Current status and pathogenesis. Alc Clin Exp Res, 14: 635–647, 1990

Smith DW, Jones KL, Hanson JW: Perspectives on the cause and frequency of Fetal Alcohol Syndrome. Ann N.Y. Acad Sci, 173: 138 1976

Smith DW: Alcohol effects in fetus. In: Fetal Drug Syndrome; Effects of Ethanol and Hydantoins. Pediatrics I Review 1, American Academy of Pediatrics, 1979

Smith DW: *Mothering your Unborn Baby*. W.B. Saunders Co, Philadelphia, 1979

Spohr HL, Steinhausen HC: Follow-up studies of children with Fetal Alcohol Syndrome. Neuropediatrics, 18: 13–17, 1987

Spohr H-L, Williams J, Steinhausen H-C,: Prenatal alcohol exposure and long-term development consequences. *The Lancet*, 341: 908–910, 1993

Stock DL, Streissguth AP, Martin DC: Neonatal sucking as an outcome variable: Comparison of quantitive and clinical assessments. Early Human Development, 10: 273–278, 1985

Streissguth AP, Aase JM, Sterling MD, Clarren K et al: Fetal Alcohol Syndrome in adolescents and adults. JAMA, 265(15): 1961–1967, 1991

Streissguth AP, Barr HM, Martin DC, Herman CS: Effects of maternal alcohol, nicotine and caffeine use during pregnancy on infant mental and motor development at 8 months. Alc Clin Exp Res, 4(2): 152–164, 1980

Streissguth AP, Barr HM, Martin DC: Alcohol exposure in utero and functional deficits in children during the first four years of life. In: Mechanism of alcohol damage in utero, Eds: R Porter, M O'Connor, J Whelan, Ciba Foundation Symposium 105, London, Pitman Publishing, 1984

Streissguth AP, Barr HM, Sampson PD, Bookstein FL, Darby BL: Neurobehavioural effects of prenatal alcohol; Part 1, Research Strategy. (Review of the literature) Neurotoxicology and Teratology, 11; 461–476, 1989

Streissguth AP, Barr HM, Sampson PD, Darby BL, Martin DC: IQ at age four in relation to maternal alcohol use and smoking during pregnancy. Dev Psychol, 25(1): 3–11, 1989

Streissguth AP, Barr HM, Sampson PD, Parrish-Johnson J et al.: Attention, distraction and reaction time at age 7 years and prenatal alcohol exposure. Neurobehav Toxicol Tereatol, 8(6): 717–725, 1986

Streissguth AP, Barr HM, Sampson PD: Moderate prenatal alcohol exposure; Effects on child IQ and learning problems at age 7½ years. Alco Clin Exp Res, 14(5): 66269, 1990

Streissguth AP, Bookstein FL, Sampson PD, Barr HM: Neurobehavioural effects of prenatal alcohol; Part III, PLS analyses of neuropsychologic tests. Neurotoxicology and Teratology, 11: 493–507, 1989

Streissguth AP, Herman CS, Smith DW: Intelligence, behaviour and dysmorphongenesis in Fetal Alcohol Syndrome: A report on 20 patients. J Pediatr, 92: 363–367, 1978

Streissguth AP, Herman CS, Smith DW: Stability of intelligence in Fetal Alcohol Syndrome. Alc Clin Exp Res, 2: 165–170, 1978

Streissguth AP, LaDue RA: Fetal Alcohol Syndrome and Fetal Alcohol Effects: Teratogenic causes of mental retardation and developmental disabilities. In: Toxic substances and mental retardation, Ed SR Schroeder. Washington DC, American Association on Mental Deficiency, 1–32 1987

Streissguth AP, Martin DC, Barr HM, Sandman BM et al.: Intrauterine alcohol and nicotine exposure; Attention and reaction in 4 year old children. Dev Psychol, 20: 533–541, 1984

Streissguth AP, Martin DC, Martin JC, Barr HM: The Seattle longitudial prospective study on alcohol and pregnancy. Neurobehav Toxicol Teratol, 3: 223–233, 1981

Streissguth AP, Sampson PS, Barr HM:Neurobehavioural dose-response effects of prenatal alcohol exposure in humans from infancy to adulthood. In: Prenatal Abuse of Licit and Illicit Drugs, Ed, DE Hutchings, New York Academy of Sciences, 562: 145–158, 1989

Streissguth AP: Fetal Alcohol syndrome: An epidemiological perspective. Am J Epidemiol, 107(6): 467–478, 1978

Streissguth AP: Fetal Alcohol Syndrome: Early and long-term consequences. In: Problems of the 53rd Annual Scientific Meeting

(NIDA Research Monograph No: 119) Ed, L Harris, Rockville, MD, U.S. Department of Health and Human Services. 1991

Streissguth AP: Prenatal alcohol-induced brain damage and long term postnatal consequences. Alc Clin Exp Res, 14(5): 648–649, 1990

Streissguth AP: Psychologic handicaps in children with Fetal Alcohol Syndrome. Ann N.Y. Acad Sci, 273: 140 1976

Streissguth AP: The 1990 Betty Ford Lecture: What every community should know about drinking during pregnancy and the lifelong consequences for society. Substance Abuse, 12(3): 114–127, 1991

Streissguth AP: The behavioural teratology of alcohol; performance, behavioural and intellectual deficits in prenatally exposed children. In: Alcohol and brain development, Ed:JR West pp3–44, New Oxford, Oxford University Press, 1986

Streissguth P, Barr HM, Martin DC: Maternal alcohol use and neonatal habituation assessed with Brazelton Scale. Child Development, 54: 1109–1118, 1983

Streissguth, A P (1992) Foetal Alcohol Syndrome: Early and Long Term Consequences.

Streissguth, A P, Aase, J M, Clarren, S K, Randels, S P, LaDue, R A, and Smith, D F. Foetal Alcohol Syndrome in Adolescents and Adults. The Journal of the American Medical Association 265 (15): 1961–1967, 1991.

Streissguth, A P, Clarren, S K, and Jones, K L (1985) Natural History of the Foetal Alcohol Syndrome: A Ten-Year Follow Up of Eleven Patients. Lancet 2, 85–92

Sullivan JF and Lankford HG: Urinary excretion of zinc in alcoholic and post-alcoholic cirrhosis. Am J Clin Nutr, 10: 153–157, 1962

Tenbrink MS and Buchin SY: Fetal Alcohol Syndrome: Report of a case. JAMA, 232(11):1144, 1975

The Foetal Alcohol Syndrome and Placental Transport of Valine, From Nutrition Reviews, Vol 40, No. 2/February 1982.

The Lancet, March 14th 1981. Zinc Status of Pregnant Alcoholic Women: A Determinant of Foetal Outcome.

The Role of Zinc Deficiency in Foetal Alcohol Syndrome, From Nutrition Reviews, Vol 40, No. 2/February 1982.

The Role of Zinc Deficiency in Foetal Alcohol Syndrome. Nutrition Reviews 40: 43–45, 1981.

Tittmar H-G: Some effects of alcohol in reproduction. Br J Alcohol and Alcoholism, 13: 3 1978

Tze WJ and Lee M: Adverse Effects of Maternal Alcohol Consumption on Pregnancy and Foetal Growth in Rats. *Nature*, 257: 479–480, 1975

Vallee BL, Wacker WE, Bartholonay AF, Robin ED: Zinc metabolism in hepatic dysfunction; serum Zinc concentrations in Laenne's cirrhosis and their validation by sequential analysis. New Engl J Med, 135: 403–408, 1956

van Thiel DM, Lester R, Sherins RJ (1974) Hypogonadism in alcoholic liver disease: Evidence for a double defect. Gastroenterology, 67:1188–1199

van Thiel OH, Gavaler JS, Lester R, Goodman MD (1975) Alcohol induced testicular atrophy: An experimental model for hypogonadism occurring in chronic alcoholic man. Gastroenterology, 69:326–332

Vorhees CV, Mollnow E: Behavioural teratogenesis; Long term influences on behaviour from early exposure to environmental agents. In: *Handbook on infant development*, 2nd edition, Ed: JD Osofsky, pp913–971, New York, Wiley, 1987

Weinberg J: Effects of ethanol and maternal nutrition status on fetal development. Alc Clin Exp Res, 9: 49–55, 1985

West JR, Dewey SL, Pierce DR, Black AC: Prenatal and early postnatal exposure to ethanol permanently alters the rat hippocampus. In: Mechanisms of alcohol damage in utero. CIBA Foundation Symposium, 105. London, Pitman, 1984

Wichman L: The value of semen analysis in predicting pregnancy. Acta Universitatis, ser A Vol 346, p5, 1992

Woollam DHM: Alcohol and the safety of the unborn child. R.S.H. 6: 241–244, 1981

Wright JT, Waterson EJ, Barrison IG et al.: Alcohol consumption, pregnancy and low birth weight. *The Lancet*, 663–665, March 26, 1983

Ylikahri R, Huttunen M, Harkonen M, Adlercreutz H (1974) Hangover and testosterone. Br Med J, 2:445

Chapter 5: Contraception

Bostoff J, Gamlin L, 1989, *The Complete Guide to Food Allergy and Intolerance*, New York Crown Publishers

Bryce-Smith D, 1981, Environmental Influences on Parental Development, Thessaloniks Conference

Grant ECG, 1994, *Sexual Chemistry, Understanding Our Hormones, the Pill and HRT*, London, Cedar. ISBN 0-7493-1363-3

Oberleas D, Caldwell DF, Prasad AS, 1972 International Journal of Neurobiology, Academic Press

Passwater R and Cranton E, 1983, *Trace Elements, Hair Analysis and Nutrition*, New Conran Keats Publishing. ISBN 0-87983-265-7

Pfeiffer, *Zinc and Other Micronutrients*, 1978. New Conran, Keats Publishing Co. LCCC No. 77–91327

Saner G et al, 1985, Hair manganese concentrations in newborns and their mothers. *American Journal of Clinical Nutrition* 41

Scheibner V, 2000, Behavioral Problems in Childhood, the Link to Vaccination, Griffin Press, Netley, South Australia. ISBN 0-9578007-0-3

Underwood EJ, 1977, Trace Elements in Human and Animal Nutrition, *New York Academic Press*. ISBN 0-12-709065-7

Vallee B, 1965, Chapter Zinc, Mineral Metabolism, Vol II B., London Academic Press

Ward NI, 1995, Preconceptual Care and Pregnancy Outcome, *Journal of Nutritional and Environmental Medicine* 5

Williams RJ, 1973, *Nutrition Against Disease*, London, Bantam LCCCN 70–166201

Chapter 6: Genitourinary Infections

Acheson, D (1989) Letter from the Chief Medical Officer on listeria and food. Department of Health and Social Security. Letter ref PL/CMo (89) 3, 16 February

Alani MD, Darougar S, Mac D, Burns DC.et al (1977) Isolation of Chlamydia trachomatis from the male urethra. Br J Vener Dis, 53:88–92

Alary, Michael, Roly, Jean R., et al., 'Strategy for screening pregnant women for chlamydial infection in a low prevalence area'. Obstet Gynecol 1993, 82: 399–404

Alder, M.W., ABC of Sexually Transmitted Diseases, London, BMA, 1984, 48

Alexander ER, Chandler JW, Pheiffer TA et al (1977) Prospective study of perinatal Chlamydia trachomatis infection. In: Hobson DC, Holmes KK, Eds. Nongonococcal urethritis and related infections. Am Soc Microbiology Washington D.C. 148

Arth C, Von Schmidt B, Grossman M, Schachter J (1978) Chlamydial pneumonitis. J Pediatrics, 93: 447–449

Aspock, H., 'Toxoplasmosis'. In: Prenatal and perinatal infections. EURO reports and Studies, 93, 43–51

Barbacci MB, Spence MR, Kappus EW et al (1986) Post-abortal endometritis and isolation of Chlamydia trachomatis. Obstet Gynecol, 68:686–690

Beem MO, Saxon EM (1977) Respiratory tract colonization and a distinctive pneumonia syndrome in infants infected with Chlamydia trachomatis. N Engl J Mod, 296: 306–310

Berger RE, Alexander ER, Monda GD, Ansell J et al (1978) Chlamydia trachomatis as a cause of acute "idiopathic" epididymitis. N Engl J Med, 298: 301–304

Blackwell, Anona L., Thomas, Philip D., et al., 'Health gains from screening for infection of the lower genital tract in women attending for termination of pregnancy', Lancet, 1993, 342: 206–210

Blattner, Russel J. 'The role of viruses in congenital defects', Am J Dis Child, 1974, 128, 781–786

Bowie WR, Wang SP, Alexander ER, Floyd J et al (1977) Etiology of nongonococcal urethritis: Evidence of Chlamydia trachomatis and Ureaplasma urealyticum. J Clin Invest, 59: 735–742

Braun P, Lee YH, Kiem JO et al (1971) Birth weight and genital mycoplasmas in pregnancy. N Engl J Med, 284: 167–171

Brooks, Geoffrey F., 'Neisseria gonorrhea infections in children'. In: Gonaccal Infections, Geoffrey F, Brooks and Elizabeth A. Donegan, eds. E. Arnold, 1985, 132

Brooks, op. cit., 133–134

Brown, Zane A., et al., 'Effects on infants of a first episode of genital herpes during pregnancy', New Eng J Med 1987, 317, 1246–1251

Brunham RC, Binns B, McDowell J, Paraskevas M (1986) Chlamydia trachomatis infection in women with ectopic pregnancy. Obstet Gynecol, 67: 722–726

Brunham RC, MacLean IW, Binns B et al (1985) Chlamydia trachomatis: its role in tubal infertility. J Infect Dis, 152: 1275–1282

Cassell, Gail, ed. 'Ureaplasmas of humans: with emphasis on maternal and neonatal infections'. Pediatric Infectious Disease, 1986, 5, 6, Suppl

Cates W, Rolfs RT, Aral SO (1990) Sexually transmitted diseases, pelvic inflammatory disease and infertility: an epidemiologic update. Epidemiol Rev, 12: 199–220

Cates W., Wasserheit JN (1991) Genital chlamydial infections: Epidemiology and Reproductive sequelae. Am J Obstet Gynecol. 164:1771–1781

Catterall RD (1981) Biological effects of sexual freedom. The Lancet, 315–319, February 7

Cengiz, Dincer, Rotc, Firat, Soylemez, Firide, 'Tackling the threat of toxoplasmosis', Midwife Health Visitor and Community Nurse, 1991, 27(7): 199–20

Chaim W, Sarov B, Sarov I, Piura B et al (1989) Serum IgH and IgA antibodies to chlamydia in ectopic pregnancies. Contraception, 40: 59–71

Chandler JW, Alexander ER, Pheiffer TA et al (1977) Opthalmia neonatorum associated with maternal chlamydial infection. Trans Am Acad Opthalmol Otolaryngol, 83: 302–308

Chang MJ, Rodriquez WD, Mohla C (1982) Chlamydia trachomatis in otitis media. Pediatr Infect Dis, 1: 95–97

Cherry, Sheldon H., Planning Ahead for Pregnancy, London, Viking, 1987, 75

Chow JM, Yonekura MU, Richwald GA et al (1990) The association between Chlamydia trachomatis and ectopic pregnancy: A matched-pair, case-control study. JAMA, 263: 3164–3167

Chrystie, Ian, Summer, Debsorah, et al., 'Screening of pregnant women for evidence of current hepatitis B infection: selective or universal?', Health Trends 1992, 24(1): 13–15

Corbett, Margaret-Ann and Jerrilyn, H. Meyer, *The Adolescent and Pregnancy*, 1987, Boston, Oxford, Blackwell Scientific Publications, 1987

Crook, William G. (1983) *The Yeast Connection*, Professional Books

Dahle, A.J., et al., 'Progressive hearing impairment in children with congenital cytomegalovirus, infection', J Speech Hear Dis, 1970, 44, 220

Davies, Stephen and Stewart, Alan, Nutritional Medicine, London, Pan, 1987, 360

Department of Health and Social Security: Sexually transmitted diseases. In: On the state of public health: The annual report of the Chief Medical Officer of the DHSS for the year 1978, London HMSO, 6, 1980

Dunlop EMC (1980) Chlamydial infection; terminology, disease and treatment. Recent advances in sexually transmitted diseases, Churchill Livingstone, Edinburgh, London, New York, 101–119

Dunlop EMC, Waughan-Jackson JD, Darougar S, Jones Chlamydial infection: incidence in "non-specific" urethritis. Br J Vener Dis, 48: 425–428, 1972

Eliard T, Brorsson JE, Hamark B et al (1976) Isolation of chlamydia trachomatis infection in patients with acute salpingitis. Scand J Infect Dis., 9: 82–85

Embil JA, Ozere RU, MacDonald SW (1978) Chlamydia trachomatis and pneumonia in infants: report of two cases. Canad Med Assoc J, 119: 1199

Embree JE, Krause VW, Embil JA, MacDonald S (1980) Placental infection with Mycoplasma hominis and Ureaplasma urealyticum: Clinical correlation. Obstet Gynecol, 56: 475

Fine, P.E.M., et al. (1985) 'Infectious diseases during pregnancy: a follow-up study of the long-term effects of exposure to viral infection in utero. Studies on medical and population subjects'. HMSO

Foster RK, Dawson CR, Schachter J (1970) Late follow-up of patients with neonatal inclusion conjunctivitis. Am J Opthalmol, 69: 467

Friberg J, Gnarpe I: Mycoplasma in human reproductive failure. Am J Obstet Gynecol, 23–26 May, 1973

Friberg, J., Gnarpe, H., 'Mycoplasma and human reproductive failure', Am J Obstet Gynaecol, 1973, 116, 23–26

Frommell CT, Bruhn FW, Schwatzman DJ (1977) Isolation of Chlamydia trachomatis in infant lung tissues. N Engl J Mod, 296: 1150–1152

Frommell GT, Rothenberg R, Wang SP et al (1979) Chlamydial infection of mothers and their infants. J Pediatrics, 95: 28–32

Gellin, B.G.B., Broome, C.V., 'Listeriosis' JAMA, 1989, 261: 1313–1319

Gibbs, Ronald S., 'Microbiology of the female genital tract', Am J Obstet and Gynecol, 1987, 156, 491–495

Grant, Ellen, Personal Communication, April 1988

Grant, Ellen, The Bitter Pill, London, Corgi, 1975, 174

Hallberg A, MUrdh P-A, Persson K, Ripa T (1979) Pneumonia associated with Chlamydia trachomatis infection in an infant. Acta Paediatr Scand, 68: 765–767

Hammerschlag MR. Anderka M, Semine DZ et al (1979) Prospective study of maternal and infantile infection with Chlamydia trachomatis. Pediatrics, 64:142–148

Hammerschlag MR. Hammerschlag PE, Alexander ER (1980) The role of Chlamydia trachomatis in middle ear effusion in children. Pediatrics, 66: 615–617

Hammerschlag MR: Chlamydial pneumonia in infants.

Hanshaw, J.B., 'Developmental abnormalities associated with congenital cytomegalovirus infection', Adv Teratology, 1970, 4, 62

Hardy, P.H., et al., 'Prevalence of six sexually transmitted disease agents among pregnant inner-city adolescents and pregnancy outome', Lancet. 1984, 2, 333–337

Harrison HR, English MG, Lee CK, Alexander ER (1978) Chlamydia trachomatis infant pneumonitis: comparison with matched controls and other infant pneumonitis. N Engl J Med, 298: 702–708

Harrison HR, Taussing LM, Fulginitis V (1982) Chlamydia trachomatis and chronic respiratory disease in children. Pediatr Infect Dis, 1: 29–33

Harrison RF, Hurley R, deLouvois J (1979) Genital mycoplasmas and birth weight in offspring of primigravid women. Am J Obstet Gynecol, 133: 201–203

Hartford SL, Silva PD, DiZehera GS et al (1987) Serologic evidence of prior chlamydial infection in patients with tubal ectopic pregnancy and contralateral tubal disease. Fertil Steril, 47: 118–121

Hay, M., 'Neonatal listeriosis and ventriculomegaly: two case reports', Maternal and Child Health, 1989, 14(1): 14–15

Hay, Pillip E., Lamont, Ronald F., et al., 'Abnormal bacterial colonisation of the genital tract and subsequent preterm delivery and late miscarriage', BMJ 1994, 308: 295–8

Health Education Council, 'Herpes. What it is and how to Cope', Health Education Council 1985

Health Education Council, Guide to a Healthy Sex Life, 1985, 22

Heggie AD, Lumicao GG, Stuart LA et al (1981) Chlamydia trachomatis infection in mothers and infants. AJDC, 135: 507–511

Hollingworth, Barton, et al., 'Colposcopy of women with cervical HPV type 16 infection but normal cytology', Lancet, 1987, 2, 1148

Holmes KK, Hansfield HH, Wang SF, Wentworth BB et al (1975) Etiology of non-gonococcal urethritis. N Engl J Med, 292: 1199–2005

Hurley, Rosalind. Reported in Davies, S., op. cit., 364

Israel, K.S., et al., 'Neonatal and childhood gonococcal infections', Clin Obs Gyn, 1975, 18, 143–151

Jacob, Martha, et al., 'A forgotten factor in pelvic inflammatory disease: infection in the male partner', British Medical Journal, 1987, 294, 869

Jacobs NF, Arum ES, Krauss SJ (1977) Nongonococcal urethritis: the role of Chlamydia trachomatis. Ann of Int Med, 86: 313–314

Kane JL, Woodland RM, Forsey T et al (1984) Evidence of chiamydial infection in infertile women with and without fallopian tube obstruction. Fertil Steril, 42:832–838

Kelver ME, Ngamani M (1989) Chlamydial serology in women with tubal infertility. Int J Fertil, 43: 42–45

Kudsin, RB, Driscoll SC, Pelletier PA (1981) Ureaplasma urealyticum incriminated perinatal morbidity and mortality. Science, 213:474

Lindsay, S., Alger, Farley, John J., et al., 'Interactions of human immunodeficiency virus infection and pregnancy', Obstet Gynaecol 1993, 82: 787–96

Mardh, P.H., 'Medical chlamydiology: a position paper'. Scandinavian Journal of Infectious Diseases (supp 32), 1981, 3–8

Mardh, P.H., et al., 'Endometriosis caused by chlamydia trachomatis'. Br J Vener Dis, 1981, 57–191

Martin DH, Koutsky L, Eschenbach DA et al (1982) Prematurity and perinatal mortality in pregnancies complicated by maternal Chlamydia trachomatis infections. JAMA, 247: 1585–1588

McCormick WM, Rosner B, Lee YH (1973) Colonization with genital mycoplasmas in women. Am J Epidemiol 97: 240–245

Miller Br, Ahrons S, Laurin J, MUrdh P-a (1982) Pelvic infection after elective abortion associated with Chlamydia trachomatis. Obstet Gynecol., 59:210–13

Miller PR. Taylor-Robinson D, Furr PM, Toft B, Allen J (1985) Serological evidence that chlamydia and mycoplasmas are involved in infertility of women. J Reprod Fertil, 73:237–240

Minassian SS, Wu CH, Jungkind D, Gorcial B et al (1990) Chlamydial antibody as determined with an enzyme-linked immunosorbent assay, in tubal factor infertility. J Reprod Med, 35: 141–145

Minkoff, H., Nanda, D., et al., 'AIDS-related complex: follow-up of mothers, children and subsequently born siblings', Obstet Gynaecol, 1987, 69: 288–91

Moore, D.E., et al., 'Association of Chlamydia trachomatis with tubal infertility', Fert Ster, 1980, 32, 303–304

N Engl J Med, 298: 1083 1978

Nevison, Jenny. Unpublished paper. Details available through Foresight.

Nicholas, N.S., Urinary tract infections in pregnancy, Maternal and Child Health, October, 294–297

Noritoshi, Takei, Sham, Pak, et al., 'Prenatal exposure to influenza and the development

Oriel JD, Reeve P, Wright JT, Owen J (1976) Chlamydial infection in male urethra. Br J Vener Dis, 52: 46–51

Osser J, Persson K (1984) Post-abortal pelvic infection associated with Chlamydia trachomatis and the influence of humoral immunity. Am J Obstet Gynecol: 150;699–703

Ovigstad E, Skang K, Jerve F et al (1983) Pelvic inflammatory disease associated with Chlamydia trachomatis infection after therapeutic abortion. Br J Vener Dis, 59:189–192

Padjen A, Nash LD, Fiscelli T (1984) The relationship between chlamydial antibodies and involuntary infertility. Fertil Steril, 41: 975–985

Pierroud HM, Miedzbrodzka K (1978) Chlamydial infection of the urethra in men. Br J Vener Dis, 54: 45–49

Quinn PA, Shewchuck MD, Shuber J et al (1983) Serologic evidence of urealyticum infection in women with spontaneous pregnancy loss. Am J Obstet Gynecol, 145:245–249

Rees E, Tait IA, Hobson D, Byng RE, Johnson FWA (1977) Neonatal conjunctivitis caused by Neisseria gonorrhea and Chlamydia trachomatis. Br J Vener Dis, 53: 173–179

Rees E, Tait IA, Hobson D, Karayiarinis P, Lee N (1981) Persistence of chlamydial infection after treatment for neonatal conjunctivitis. Arch Dis in Childhood, 56: 193–198

Reniers J, Collet M, Frost E et al (1989) Chlamydial antibodies and tubal infertility. Int j Epidemiol, 18: 261–263

Ross JM, Furr PM, Taylor-Robinson D et al (1981) The effect of genital mycoplasmas on human growth. Br J Obstet Gynaecol, 88: 749–755

Royal College of Physicians Committee on Genitourinary Medicine (1987) Chlamydial diagnostic services in the United Kingdom and Eire: current facilities and perceived needs. Genitourin Med 63: 371–374

Sack, Stephen L., *The Truth About Herpes*, Vancouver, Verdant Press, 1986, 87

Sacks, op. cit., 78–80

Scarrel, P.M., Pratt, K.A. 'Symptomatic gonorrhea during pregnancy', Obstet Gynaecol, 1968, 32, 670–673

Schachter J, Grossman M, Holt J et al (1979) Infection with Chlamydia trachomatis: Involvement of multiple anatomic sites in neonates.J Infect Dis, 139: 232–234

SchachterJ, Grossman M, Holt J et al: Prospective study of chlamydial infections in neonates. *The Lancet*, 377–380, August 25, 1979

Schacter, Julius and Grossman, Moses, 'Chlamydia', Infectious Diseases of the Foetus and Newborn Infant, Jack Remington and Jerome O., Klein, eds. W.B. Saunders Co., 1983

Schaefer C, Harrison R, Boyce T, Lewis M: Illnesses in infants born to women with Chlamydia trachomatis infection. AJDC, 139: 127–133, February, 1985

Schneider, A., et al., 'Colposcopy is superior to cytology for the detection of early genital human papillomavirus infection', Obstet Gynaecol, 1988, 71, 236–241

Schofield, C.B.S, *Sexually Transmitted Diseases*, London, Churchill Livingstone, 1972

Sellors JW, Mahony JB, Chrnesky MA et al (1988) Tubal factor infertility: an association with prior chlamydial infection and asymptomatic salpingitis. Fertil Steril, 49: 451–457

Shermark I, Daling J, Stergachis A et al (1990) Sexually transmitted disease and tubal pregnancy. Sex Trans Dis, 17: 115–121

Shurin PA, Albert S, Rosner B et al (1975) Chorioamnionitis and colonization of the newborn infant with genital mycoplasmas. N Engl J Med, 293: 5–8

Simpson, Joe Leigh, 'Foetal Wastage'. In: Obstetrics, Normal and Problem Pregnancies, Gabbe, Steven, et al., eds., New York, Churchil Livingstone, 1986, 665

Southgate LJ, Treharne JD, Williams R (1989) Detection and treatment and follow-up of women with Chlamydia trachomatis infection seeking abortion in inner city general practices. Br Med J, 299: 1136–1137

Stamm WE, Cole B (1986) Asymptomatic Chlamydia trachomatis urethritis in men. Sex Transm Dis, 13: 163–165

Stamm WE, Koutsky LA, Benedetti JK, Jourden JL et al (1984) Chlamydia trachomatis urethral infections in men: Prevalence, risk factors and clinical manifestations. Ann Intern Med, 100:47–51

Suominen J., Gronroos M., Terho P., Wichmann L. (1983) Chronic prostatitis, Chlamydia trachomatis and infertility. Int J Andrology, 6:405–413.

Sutton, Grahame, 'Genital Infections', Midwife, Health Visitor and Community Nurse, 1982, 18(2), 42–45

Svensson L, MUrdh P-A, Ahlgren M, Nordenskjold F (1985) Ectopic pregnancy and antibodies to Chlamydia trachomatis. Fertil Steril, 44: 313–317

Terho F (1978) Chlamydia trachomatis in nonspecific urethritis. Br J Vener Dis, 54: 251–256

Tipple MA, Beem MO, Saxon EM (1979) Clinical characteristics of the afebrile pneumonia associated with Chlamydia trachomatis infection in infants of less than six months of age. Pediatrics, 63: 192–197

Tipple MA, Saxon EM, Radkowski MA, Beem MO (1977) Clinical characteristics of Chlamydia trachomatis pneumonia. Podiatric Res, 11:508

Truss, C., Orion, Missing Diagnosis, MD Inc., 1983

Walters MD, Eddy CA, Gibbs RS, Schachter J et al (1988) Antibodies to Chlamydia trachomatis and the risk of tubal pregnancy. Am J Obstet Gynecol, 159: 942–946

Walton, Pauline, 'New antibiotics in fight against genital disease', Doctor, 11 September 1980.

Watson PC, Gaidner D: TRIC agent as a cause of neonatal eye sepsis. Br Med J, 3: 527 1968

Waughan-Jackson JD, Dunlop EMC, Darougar S et al (1977) Urethritis due to Chlamydia trachomatis. Br J Vener Dis, 53: 180–183

Westergaard L, Philipson T, Scheibel J (1982) Significance of cervical Chlamydia trachomatis infection in postabortal pelvic inflammatory disease. Obstet Gynecol, 60;322–325

Westrom, L., 'Effect of acute pelvic infectious disease on fertility', Am J Obstet Gynaecol, 1975, 121, 707–713

Wong JL, Hines PA, Brasher MD, Rogers GT et al (1977) The etiology of nongonococcal urethritis in men attending a venereal disease clinic.J Am Vener Dis Assoc, 4:4–8

Zuher M, Naib MD (1970) Cytology of TRIC agent infection of the eye of newborn infants and their mothers' genital tracts. Acta Gytologica, Vol:14, No:7, 390–395

Chapter 7: Allergies and Intestinal Parasites

A case of functional hyperglycaemia – a medicolegal problem. Br J Psychiatry, 123: 353–358, 1973

A Shennan et al, A randomised controlled trial of metronidazole for the prevention of preterm birth in women positive for cervicovaginal foetal fibronectin: the PREMET Study: British Journal of Obstetrics and Gynaecology January 2006 113 (1), 65–74

Adverse Reactions to Food, Topical Update – 2 A National Dairy Council publication, 5/7 John Princes Street, London, W1M 0AP, 1994

Anon., 'Oregon Enacts America's First Law to Diagnose Underlying Organic Causes of Mental Illness', *Int J Biosocial Res*, 1984, 6(1), 13

Barker DJP et al: Foetal nutrition and cardiovascular disease in adult life. *The Lancet*: 1: 938–941, 1993

Barker DJP: Foetal and Infant Origins of Adult Disease. British Medical Journal Publication, 1982

Bolton R: Hostility in fantasy: a further test of the hyperglycaemia-aggression hypothesis. Aggressive Beh, 2: 257–274, 1976

Bolton R: The hypoglycaemia-aggression hypothesis; an overview of research. In: Biosocial Bases of Antisocial Behaviour, Ed: SA Mendick, Cambridge University Press, New York, 1985

Brenner AA: A study of the efficacy of the Feingold diet on hyperkinetic children. Clin Pediatr, 16: 652–656, 1977

Bryce-Smith D: Environmental and chemical influences on behaviour and mentation. (John Leys Lecture) Chem Soc Rev, 15: 93–123, 1986

Bryce-Smith D: The Third Leg: Lecture in the Power of Prevention Conference, 24 June, Oxford, UK, 1994

Buckley RE: Hypoglycaemia temporal lobe disturbances in aggressive behaviour. J Orthomolecular Psychiatry, 8(3): 188–192, 1979

Collins-Williams C: Intolerance to additives. Ann Allergy 51: 315–316, 1983

Connors CK and Blouin AG: Nutritional effects on behaviour of children. J Psychiatr Res, 17: 193–201, 1983

Connors CK: *Food Additives and Hyperactive Children*. Pienum Press, New York, 1980

Cook PS and Woodhill JM: The Feingold dietary treatment of the hyperkinetic syndrome. Med J Austr, 2: 85–90, 1976

Crook WG: Food additives and hyperactivity. *The Lancet*, p1128, May 15 1982

Dickerson JWT: Diet and Hyperactivity. J Human Nutr, 31: 167–174, 1980

Doyle W et al: Maternal nutrient intake and birth weight. J Human Nutr and Dietetics, 2: 415–422, 1989

Durlach J: Clinical aspects of chronic magnesium deficiency. In: Magnesium in Health, Ed: MS Seeling, Spectrum Publications, New York, 1980

Eagle, Robert, *Eating and Allergy*, Wellingborough, Thorsons, 1986. This book gives an excellent survey of food allergy, including useful sections on diagnosis and desensitisation.

Egger, J, et al., 'Controlled Trial of Oliantigenic Treatment in the Hyperkinetic Syndrome', *Lancet*, 1985, 1, 540–545

Eysenck HJ and Eysenck SBG, Eds: Improvement of IQ and Behaviour as a function of dietary Supplementation: A symposium, Pergamon Press, 1991

Feingold BF. Hyperkinesis and learning disabilities linked to the ingestion of artificial food colours and flavours. J Lear Disabilities, 9: 19–27, 1976

Feingold BF: Adverse Reactions to Hyperkinesis and Learning Disabilities(H-LD) Congressional Record, S-1973, 39–42, 1973

Feingold BF: Dietary Management of Behaviour and Learning Disabilities. In: Nutrition and Behaviour, Ed: SA Miller, p37 Franklin Institute Press, Philadelphia, Pennsylvania, USA, 1981

Feingold BF: Food additives and child development. Hospital Practice, 21, 11–12, 17–18, 1973

Feingold BF: Hyperkinesis and learning disabilities linked to artificial food flavours and colours. AM J Nutr, 75: 797–803, 1975

Feingold BF: Recognition of food additives as a cause of symptoms of allergy. Ann of Allergy, 26: 309, 1968

Feingold BF: Why Your Child is Hyperactive. Random House, New York, 1975

Food Allergy: How Much in the Mind', *Lancet*, 1983, 1, 1259–1261

Galler JR: Malnutrition – a neglected cause of learning failure. Postgrad Med: 80: 224–230, 1986

Goldman JA et al: Behavioural effects of sucrose in preschool children. J Abnorm Child Psychol, 14(4): 565–577, 1986

Goyette CH, Connors CK, Petti TA et al: Effects of artificial food colours on hyperkinetic children: A double-blind challenge study. Psychopharmacology Bull, 14: 39–40, 1978

Grant, ECG, 'Food Allergies and Migraine', *Lancet,* 1979, 1, 966–968

Gray J and Buttriss J: Maternal and Foetal Nutrition. National Dairy Council Nutrition Service, Fact File Number 11, 1994

Guidance on Assessing Risk from Cryptosporidium Oocysts in Treated Water Supplies – Drinking Water Inspectorate www.dwi.gov.uk

Hare, Francis, *The Food Factor in Disease*, 1905

Jameson S: Effects of zinc deficiency on human reproduction. Acta Medica Scand, 197A, Suppl. 593, 3–89, 1976

Juhlin L: Incidence of intolerance to food additives. Int J Dermatology, 19: 548–551, 1980

King DS: Can allergic exposure provoke psychological symptoms? A double-blind test. Biological Psychiatry, 16(1): 3–19, 1981

King DS: Food additives and behavioural effects of food and chemical exposure to sensitive individuals. Nutrition and Health, 3: 137–151, 1984

Latham MC and Cobos F: The effects of malnutrition on intellectual development and learning. Am J Public Health, 61: 1307–1324, 1971

Laurence KM et al: Double-blind randomised controlled trial of folate treatment before conception to prevent recurrence of neural tube defects. Br Med J, 282: 1509–1511, 1981

Levy F, Dumbrell S, Hobbes G, Ryan M, et al: Hyperkinesis and diet: a double-blind crossover trail with a tartrazine challenge. Med J Austr, 1: 61–64, 1978

Lipton MA, Nemeroff CB, Mailman RB: Hyperkinesis and food additives. In: RJ Wurtman & JJ Wurtman, Eds. Nutrition and Brain, New York, Raven Press, 1979

MAFF, Food Allergy and Other Unpleasant Reactions to Food. A Guide from the Food Safety Directorate, available free from Food Sense, London, SE99 7TT

Mansfield, Peter, and Jean Munro, *Chemical Children*, London, Century, 1987. This book gives an overview of how harmful pollutants, including chemicals, can affect children.

Masefield, Jennifer, 'Psychiatric Illness caused or exacerbated by Food Allergies', 1988 (unpublished paper)

Menkes MM, Rowe J, Menkes J: A 25-year follow-up on the hyperactive child with minimal brain dysfunction. Pediatrics 39: 398–399, 1967

Menzies IC: Disturbed children: The role of food and chemical sensitivities. Nutrition and Health, 3: 39–54, 1984

Miller M and Millstone E: Food Additives Campaign Team: Report on colour Additives. FACT, 25 Horsell Road, London N5 1XL, June 1987

Miller M: Danger! Additives at Work, London Food Commission, London 1985

Moynahan EJ: Zinc deficiency and disturbances of mood and visual behaviour. *The Lancet*, 1: 91, 1976

Mozer K: *Physiology of hostility*. Markham Publishing Co, Chicago, III, 1971

O'Banion DR: *An Ecological and Nutritional Approach to Behavioural Medicine*. Charles C Thomas, Springfield, Illinois, USA, 1981

Pollitt E and Liebel R: Iron deficiency anaemia and scholastic achievement in young adolescents. JmPediatrics, 88: 372–381, 1976

Pollitt E et al: Fasting and cognitive function. J Psychiatr Res, 17: 169–174,1983

Pollitt et al: Brief fasting, stress and cognition in children. Am J Clin Nutr, 34: 1526–1533, 1981

Prinz RJ, Roberts Hantman E: Dietary correlates of hyperactive behaviour in children. J Consult Clin Psychol, 48(6): 760–769, 1980

SCF Report of the Scientific Committee for Food, 12th series, Commission of the European communities, EUR 7823, Brussels, 1982

Schoenthaler S and Doraz W: Types of offences which can be reduced in an institutional setting using nutritional intervention: A preliminary empirical evaluation. Int J biosocial Res, 4(2): 74–84, 1983

Schoenthaler S: Diet and crime: An empirical examination of the value of nutrition in the control and treatment of incarcerated juvenile offenders. Int J Biosocial Res, 4(1): 25–39, 1983

Schoenthaler S: The Los Angeles probation department diet-behaviour program: An empirical evaluation of six institutions. Int J Biosocial Res, 5(2): 88–98, 1983

Schoenthaler SJ, Doraz WE, Wakefield JA: The impact of a low additive and sucrose diet on academic performance in 803 New York City public schools. Int J Biosocial Res, 8(2): 138–148, 185–195, 1986

Sever LE and Emanuel I: Is there a connection between maternal zinc deficiency and congenital malformations in the central nervous system in man? Teratology, 7: 117–118, 1973

Silbergeld EK and Anderson SM: Artificial food colours and childhood behaviour disorders. Bull New York Acad Med, Second Series, Vol:58, No:3, pp275–295, April 1982

Simmer K et al: A double-blind trial of zinc supplementation in pregnancy. European J Clin Nutr, 45: 139–144, 1991

Smith JM: Adverse reactions to food and drug additives. European J Clin Nutr, 45 (Suppl.1): 17–21, 1991

Smithells RW et al: Possible prevention of neural tube defects by preconceptional vitamin supplementation. The Lancet, ii: 339–340, 1980

Sprague R, Cohen M, Eichiseder W: Are there hyperactive children in Europe and the South Pacific? American Psychological Association Conference, San Francisco, 1977

Sprague R, Cohen M, Werry J: Normative Data on the Connors' Teacher Rating Scale and Abbreviated Scale: Technical Report. Institute on Child Behaviour and Development, University of Illinois at Urbana-Campaign, 1974

Swanson JM and Kinsbourne M: Food dyes impair performance of hyperactive children on laboratory learning tests. Science, 207: 1485–1487, 1980

Taylor RJ: Food Additives. John Wiley, Chichester, 1980

The Gardner Merchant School Meals survey – 'What Are Our Children Eating?' Gardner Merchant, Educational Services, Kenley House, Kenley Lane, Kenley, CR8 5ED, 1994

The Journal of The Hyperactive Children's Support Group, No:43, p16, Summer, 1992, No:45, p15, 1993

Tryphonas J and Trites R: Food allergy in children with hyperactivity, learning disabilities and/or minimal brain dysfunction. Ann of allergy, 42: 22–27, 1979

Virkkunen M and Huttunen MO: Evidence of abnormal glucose tolerance test among violent offenders. Neuropsychobiology, 8: 30–34, 1982

Virkkunen M: Reactive hypoglycaemic tendency among habitually violent offenders: a further study by means of the glucose tolerance test. Neuropsychobiology, 8: 35–40, 1982

Von Pirquet, Clement, 1906

Webb T and Oski F: Behavioural status of young adolescents with iron deficiency anaemia. J Spec Education, 8(2): 153–156, 1974

Weiss B: *Food Safety and Evaluation: The Link to Behavioural Disorders in Children,* pp 221–250, Pienum Publishing Corporation, 1984

Weiss G and Hechtman L: The hyperactive child syndrome. Science, 205: 1348–1353, 1979

WeissB, Williams JH, Margen S, Abrams B, Caan B, et al: Behavioural responses to artificial food colours. Scienc, 207: 1487–1489, 1980.

Wender PH: Minimal brain dysfunction syndrome in children. New York, Wiley, 1971

Williams JI and Cram DM: Diet in the management of Hyperkinesis: A review of the tests of Feingold hypotheses. Canadian Psych. Assoc. J, 23: 241–248, 1978

www.physchem.ox.ac.uk Safety data – Metronidazole – Harmful if swallowed(!), may act as a carcinogen.

Wynn SW et al: The association of maternal social class with maternal diet and the dimensions of babies in the population of London women. Nutrition and Health, 9: 303–315, 1994

Yarura-Tobias JA and Neziroglu FA: Violent behaviour, brain dysrhythmia and glucose dysfunction: a new syndrome. J Orthomolecular Psychiatry, 4: 128–188, 1975

Young E et al: A population study of food intolerance. The Lancet, 343: 1127–1129, 1994

Chapter 8: Electromagnetic pollution

Andrews, Lori, B., *New Conceptions*, New York, St Martin's Press, 1984, 23

Anon, 'Power Lines Cancer Link', *Today*, 18 March 1988

Anon. The Bulletin of the Atomic Commission. 1992, 48(1)

Becker, Robert, *Cross Currents*, Bloomsbury, London, 1990, 276

Bertell, Rosalie, *No Immediate Danger*. 1988

Bertell, Rosalie. In: Toynbee, Polly, 'Behind the Lines', *Guardian*, 15 December 1986, 12

Bithell, J.F., Stewart A.M., 'Prenatal irradiation and childhood malignancy: a review of British data from the Oxford Survey', Br J Cancer, 1975, 31, 271–287

Ferreira, Antonio J., Prenatal Environmental, Springfield, Ill, Charles C. Thomas 1969

Franc, M.C., Meunier, A., et al., Archives du malades professionelles, du medicin du travail et due securite sociale. 1981, 42(3): 183–194

Gabby, Samuel Lee, 'Observations on the effects of artificial light on the health and development of mice'. In: Ott, John N., op. cit., 100

Herzog,P & Rieger,CT., Risk of Cancer from diagnostic X-rays, Lancet 2004 Jan 31: 363(9406):345–51, 2004

Hollwich, Fritz, The Influence of Ocular Light Perception on Metabolism in Man and Animals, New York, Springer-Verlag, 1980, Preface

Kime, Zane R., op. cit., 92

Kime, Zane R., Sunlight, Penryn, World Health Publication, 1980, 199

Kirk, K.M., Lyon, M.F., 'Induction of congenital malformations in the offspring of male mice treated with X-Rays at premeiotic and post-meiotic Electromagnetic Pollution stages', Mutation Research, 1984, 125, 75–85

Li,D.K. et.al, A population based prospective cohort study of personal exposure to magnetic fields during pregnancy and the risk of miscarriage,. Epidemiology, Jan: 13(1) :9–20, 2002

McCarthy, Paul, Health, February 1988, 32

McCree, Donald. In: Gold, Michael, 'Additional findings at low exposures have prompted serious second thoughts about US safeguards', Science 80, Premier Issue, 81

Nomura, T., 'Parental exposure to X-Rays and chemicals induces heritable tumours and anomalies in mice', Nature, 1982, 296, 575–577

Nordstrom, S., et al., 'Genetic defects in offspring of power-frequency workers', Bioelectromagnetics, 1983, 4: 91

Nordstrom, S., et al., 'Reproductive hazards among workers at high-voltage systems', Bioelectromagnetics, 1981, 4, 91–101

Ott, John N., Light Radiation and You, Greenwich, CN, 1985, 78–139. These two chapters give some interesting examples

Rosenthal, Norman E., et al., 'Antidepressant Effects of Light in Seasonal Effective Disorder', Am J Psychiatr, 1985, 2, 163–170

Schauss, Alexander G., 'Body Chemistry and Human Behaviour'.
Course: Oxford, 18 November 1986

Smith, David W., *Mothering Your Unborn Baby*, Philadelphia, W.B.
Saunders, 1979, 67

Stellman, Jeanne, Daum, Susan M., *Work is Dangerous to your
Health*, Vintage Books, 1979, 141

Teymor, Melvin L., *Infertility*, New York, Grune and Stratton Inc, 1978

Wright, Pearce, 'Claims that power cables cause Cancer to be
investigated', *The Times*, 18 March 1988

Chapter 9: Chemical Hazards

VACCINES

Beattie, Greg,*Vaccinations, A Parent's Dilemma, 1997*, published by
the Informed Parent, P.O. Box 870, Harrow, Middlesex HA3 7UW,
ISBN 1-876308-00-1

Blaylock, Russell, Dr, See Dr Blaybock's website for more papers on
vaccines: http://www.russellblaylockmd.com

Buchwald, Gerhard, Dr.med. *The Vaccination Nonsense*, 2005,
translated from the German edition, published by Books on
Demand GmbH, Norderstedt, ISBN 3-8334-2508-3

Buttram, Harold, MD, *A Commentary on Current Childhood Vaccine
Programmes*, Philosophical Publishing Company,
www.soul.org/ppc, P.O. Box 77, Quakertown PA 18951, USA,
ISBN 1-891485-30-X

Coulter, Harris L, *Vaccination, Social Violence and Criminality*,
ISBN-10 15556430841

Curtis, Susan, *Handbook of Homeopathic Alternatives to
Immunisation*, ISBN-10 1874581029

Fisher, Barbara Loe, *The Consumer's Guide to Childhood Vaccines,*
1997, published by the national Vaccine Information Centre,
512 West Maple Avenue, Suite 206, Vienna, Virginia 22180, USA,
ISBN 1-88920-01-3

Gunn, Trevor, *Mass Immunisation: A Point in Question*,
ISBN-10 095176571X

Halvorsen, Richard, *The Truth about Vaccines: How we are used as
guinea pigs without knowing it*, ISBN-10 1903933923

Kirby, David, *Evidence of Harm: Mercury in Vaccines and the Autism
Epidemic: a Medical Controversy*, ISBN-10 0312326459

Lydall, Wendy *Raising a Vaccine-Free Child*, 2005, Author House, Australia, ISBN 1-4184-5017-0

McBride, Natasha, *Gut and Psychology Syndrome*: *Natural Treatment for Autism, ADD/ADHD, Dyslexia, Dyspraxia, Depression,Schizophrenia*, ISBN-10 0954852028

McTaggart, Lynne, *What Doctors Don't Tell You*,Thorsons, 77–85 Fulham Palace Road, London W6 8JB, , ISBN 0-7225-3024-2

McTaggart, Lynne *The Vaccination Bible*, ISBN 0-9534734-0-6

Miller, Neil Z, *Vaccines, Autism and Childhood Disorders: Crucial Data That Could Save Your Child's Life*, New Atlantean Press, P.O. Box 9638, Santa Fe, New Mexico, 87504, ISBN 1-881217329, www.thinktwice.com

Miller, Neil Z, *Vaccines: Are They Really Safe and Effective?* New Atlantean Press, ISBN 1-881217-302

Moritz, Andreas, *Vaccine-nation, Poisoning the Population,* Ener-Chi, Wellness Press, ISBN 978-0-9845954-2-6, www.ener-chi.com

Neustaedter, Randall, *The Vaccine Guide: Risks and Benefits for Children and Adults,* 1996, North Atlantic Books, P.O. Box 12327, Berkeley, California 94712, ISBN 978-1-55643-423-5

O'Shea, Tim, *The Sanctity of Human Blood: Vaccination Is Not Immunization*, ISBN-10 1929487088

Roberts, Janine, *Fear of the Invisible*, Impact Investigtive Media Productions, ISBN 978-0-9559177-2-1

Scheibner, Viera, Behavioural Problems in Childhood: The Link to Vaccination, March 2000, Griffin Press, Netley, South Australia, ISBN 0957800703

Smits, Tinus, *Autism – Beyond* Despair, ISBN-10 9076189285

Sussman, Lara, *Understanding MMR – the Facts, Choices and Alternatives: Helping You Make the Right Choice for Your Family,* ISBN-10 1905830041

Wakefield, Andrew J. *Callous Disregard: Autism and Vaccines: The Truth Behind a Tragedy,* ISBN-10 1616081694

Walker, Martin, *Silenced Witnesses, Vol. I & II,* Slingshot Publications, BM Box 8314, London, www.slingshotpublications.com, ISBN 978-0-9519646-6-8

Walker, Martin *Dirty Medicine*, Slingshot Publications, ISBN 978-0-9564093-1-7

APPENDIX 3

Specific Anomalies and some relevant Research

From the Foresight booklet written in the mid-1980s by Belinda Barnes and approved by Professor John Dickerson, BSc (Lond.), PhD (Cantab.), FIBiol., FRSH, FIFST. Professor of Human Nutrition, University of Surrey.

Anorexia and poor appetite

Anorexia normally has been thought of as an affliction affecting teenage girls for psychological reasons, but it has also been recorded as affecting baby rats in animal studies, where the young are listless and have no interest in suckling. Although it is not often spoken of as 'anorexia', lack of interest in suckling is a serious problem with some babies, and many small children refuse food, making every meal a battleground.

Zinc is needed for over 90 enzyme systems in the body and shortage of this mineral has been shown to produce anorexia in young rats. Zinc absorption is enhanced by B6, folic acid and essential fatty acids.

It has been noted that vitamin A has a part to play in promoting good appetite. It has been recorded that with lack of vitamin Bi weakness of intestinal activity can cause indigestion, flatulence and constipation. Without pantothenic acid there is a shortage of digestive enzymes; slow peristaltic action (movement sending food along the digestive tract) and indigestion and constipation will follow – also food allergies. Vitamin B6 is needed by the body to make use of the essential fatty acids and many of the amino acids, and lack of this vitamin has been specifically implicated with anorexia in animal experiments.

Folic acid is essential for the utilisation of sugars and amino acids. It has been noted that without biotin animals become thin to the point of emaciation. Lack of inositol will show a slowing down of the activity of the digestive system and constipation.

It has been noted that without vitamin E babies will be listless and anaemia and jaundice can develop. The essential fatty acids, linolenic, linoleic and arachidonic acid, are all needed to furbish the intestinal bacteria necessary for normal breakdown and digestion of foods.

Magnesium is needed for protein synthesis and to assist the function of many enzymes. It has been noted in animal studies that, without it, anorexia will develop. Manganese is needed for numerous enzymes and, to help in the utilisation of fats, it is necessary for lipid metabolism.

Chromium is needed by the body for the utilisation of glucose. Nickel and vanadium are both thought to also be involved in lipid metabolism.

Repletion of essential vitamins and minerals and fatty acids during pregnancy and lactation should maximise the chance of a baby with a healthy normal appetite and an abundant supply of good quality breast milk.

Appetite in the reluctant breast-feeder has often been seen to improve after supplementation of the mother with 3 Foresight Vitamin Supplements, 3 Foresight Mineral Supplements and 3 Zinc Plus per day.

Ataxia, tremor and spasticity

Studies from Wayne State University show that, in rats whose mothers were deprived of copper before birth, ataxia was seen in the newborn. Those deprived of manganese in the womb had involuntary movements, gross tremor and twitching, malformation of the inner ear (which controls balance), lack of coordination, head retraction, ataxia and loss of righting reflexes. Manganese carries oxygen in the blood to the brain, so lack of manganese could be a factor in oxygen insufficiency at birth. Manganese is also necessary for the utilization of fats, which could affect brain development.

Nickel and vanadium are two more essential elements which are involved in lipid metabolism and therefore, presumably, in brain development.

While understanding that these problems are often due to a birth injury (e.g. caused by not enough oxygen at a crucial moment), we feel it might be helpful to look at some of the observations made regarding similar problems during animal studies.

In studies conducted at University of Cambridge in the 1960s, Isobel Jennings recorded that rats born to mothers who were deprived of pantothenic acid during the pregnancy suffered tremor and damage to the nervous system.

In human adults B6 deficiency has been found to cause twitching and tremors; B12 deficiency has been found to cause deterioration of nervous tissue and deterioration of the spinal cord until paralysis may ensue. Another B vitamin, choline, is used in normal muscle contractions, and is also needed in lipid metabolism.

Essential fatty acids (such as linoleic, linolenic and arachidonic acid) are needed for the health and function of nerve cells.

Carl Pfeiffer in his book *Zinc and Other Micronutrients* states that calcium is needed to control the irritability of nerves, and magnesium to allow muscle contraction and nerve excitability. Potassium is also needed for all nerve conduction and muscle conduction.

See the Foresight literature for further information on how to mitigate against nutritional deficiencies during pregnancy.

Brain damage, fits, convulsions and mental impairment

In animal studies conducted at Cambridge in the 1960s by Isobel Jennings, it was noted that rats born to mothers kept short of vitamin A since birth were at risk of hydrocephalus. In some cases the rats were found to have high levels of carotene accumulated in the liver. This is a phenomenon seen in cases of zinc deficiency recorded in three separate studies. (Smith JC, Barn T, Smith JC)

In the same series of studies at Cambridge it was noted that rats that had been kept short of vitamin Bi in the womb were slow to learn. Those whose mothers had been deprived of pantothenic acid were found to suffer from lack of myelination and damage to the nervous system. Where the mother was kept short of folic acid there were deformities of the brain. Many of those who were deprived of vitamin E suffered neural tube defects such as anencephaly and hydrocephaly, and those who were born without obvious deformity were seen to be backward in development. Those whose mothers were short of essential fatty acids were seen to lack brain development. High carotene in the liver and low plasma vitamin A was recorded at Queen Charlotte's Maternity Hospital by Gal and Parkinson in studies on stillborn babies with neural tube defects.

It is well known that lack of vitamin Bi 2 will cause deterioration of the spinal cord in humans. Lack of vitamin D and calcium may cause skeletal deformities, including deformities of the skull. An asymmetrical or 'odd shaped' skull is often noted in the retarded. In some cases fusion of platelets may occlude blood supply to brain cells, thus starving them of nutrients and oxygen.

In studies at Wayne State University, USA, where paucities of a number of different trace minerals were induced it was noted that rats deprived of magnesium suffered convulsions. Those deprived of copper were born with small brains; those short of iron had brain defects, as did those who were kept short of zinc.

Manganese deficiency in the foetus caused malformation of the inner ear, ataxia, uncoordination, head retraction, tremor, loss of righting reflexes, hyper-irritability and learning difficulties. Other research from USA has tested manganese deficiency and epilepsy.

It has been known for a long time that lack of iodine may disturb thyroid function, which can cause serious mental retardation. Recently lack of selenium has been linked, in vitro, with splitting of the chromosome Trisomy 21 that is involved in the causation of Down's syndrome.

The full Foresight programme is designed to maximise the chances of the foetus having every nutrient necessary for optimal development.

Cleft lip and/or palate

Over 800 children are still being born each year with cleft palate, and some research into causes has been done – mainly by Isobel

Jennings at Cambridge University in the 1960s and early 1970s, and by Dr Weston Price in the 1930s.

At Cambridge, animal experiments revealed that lack of vitamins B2 (riboflavin), nicotinamide, pantothenic acid and folic acid in the mother's diet caused animals to be born with a cleft palate.

The work of Dr Weston Price revealed that a diet high in refined and processed foods (as against fresh and raw foods) produced all manner of deformities among which were a number of different deformities of the skull, palate and jaw. His work included observation of primitive tribes who eat fresh fruits, grains and vegetables as they are grown, and a study of Westernised people who ate only refined flour, cooked foods etc. His work is all contained in his very detailed book *Nutrition and Physical Degeneration*.

The work of Dr Price in no way conflicts with the experimental findings of Mrs Jennings, as all the B vitamin deficiencies she incriminated are the B vitamins that are removed from refined grains during processing.

B2 is also destroyed by light – e.g. in milk in glass milk bottles; nicotinamide is made in the body with the help of B1, B2 and B6, vitamins that can be destroyed by heat (i.e. cooking) and removed from the body by alcohol, smoking and the contraceptive pill; extra pantothenic acid may be used by the body in the case of allergic illness or during emotional stress; folic acid may be destroyed by alcohol, the contraceptive pill and some medications used for epilepsy.

The Foresight programme & supplements help to ensure B-vitamin status.

Damaged blood vessels and blood disorders

It is known that vitamin A has a part to play in the formation of red and white blood cells. In animal studies conducted at Cambridge in the early 1970s, lack of vitamin B2 (which is a vitamin involved in vitamin A metabolism) was found to cause broken capillaries, blood disorders and oedema and anaemia in young rats. (Jennings I)

Lack of pantothenic acid causes low blood pressure and low blood sugar. Lack of vitamin B6 can be involved in anaemia – as can deficiencies of a number of other nutrients, including iron, copper, vitamin E and vitamin B12.

Folic acid has a part to play in the formation of the red blood cells in the bone marrow. In the same series of animal studies, lack of this vitamin was found to cause malformation of the blood vessels, oedema and anaemia in the young rats. Sufficient folic acid and vitamin B12 are needed for the prevention of pernicious anaemia.

Lack of biotin was found to cause damage to the blood vessels of the young rats. In other studies too little choline has been found to result in haemorrhages in the eye, the heart muscle and the adrenal gland in adult humans – also high blood pressure and oedema. Inositol is needed to transport the fat-soluble vitamins found in the blood (vitamins A, D, E and K).

Enough vitamin C is needed to keep capillary walls intact. Lack of this vitamin may result in perifollicular haemorrhages in thighs, buttocks and abdomen.

Lack of vitamin E can cause anaemia, oedema and retarded heart development. Lack of essential fatty acids can lead to degenerative changes in the blood vessels.

Calcium is needed for controlling blood-clotting mechanisms. Potassium is needed to regulate the blood pH and to keep the water balance. Lack of copper can cause anaemia (but lack of copper is quite rare since the advent of copper water pipes). Iron is needed to make haemoglobin, the substance which carries oxygen in the blood.

Manganese is also involved in the transport of oxygen in the blood. Chromium is required for the preservation of the blood vessel walls and without it arteriosclerosis and hypertension may develop. Selenium, cobalt nickel and iodine are also needed by the blood.

Diaphragmatic hernia

The problem has been connected with just two nutritional deficiencies, vitamin A and folic acid. In Cambridge in the 1960s, in animal studies conducted by Isobel Jennings, rat mothers were deprived of vitamin A during the pregnancy and hernia of the diaphragm was among the anomalies found in the young. In another study, other rat mothers were deprived of folic acid and deformity of the diaphragm was noted in some of the young.

The element zinc is required to convert carotene into plasma vitamin A – the type of A which is available to the baby. Lack of zinc would inhibit this process. A number of factors may reduce the level of zinc in the body including infections, injury, the contraceptive pill, alcohol and smoking. These last three also lower the levels of folic acid.

The Foresight programme and supplements help to ensure vitamin status.

Down's syndrome

In very recent experiments in USA cells were grown in vitro (in a test-tube). When the medium they were grown in was kept short of selenium, they were affected in a characteristic way. The relevant chromosome split, making the Trisomy 21 phenomenon that is found in the cells of those suffering from Down's syndrome.

When I heard of this experiment I took from my files the hair analyses of the youngest three Down's syndrome children I had tested (aged 11 months to 2½ years). All three had no measurable selenium in the hair. I then looked at the hair analyses of three mothers who had previously given birth to Down's syndrome babies. Two had almost no measurable selenium; the third had a low level of selenium, but her child was by then seven years old, so she had possibly had time to make up some of the deficiency.

Another finding we seem to make quite consistently with the Down's syndrome children when they are tiny is that they have a high level of toxic metals. This is usually lead, cadmium or aluminium, but I have seen one over-high copper. Any of these metals, if way out of line, could use up the selenium, as the body uses selenium to clear the toxic metals.

I have heard of three half-Chinese Merseyside children with Down's syndrome whose Chinese fathers all came from a part of China where the soil is lacking in selenium. The mothers in each case were English.

This evidence is anecdotal, but all points to the involvement of selenium deficiency compounded/caused by a high level of toxic metal in the body.

Eye defects, malformations of the eye, cataracts and squints

Research done at Cambridge University in the 1960s by Isobel Jennings showed that animals deprived of vitamin A, pantothenic acid and folic acid in the womb were born with eye defects. (Jennings I)

Work from a variety of sources in USA has correlated eye defects with lack of iron, zinc and chromium in the mother's diet during the pregnancy. (Caldwell D, Oberleas D)

Lack of vitamin B2 and lack of selenium have both been connected with cataracts – possibly because B2 is involved in vitamin A metabolism. Selenium is essential for preserving vitamin E in the cells.

Lack of vitamin E has been connected with squints, which are five times as common in the children of mothers who smoke. This may be because the lungs of smokers use up the vitamin E to protect tissues.

Deficiencies of vitamin A may be found in people lacking in zinc, as zinc controls the conversion of carotene to plasma vitamin A. Zinc may be deficient due to the use of the contraceptive pill, the coil, alcohol and/or smoking. Extra zinc is also used for healing in cases of infection, injury and all kinds of stress. Lack of zinc and the other micro-nutrients chromium and selenium may be due to the modern refined diet, and/or high consumption of sugar. Fluoride is known to be antagonistic to selenium. Iron may be squandered by very heavy periods, and/or donating blood.

Lack of vitamin B2 may be induced by the contraceptive pill, by alcohol, smoking and possibly the supplementation of vitamin A without the supplementation of B2. Light destroys B2 so milk in glass bottles would have lost much of the B2 content. Pantothenate may be used up in times of stress. Folic acid may be squandered by the contraceptive pill, smoking, alcohol and many medications used for treating epilepsy.

Comparatively little has been turned up in animal studies to help our search, but it has been noted that the inner ear is malformed in young rats whose mothers have been deprived of manganese during the pregnancy. The inner ear is the part of the ear that is used for balance, but it is so close to the middle ear that any malformation may well distort the shape of the middle ear as well. The fine bones of the middle ear are formed almost entirely of manganese, so any shortage of manganese must presumably be to their disadvantage.

Manganese is carried in the blood by the B-complex vitamin choline. Certain types of insecticide of the DDT (organophosphate preparations) variety kill the insect by destroying choline in its body, thus making the uptake of manganese impossible. The insect then spins to his death. It is interesting to note that although DDT is illegal on food crops in this country, from a sample of 143 foods studied in 1985 by Pesticides Action Network, 19 were contaminated by DDT. The legal component DEE is still present in many foods, and is very similar in action.

Liming of the soil (to prevent club-root and other plant diseases) may prevent the uptake of manganese from the soil. So may treatment with certain types of herbicides which destroy the macrobacteria of the topsoil. These bacteria normally provide the protein used by the plant to metabolise the manganese.

'Rust' on lettuces and split cabbage stalks are signs of manganese deficiency, and how often do we see this in the food we eat? Only 9% of manganese is still present in refined flour – 91% of the original quota is thrown away or fed to the animals!

Ben Feingold of USA queried whether some food colourings and other chemicals were removed from the body by some mechanism involving manganese. Foresight doctors have noted empirically that high levels of lead and other toxic metals seem to take manganese with them when they are removed from the body. Children with high levels of toxic metal often have little manganese left. These observations have been made over a long period of time by people regularly reading hair analysis.

For details of manganese supplementation contact Foresight.

Heart, liver and kidney defects

Heart defects have been detected in the young of animals deprived of vitamin A, pantothenic acid, folic acid, biotin and vitamin E in work done at the University of Cambridge in the 1960s, in animals deprived of manganese and zinc in work done at Wayne State University, USA, and in farm animals who were short of nickel in Hungary.

Foresight doctors have noted no measurable nickel in hair samples from seven mothers each of whom gave birth to a baby with a heart defect before coming to Foresight.

Kidney defects were found in animal studies at Cambridge in rats born to mothers deprived of vitamin B2, pantothenic acid, folic acid, choline, vitamin E and essential fatty acids. In USA kidney defects have been related to zinc deficiency, and in Hungary to lack of nickel in farm animals.

Liver defects have been detected in animals deprived of biotin, B2, choline and again nickel by the same sources of information as above.

Vitamin B2 may be destroyed by light (e.g. in milk in glass milk bottles) and is also found to be lowered in the body by the contraceptive pill, by smoking and by alcohol. As it is involved with vitamin A metabolism it is possible that eyestrain and sunbathing may add to the need for this vitamin. Taking vitamin A without extra B2 may also squander this vitamin. Pantothenate may be used up by emotional stress or by allergic illness. Folate is used up by the contraceptive pill, by alcohol and smoking and by some medications given for epilepsy. Choline may be destroyed by certain types of insecticide; vitamin E and essential fatty acids are removed from much processed and refined food to improve shelf life. Zinc and other essential trace minerals may be lowered by the contraceptive pill and by smoking, alcohol, and infections or injury. All stress, whether physical or mental, can increase the need for nutrients.

Jaundice

Not very much is known about the source of this problem, although many theories are put forward, but we felt it might be helpful to parents if we ran over the list of deficiencies etc. known to adversely affect liver function. Hopefully by mothers avoiding these deficiencies and toxins during the pregnancy the baby may be given every chance of a smooth passage.

In a series of animal studies at Cambridge University in the 1960s conducted by Isobel Jennings, it was observed that the young of rat mothers who had been deprived of vitamin B2 during pregnancy had reduced oxygen consumption in the liver.

Those whose mothers were deprived of biotin were born with damage to the liver.

It has been recorded that people who lack choline have a fatty liver and that inositol, another of the B-complex vitamins, is needed by human liver cells for normal function.

It has been noted by the Shute brothers of Canada that babies who are short of vitamin E will be listless and anaemic and jaundice can develop. Essential fatty acids (linoleic, linolenic and arachidonic acid) stimulate the flow of bile. These fatty acids are found more in human milk than in cow's milk.

Of the trace minerals, selenium, nickel and zinc are known to be essential for liver function. It is possible this list is not complete, but problems are known to develop with shortages of these three.

It is also likely that a body burden of toxic metals could put an extra strain on the infant liver.

Foresight makes every possible effort to cleanse lead, mercury, cadmium, aluminium and over-high levels of copper from the mother's system before the start of the pregnancy. Also they ensure the mother has no nutritional deficiencies.

Also, of course, we advise no smoking or drinking during the course of the pregnancy and nursing.

Lack of myelination

In different animal studies, five nutrients have been found to cause demyelination where they are in short supply.

At Cambridge in the 1960s in a series of animal studies involving breeding baby rats, it was observed that rats whose mothers were deprived of pantothenic acid during the pregnancy suffered lack of myelination and damage to the nervous system.

Other workers noted that lecithin was essential to the integrity of the myelin sheath. This can be made in the body from methionine, choline and inositol.

Workers at Wayne State University in the 1970s conducted a series of animal studies in which mother rats were deprived of trace minerals. It was observed that the young from mothers deprived of copper suffered demyelination.

Skin disorders, uneven pigmentation, cradle cap

Vitamin A is known to be essential for a healthy skin, and lack of nicotinamide is known to result in dermatitis. Lack of B6 has been implicated in dermatitis of the head, in the eyebrows and behind the ears, sore lips and tongue, a rash round the base of the nose and behind the ears, also a rash around the genitals, and hands can become cracked and sore.

Lack of PABA (para-aminobenzoic acid) is recorded as resulting in greying of the hair in adults and uneven pigmentation of the skin; also a skin condition which makes it impossible to be in the sun without burning.

Lack of biotin may result in dry, peeling skin. Lack of essential fatty acids (linoleic, linolenic and arachidonic acid) may result in the hair going dry and thin, and the skin becoming thick, dry and scaly. These fatty acids are present in breast milk and evening primrose oil (EPO) in large quantities. Goat's milk contains more than cow's milk. Safflower oil (90% unsaturated) and sunflower oil (20% unsaturated) are the best cooking oils.

In animal studies in USA it has been recorded that lack of copper can cause depigmentation, and zinc deficiency can result in seborrhoea, loss of hair, lank lifeless hair and acne.

369

Folic acid and vitamin E are known to be helpful in all forms of healing, and vitamin E and selenium will contribute to a youthful skin.

Empirically, the Foresight clinicians have found that children with skin disorders often have high levels of one or other of the toxic metals and the condition often responds to this metal being cleansed from the system, and essential minerals restored. Drinking water should be filtered through a Brita water filter.

Again, many skin conditions respond to the removal of allergens: either foods from the diet, or factors from the surrounding environment. A combination of approaches is probably likely to be the most successful.

Before the next pregnancy it would probably help for the mother to ensure repletion of all the dietary components known to help skin conditions, and to ensure the removal of all known toxic metals from the system. Also to detect and eliminate allergenic substances from her diet/environment. One little boy I know recovered from eczema when his bath water was filtered!

Small-for-dates, premature and failure to thrive

44,355 babies were born in 1983 with a weight of under 2,500 gms, 1 in every 14 births. A number of studies have been done to detect the causes of small birth weight.

Animal studies conducted by Isobel Jennings at Cambridge in the 1960s showed that in animals whose diets were deficient in vitamins B1, B2, pantothenic acid, folic acid, E and in essential fatty acids the foetus might be small or fail to develop normally.

Studies at Wayne State University by Caldwell and Oberleas in the 1970s showed that diets deficient in copper, zinc and manganese would produce small offspring in rats. Other studies have related small birth weight in animals to lack of nickel, vanadium and iodine.

Work by Professor Bryce-Smith at Reading University has correlated high levels of lead and/or cadmium in the placental blood and tissue with low birth weight.

In the course of the same study it was noted that where the placental blood and tissue contained high levels of aluminium and mercury, problems with the placenta tended to cause early births.

The Reading studies have also shown that where copper was too high in relation to the amount of zinc in placental blood and tissue, the baby tended to be born early. Cambridge work also related lack of biotin, B2, pantothenic acid and folic acid to premature birth.

In his book *Nutrition and Physical Degeneration*, Dr Weston Price revealed many birth problems were related to our inadequate Western diet of refined and processed foods.

All these findings in no way conflict, as a wholefood diet rich in raw, fresh foods contains the vitamins and minerals described. These are largely removed in modern processed foods, and by excessive slimming diets which constrict the diet. Many trace minerals are removed from the body by heavy metals such as lead, cadmium, mercury and aluminium. Copper in excess can drive down zinc and manganese.

Despite unpropitious histories only 1 Foresight baby in 75 has had a small birth-weight. Two were premature for special reasons.

Spina bifida, hydrocephalus, anencephalus and exencephalus

In animal studies conducted at Cambridge in the 1970s it was found that hydrocephalus may result if the mother rat is kept short of vitamin A, and/or vitamin E. In rats short of vitamin E exencephalus was also seen.

Spina bifida was seen in young rats whose mothers were kept short of folic acid.

In studies at University of California, Wayne State University, Harvard University Medical School and University of Kentucky rat mothers were deprived of zinc and/or manganese. Neural tube defects arose with a shortage of either of these minerals.

In a study at Queen Charlotte's Hospital, London, post-mortems were performed on neural tube defect babies who had died. These revealed high vitamin A stored in the livers of affected babies. Zinc is needed to convert the basic carotene, which is stored in the liver, to plasma vitamin A. So these findings would be consistent with the findings in USA that low zinc is a factor.

Professor Smithalls in Leeds found he could significantly reduce the expected rate of second spina bifida births by giving supplements of a multivitamin compound containing vitamin A and folic acid.

In South Wales, Lawrence significantly reduced neural tube defects by counselling on diet, and by supplementing folic acid. Folic acid is involved in zinc metabolism.

At University of Aston in Birmingham, Wibberley found that cord and placental blood from births where the baby had a neural tube defect contained high lead and/or cadmium. This is consistent with other findings as lead and/or cadmium will chase zinc and/or manganese from the body.

Low vitamin A in the plasma may result from a paucity of zinc. Also vitamin E helps to preserve vitamin A in the tissues so where there was a shortage of E, a shortage of A would occur sooner and be more marked.

Foresight care eliminates toxic metals such as lead and cadmium, and ensures repletion in zinc, manganese, vitamins A and E, and folic acid.

Talipes or club foot, and limb reduction deformities

In animal studies conducted at Cambridge in the 1970s, rats born to mothers who had been kept short of B2 were born with abnormally short limbs and some with claws joined together. Rats born to mothers kept short of nicotinamide were found to have hind limb defects. Those whose mothers were kept short of pantothenic acid were found to be born with club foot, and the offspring whose mothers were short of folic acid were born with deformed limbs. Ratlings who were short of vitamin E in the womb were reported to have joined claws.

In work done in Wayne State University in the early 1970s by Oberleas and Caldwell, lack of iron was found to cause bone defects. Lack of manganese, observed in the same series of studies, was found to cause bone matrix malformation. Lack of zinc was also recorded and was found to cause faulty trunk and limb development and fusion of limbs.

Refining of sugar reduces the content of the B-complex vitamins to practically nil (B2, nicotinamide, pantothenic acid and folic acid). Likewise the refining of grain removes all but a fraction from white flour and white flour products. Vitamin B2 is also reduced by the contraceptive pill, and by smoking and alcohol.

Nicotinamide and pantothenic acid are used up during stress, and by allergic illness. Folic acid is also squandered by the contraceptive pill, as are zinc and manganese.

The uptake of manganese by the body is inhibited in the absence of choline and many of the insecticides in common use destroy choline in the insect's body. This is how the insect is killed. Also there may be a connection with the much increased use of the organophosphate insecticides for warble-fly in cattle in recent years. After their mothers had treatment, calves have been born without hooves.

Limb reductions have risen enormously in the last few years and Foresight doctors are wondering if this is also possibly due to breakthrough pregnancies to women on the contraceptive pill (the mini-pill now in common use has a 3% failure rate) as use of the contraceptive pill is known to reduce B2 levels in the body, also folate, zinc and manganese.

We have had two letters from couples who have had children born with limb reduction deformities after exposure to woodworm treatment chemicals.

Underdevelopment of the lung

In animal studies done in the 1960s at University of Cambridge by Isobel Jennings, underdevelopment of the lungs was found in young rats born to mothers who had been deprived of folic acid during pregnancy, and again in those whose mothers had been deprived of vitamin E.

Modern refined and processed foods are often short of these essential nutrients. In white flour the folic acid content is down to

33% of that found in wholewheat, and the vitamin E is down to 14%.

Folic acid is removed from the body by the contraceptive pill, by alcohol, by smoking and by some medications given to control epilepsy.

Vitamin E is used up by the body in wound healing, by smoking and inhaled allergens, and by sunburn and accidental burns.

In USA allergic conditions involving the lungs have been found to respond to supplementation of selenium. Selenium is said to be involved with retaining vitamin E in the cell, so this may also be relevant.

Urogenital problems and deformity of the ureters

Studies in the 1960s at Cambridge University found that rats were born with urogenital problems, and with deformed penis and undescended testicles in the males, where the mother was deprived of vitamin A. Lack of folic acid can also cause deformities of the urogenital system, and lack of pantothenic acid was reported to cause damage to the ureters.

Urogenital problems have been found to be more common following the use of the contraceptive pill. This may be a direct hormonal influence or may be due to lack of zinc (which is removed by the pill) causing an inhibition of the conversion of carotene to plasma vitamin A. Folate metabolism may also be inhibited by lack of zinc.

Folic acid is removed from the baby by the contraceptive pill, by alcohol, by smoking and by some medications given to control epilepsy.

Zinc is also squandered by the pill, alcohol and smoking.

* * *

NB: I hope the last twelve pages have been helpful. You will be able to identify the problem if you already have a misfortune in your family, and be able to avoid this happening again. Contact Foresight if you need more help.

APPENDIX 4
Article by Jean Philips from Powerwatch.org.uk

Are electromagnetic fields (EMFs) affecting your ability to have the family you want?

What on earth are electromagnetic fields (EMFs), you might ask, and what do they have to do with conceiving a child and bringing him or her to birth?

To answer these questions, we include a little information to put them into context.

We have evolved with a background level of natural EMFs generated by the earth herself. This had remained unchanged for millennia. Since the beginning of the 20th century all that changed.

We added powerfrequency fields from electricity generating power stations, powerlines that cross our country to supply electricity to consumers in cities, towns, villages and in rural areas. The number of electrical appliances we use at home and at work has grown enormously. We then added radiofrequency fields from radio, radar, television, mobile phones and their masts, wireless computers giving access to the internet at home and on the move, we give wireless games to the children and introduce wireless into their classrooms with interactive whiteboards and WiFi systems. All our transport is flooded with electromagnetic fields, as are our hospitals, shops and leisure venues.

We are so used to the benefits that undeniably accompany all of these innovations, that we rarely consider whether they may have disadvantages.

It was the military that first began to find occupational exposure to EMFs made some of their personnel very ill indeed. In the 1970s childhood leukaemia was linked to residential electricity supply (Wertheimer & Leeper 1979) and 'microwave sickness' was described (Silverman 1973) after people had been exposed to radiofrequency (RF) radiation. Since then there have been an ever increasing number of studies looking at the potential health effects experienced by people as a result of exposure to both powerfrequency (PF) and radiofrequency (RF) fields.

The research

The research has looked intensively at childhood leukaemia and there is international agreement that this illness is linked to PF electromagnetic fields, though the mechanisms of causation are not agreed on. In the course of the research, other illnesses have been looked at and there seems to be a growing body of evidence that illnesses other than childhood cancer may be implicated, and health effects other than those that lead to illness.

There has been a phenomenal growth in the use of equipment using RF technology. The scientists began to wonder whether this, too, might have the sort of effects on the general population as those suggested by Charlotte Silverman.

Many of you may have seen the debate in the media about whether mobile phones cause brain tumours. This is very concerning indeed, as there seems to be ever increasing evidence that these two are firmly linked.

However, that is not the focus of this article, and it is here that we look at the research that has investigated whether there are any links between PF or RF fields and reproductive problems.

The following research information is a 'snapshot in time' as research is ongoing; new papers are being published frequently and the science is still as new as our exposures.

Occupational exposure

Many studies look at occupational effects as employers have an obligation to provide safe working environments for their employees, and to minimise known risks.

Two studies (Mollerlokken 2008, Baste 2008) investigating reproductive effects in the Norwegian Navy found that exposure to RF fields produced an increased risk of infertility, and the higher the exposure, the greater the risk. Where children were born, there seemed to be a greater number of girls than boys. Occupational exposure is frequently at higher levels than those allowed for the general population, as it is assumed that workers are healthier and less vulnerable to ill health effects as a result of exposure to environmental toxins.

A study by De-Kun Li, which he presented in June 2008 to the annual meeting of the Society for Epidemiologic Research in Chicago, found that men who are exposed to levels of magnetic fields of only 0.16μT for six or more hours a day were four times as likely to have substandard sperm.

Kim (2008) found cell apoptosis (cell death) in mouse testicular germ cells from exposure to 14μT 60 Hz magnetic fields. This is a long way above typical chronic background exposure, but is also considerably below International Commission on Non-Ionizing Radiation Protection (ICNIRP) guidance levels.

Physiotherapists can be exposed to RF radiation by some of the equipment they use therapeutically. A study of pregnant physiotherapists (Ouellet-Hellstrom & Stewart 1993) found that being exposed to RF radiation increased the risk of miscarriage and the higher the exposure the greater the risk. The levels they were exposed to were not very high, similar to those which will be found in many places near mobile phone base stations and in homes and workplaces with digital DECT cordless phones and wireless Local Area Network (wLAN) systems.

Other studies have looked at residential rather than occupational exposure, or exposure as a result of lifestyle choices (e.g. mobile phone use, travel by train, etc.)

Powerfrequency fields

Powerfrequency fields occur as a result of our use of electricity. Some research is based on human exposure, some is done in laboratories or using animals. It is not always easy to say whether animal and cell studies provide information which will apply to people, but many of the experimental procedures cannot be done on people, so we are stuck with it, and the accompanying uncertainty.

The California report (Neutra 2002), which reviewed the available research studies, concluded that there was a link between miscarriage and powerfrequency magnetic fields, and two surveys carried out by local residents in Stoke on Trent, UK, found highly significant links between proximity to high-voltage powerlines and the incidence of miscarriage.

Li (2002) and Lee (2002) found that exposure to EMFs during pregnancy was linked to an increased risk of miscarriage. Lee's study found that the link was especially strong where there were high 'transient' fields, that is, where field levels changed rapidly in a short period of time. This type of exposure can happen in e.g. electric train travel; working near or passing through anti-theft pillars in shops, etc.

Experiments with mice by Hong (2003) and Cao (2006) found that low frequency EMF exposure had some adverse effects on reproduction, including miscarriage, foetal loss and malformation and developmental delay in the offspring.

Radiofrequency fields

Radiofrequency fields are produced round wireless transmitters of various types, many of which were mentioned in the introductory paragraphs. Distance from these sources is not an easy guide to determine at what point the levels are 'low' as it is not always clear how 'high' they were in the first place. Different types of transmitters give off different types of radiation (e.g. pulsed or continuous) and it is believed that different signals may have different health effects, like the 'transients' mentioned above. Whether animals and cells respond in the same ways as humans is also not known.

Dr de Pomerai found changes in growth rate and maturation in the reproductive stage of nematode worms, when the larvae were exposed to weak microwave fields (2002). In an experiment on flies, Dr Reba Goodman (Blank & Goodman 1997) of Colombia University found that 2 hours mobile phone exposure for 10 days caused significant changes in reproductive genes and cell division.

It is advisable that men should not carry a phone in their front trouser pockets, because of the potential effect this may have on their reproductive ability. A study at the University of Western Australia, published by the Royal Society in June 2005, and others (Fejes 2005, Erogul 2006, Yan 2007, Agarwal 2008) concluded that usage of mobile phones, exposure to mobile phone signals, or storage of a mobile phone close to the testes affected sperm counts, motility, viability and morphology. "In addition to these acute adverse effects of electromagnetic radiation (EMR) on sperm motility, long-term EMR exposure may lead to behavioural or structural changes of the male germ cell. These effects may be observed later in life, and they are to be investigated more seriously." This should be borne in mind by young men using a mobile phone to send text messages while holding the phone on their lap.

The graph below shows that it takes the body some time to start producing viable sperm after RF exposure.

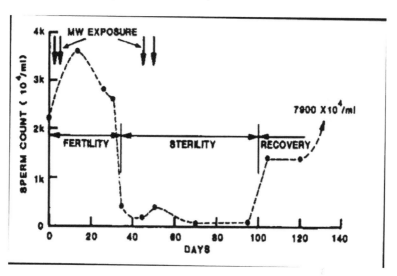

C K Chou (from article in Chinese)

At the annual meeting of the American Society for Reproductive Medicine in October 2006 in New Orleans, US researchers in Cleveland and New Orleans and doctors in Mumbai, India reported that the more that men used a mobile phone, the worse their sperm count and the poorer the quality of their sperm would be, see also Agarwal (2008). Using the phone for more than 4 hours a day caused a 25% drop in the number of sperm produced and only 20% of these looked normal. Sperm counts in UK men have fallen by 29% in the last decade. The researchers said that "many in the lowest group for sperm count would be below normal as defined by the World Health Organisation."

However, the research does not always find evidence of effects, and this could reflect sensitivity to different frequencies (Ribeiro 2007, Panagopoulos 2007).

It may be that RF radiation affects semen quality in general, or maybe sperm are affected differently as to whether they contain the XX chromosome or the XY chromosome. Where girls are born more often, perhaps there is DNA damage to the Y chromosome that makes the conception of boys less likely.

A paper (Vorobtsova 2008) looking at the history of radiobiological investigations in Russia, found that there is a possibility that the germ cells of irradiated parents may transmit genomic instability to their children, thus increasing risk of their getting cancer. This transgenerational effect has been well documented by Herbst in the 1970s who reported that diethylstilboestrol (DES), prescribed for newly pregnant women to prevent abortion, miscarriage and premature labour, resulted in a small number of cases of a rare cancer, vaginal clear-cell adenocarcinoma, in the daughters who were born as a result of the pregnancy concerned.

This was not a result of EMF exposure, but it shows the complexity of investigating the causes of reproductive problems. Individual susceptibility and exposure to other environmental pollutants further complicate the picture. For example, Cherry (2008) showed that painters and decorators, exposed to glycol solvents, were 2½ times more likely to produce fewer 'normal' sperm. RF radiation has been shown to alter the effects of relatively common drugs such as valium, anti-histamines, steroids, anti-cancer drugs such as tamoxifen, and to interact with other environmental stimuli.

Scassellati Sforzolini (2004) concluded "The possibility that ELF-MF might interfere with the genotoxic activity of xenobiotics has important implications, since human populations are likely to be exposed to a variety of genotoxic agents concomitantly with exposure to this type of physical agent." Koyama (2005) also found that EMF exposure just before or after X-ray irradiation increased mutation and altered the spectrum of mutations.

So, why are the concerns not better known about? Here we turn to politics.

The politics

Despite the increasing evidence that there are all sorts of physiological effects associated with exposure to EMFs, both high- and low-frequency, there is very little political will to make changes. Most political decisions have to be made as a result of a cost-benefit risk analysis consideration. As a lot of the research has been into relatively rare illnesses, it is considered that the cost of change would be too expensive for the amount of lives saved (family traumatisation is not included in cost benefit analysis). Pharmaceutical companies do not fund research into EMFs as any link may reduce the need for medication and thus reduce their profits.

Companies involved in the telecommunications industry provide tax income in the billions annually to government coffers, from the sale of mobile phones, calls and infrastructure development. The government would find it hard to replace this revenue. In fact, MacMillan, in the 1950s acknowledged the ill health effects from smoking, but it was not government policy to promote this, because of the income received from the tobacco industry.

Many studies partly funded by the government have put health effects down as psychosomatic (all in the mind). This absolves them from the necessity to take precautionary action.

What you can do

If you are wondering whether you, or your partner, may be affected by EMFs, that they may be playing a part in your difficulties in having the family you would like, you might decide to measure the levels of EMFs at home, as you travel, and in the workplace. There are easy to use instruments available to hire from www.emfields.org which can help you find out. If you feel you then want to take some protective measures, there are also ways of reducing your exposure, such as replacing your digital cordless phone with a landline or low emission phone; accessing broadband using a wired system rather than a wireless one; reducing the use of your mobile phone and charging it away from the bedroom. There are plenty of other possibilities that are easy and cheap to implement, as well as the more expensive ones which may not always offer the protection they claim.

Remember that electromagnetic fields are everywhere and have a lot of advantages, reasonable precautions to limit exposure are wise if you are having problems conceiving or carrying a baby to term, but worry increases tension and reduces wellbeing. Laugh a lot, do the things you enjoy, walk in nature, and eat well.

References

Agarwal A et al – 2008, *Effect of cell phone usage on semen analysis in men attending infertility clinic: an observational study* Fertil Steril 89(1):124–8

Baste V et al – 2008, *Radiofrequency electric fields; male infertility and sex ratio of offspring* Eur J Epidemiol 23(5):369–77

Blank M and Goodman R – 1997, *Do electromagnetic fields interact directly with DNA?* Bioelectromagnetics 18: 111–115

Cao YN et al – 2006, *Effects of exposure to extremely low frequency electromagnetic fields on reproduction of female mice and development of offsprings* Zhonghua Lao Dong Wei Sheng Zhi Ye Bing Za Zhi 24(8):468–70

Cherry N et al – 2008, *Occupation and male infertility: glycol ethers and other exposures* Occup Environ Med 65(10):708–14

De Pomerai D et al – 2002, *Growth and maturation of the nemaotode c. elegans following exposure to weak microwave fields*, Enzyme and Microbial Technology 30; pp 73–79

Erogul O et al – 2006, *Effects of electromagnetic radiation from a cellular phone on human sperm motility: an in vitro study*, Arch Med Research 2006 Oct;37(7):840–3.

Fejes I et al – 2005, *Is there a relationship between cell phone use and semen quality?* Arch Androl 51(5): 385–93

Herbst AL et al – 1971, *Adenocarcinoma of the vagina: Association of maternal stilbestrol therapy with tumor appearance in young women* N Engl J Med 284(15):878–881

Hong R et al – 2003, *[Effects of extremely low frequency electromagnetic fields on male reproduction in mice –article in*

Chinese] Zhonghua Lao Dong Wei Sheng Zhi Ye Bing Za Zhi 21(5): 342–5

Kim YW et al – 2008, *Effects of 60 Hz 14 microT magnetic field on the apoptosis of testicular germ cell in mice* Bioelectromagnetics Oct 6 [Epub ahead of print]

Koyama S et al – 2005, *Combined exposure of ELF magnetic fields and x-rays increased mutant yields compared with x-rays alone in pTN89 plasmids* J Radiat Res (Tokyo) 46(2):257–64

Lee GM et al – 2002, *A nested case-control study of residential and personal magnetic field measures and miscarriages* Epidemiology 13(1):21–31

Li D-K et al – 2002, *A population-based prospective cohort study of personal exposure to magnetic fields during pregnancy and the risk of miscarriage* Epidemiology 13(1):9–20

Møllerløkken OJ & BE Moen – 2008, *Is fertility reduced among men exposed to radiofrequency fields in the Norwegian Navy?* Bioelectromagnetics 29(5):345–52

Neutra RR et al – 2002, *An Evaluation of the Possible Risks From Electric and Magnetic Fields (EMFs) From Power Lines, Internal Wiring, Electrical Occupations and Appliances.* California EMF Program, California Department of Health and Human Services. http://www.ehib.org/emf/

Ouellet-Hellstrom R & WF Stewart – 1993, *Miscarriages among female physical therapists who report using radio- and microwave-frequency electromagnetic radiation* Am J Epidemiol 138(10):775–86

Panagopoulos DJ et al – 2007, *Comparison of bioactivity between GSM 900 MHz and DCS 1800 MHz mobile telephony radiation* Electromagn Biol Med 26(1):33–44

Ribeiro EP et al – 2007, *Effects of subchronic exposure to radio frequency from a conventional cellular telephone on testicular function in adult rats* J Urol 177(1):395–9

Scassellati Sforzolini et al – 2004, *[Evaluation of genotoxic and/or co-genotoxic effects in cells exposed in vitro to extremely-low frequency electromagnetic fields]* Ann Ig 16(1–2):321–40

Silverman C – 1973, *Nervous and behavioural effects of microwave radiation in humans* Am J Epidemiol 97(4):219–24

Vorobtsova IE – 2008, *Transgenerational transmission of radiation-induced genomic instability and predisposition to carcinogenesis* Vopr Onkol 54(4):490–3

Wertheimer N & E Leeper – 1979, *Electrical wiring configurations and childhood cancer* Am J Epidemiol 109(3):273–84

Yan JG et al – 2007, *Effects of cellular phone emissions on sperm motility in rats* Fertil Steril 88(4):957–64

APPENDIX 5
The Survey

A Further Survey of Foresight Results over the period of 1997–1999

Circumstances of Survey

This was an exceptionally difficult period for Foresight, as many of you may remember. The university was not able to continue doing the hair analysis for us, and it was with much difficulty that we got our own laboratory together and found Michael Cain, who then ran it. We had an interim period of seven months when we had to beg the university to cover for us, which they did, during vacations only. During the long gaps, quite understandably, couples got tired of waiting and left us to try other therapies etc. For this and other reasons, not everybody completed their supplementation programme etc. The results are therefore not quite as good as those in our first survey, but still compare very favourably with results nationwide.

We are now getting a greater ratio of couples with fertility problems than before, as this seems to be the aspect of our work that is now receiving the most media attention.

Outcomes

The most noteworthy figures are:

Out of 1,076 couples (1,061 had previous fertility or miscarriage problems), 729 couples conceived – 67.75%. These couples have given birth to 779 babies (Some were twins, some were a second birth during the study). If we counted each baby as a success (as with the HFEA), this would give us a 72.4% overall success rate! Among the couples there were 67 who were pregnant when the survey ended. Added in this would make a 78.4% success rate.

Among the 1,076 participating couples, there were 393 who had previously suffered miscarriage. From this group we had, sadly, 28 miscarriages. From those who had not miscarried previously, there were no miscarriages. There were 28 miscarriages all told.

From the 779 conceptions, the expected rate of miscarriage would be 155 to 195 (20–25%). From the particular group of 393 women who had previously miscarried, in place of 20–25% we had 7.1%. So 28, although a sad loss, was a big improvement on what might have been.

Malformations and terminations

One couple terminated twins on being told there was twin-to-twin transfusion. One lady, who had only been on the programme a short while prior to starting the pregnancy, had a Down's Syndrome baby. One foetus was terminated due to multiple deformity, but his parents did live on a landfill site. One other little boy was born with an adhesion of the intestine, but had a small operation and went home at 3 weeks old, with no further problems. In total there were 4 problems in 846 pregnancies, 1 in 211.5 (0.47%). NHS rate is 1 in 17 (6%).

Stillbirths

Tragically there were 3 stillbirths. In one case, the mother and previous Foresight baby aged 20 months were attacked by a dog and the mother was bitten while rescuing the child. Her baby was born that night, prematurely and dead (at 28 weeks).

In another case, the mother was admitted to hospital in the late evening and given a strong sedative to stop labour. Her beautiful 8 lb baby boy was born dead in the morning.

I have not got the exact circumstances of the third but know the parents concerned did not complete the full programme.

One in 282 (0.35%). National rate is 1 in 73 (1.37%).

Birth weights

Our average birth weight for single babies was 7 lb 11 oz (despite including quite a few elective caesareans with our older mothers). Our average birth weights with multiples was 5 lb 12 oz. All were twin births, except for one set of triplets.

The percentage of babies born below 5 lb 8 oz (official figure for low birth weight) was 4.6% from 779. (National rate is 9%, so just about half.) Of these babies, 20 were from multiple births. Of the 36 small birth weight babies, 9 were born between 30 and 36 weeks (mother was found to have an infection). The triplets were born by caesarean at 34 weeks.

High-tech births

Some couples went in for the Foresight programme plus high-tech and the success rates were as follows:

Couples using IUI	44.6%
Couples using IVF	47.1%
Couples using ICSI	43.1%
Couples using donors	33.3%

All told, results using all the different artificial methods: success rate = 43.5%

National average for IVF is 22.6%. I am glad to see we have almost doubled this at 43.5%.

Conclusions

From this we see that from the basic Foresight programme (even when working under difficulties) it is possible to:

- Almost double the success rate of IVF (22.6% to 43.5%)
- Raise the success rate of infertile couples overall from 22.6% to 72.4%
- Drop the miscarriage rate from 20–25% to 7.1% with those who have previously miscarried
- Drop the miscarriage rate to 0 with those who have not previously miscarried
- Drop the stillbirth rate from 1.37% to 0.35%
- Drop the malformation rate from 6% to 0.47%
- Drop the low birth-weight rate from 9% to 4.6%

APPENDIX 6
Foresight Research 2010

The Foresight charity has been running since 1978. We were founded to help achieve health in babies by natural means, thus preventing miscarriage, premature birth, malformations, and mental retardation.

Later, it was discovered how much the Foresight programme could help with fertility, and since then a lot of our work has been helping couples who were unable to conceive. The programme will either achieve a natural conception, or will hugely increase the chances of success where IVF is necessary due to blocked or absent fallopian tubes.

We have just completed a survey of our results from 2002–2009.

Group 1: 1,578 couples completed the full Foresight programme. 1,417 babies were born. 89.8% success rate. There were 52 pairs of twins and 3 sets of triplets. There were 42 miscarriages (2.96%). Only 2 of the single births were premature.

Group 2: 518 couples did a part of the programme, but did not complete it. They had 358 babies. 69.1% success rate. Of these there were 39 miscarriages (7.53%). There were 37 pairs of twins.

The average birth weight for single births was 7lb 10¾oz. Our percentage of miscarriages, both groups together, was 3.86%.

Prior to coming to Foresight our population had 2,383 failed IUI (success 162: 1 in 15.7, or 6.3%), 3,004 failed IVF (success 407: 1 in 8.4 or 11.4%) and 1,081 failed ICSI (success 211: 1 in 5 or 16.5%). They had suffered 8,939 miscarriages (the national rate for miscarriage is 16%).

The Foresight programme

- The Foresight programme's most vital component is hair mineral analysis. We supplement any needed macro minerals and trace minerals. We cleanse toxic metals such as lead, aluminium, cadmium and mercury. The deficiencies and the toxins can be dangerous to a baby and impede normal development.

- We provide a leaflet on optimising nutrition and suggest our wholefood cookbook.
- We advise against voluntary poisons such as smoking, alcohol, caffeine and drugs.
- We teach natural family planning (ovulation awareness) to avoid use of the pill.
- We check for genitourinary infection, allergies and parasites where this is necessary.
- We suggest the prospective parents have a house survey for advice on avoiding electromagnetic pollution.
- We list toxic substances in cosmetics, hair dyes, household cleaners, pesticides etc. that parents need to avoid.
- Where copper and lead contamination from plumbing is excessive we advise on water filtration.
- Our programme helps to reduce the levels of potentially harmful toxins, both inside the body and in the environment. This reduces the risk of miscarriage, premature birth, malformation or stillbirth.

Optimising the levels of needed trace minerals also assists perfect development, intelligence and, we have discovered, musicality!

Background research

The first doctor to have made a lifetime's work out of studying nutrition was Dr Weston Price of California. His book is a classic: *Nutrition and Physical Degeneration*, published in 1940. We have also studied the work of Cambridge veterinary researcher Mrs Isobel Jennings; Professor Bert Vallee of Harvard University Medical School; Dr Carl Pfeiffer of the Brain Bio Centre, New Jersey; Dr Ben Fiengold of the Kaisier Permanente Institute in California; Dr Lucille Hurley of University of California; Dr Elizabeth Lodge-Rees of California; Dr Donald Oberleas and Dr Donald Caldwell, who were at Wayne State University in the 1970s and later at Kentucky University and the Lafayette Institute in California. Professor Roger Williams of Texas University, Dr Richard Passwater and Dr Elmer Cranton were all authors of very informative books in the 1980s. In Australia, Professor EJ Underwood wrote *Trace Minerals in Human and Animal Nutrition* in 1972.

We still get information from America from Dr Harold Buttram of Pennsylvania and Dr Allan Leiberman of South Carolina, and we get papers from Dr Russell Blaylock and a number of other doctors who are well into the research.

In this country we were helped out not only by Isobel Jennings, but by Professor John Dickerson of University of Surrey and later by Dr (now Professor) Neil Ward, also at Surrey, and by Professor Derek Bryce-Smith of Reading University, who was working on the harm done by lead, and later on the benefits of zinc supplementation. We were in communication with Arthur and Margaret Wynn, and with numerous other voluntary associations, such as the Hyperactive Children's Association, the McCarrison Society, The Soil Association, Garden Organic, The Institute of Optimum Nutrition, The British School of Naturopathy and Osteopathy, the Association of Homeopaths.

We feel the time has come for our work to be more widely known and taken up. We are very willing to share all the information we have. More training courses for practitioners will be available shortly.

The present level of mainly avoidable tragedy in this country is:

- One couple in 7 is infertile. 45,000 babies each year are born prematurely; 4,500 of these are said to be permanently disabled.
- The ONS is in some confusion about the number of malformations, but it appears to be in the region of 22,000 a year.
- One baby in 16 is said to be miscarried.
- One child in 4 is said to have 'learning difficulties'. One in 5 has eczema. One in 9 has asthma.
- Recently I heard that one boy in 43 is said to be autistic.
- Cot death is still over 300 babies a year.
- Child cancer is rising year on year.

We hope that people will study our success rate. We wish to help them to avoid unnecessary suffering and we hope they will support us and our work.

APPENDIX 7

Extract of University of Surrey Research Paper results 1993 by Dr Neil Ward

Preconceptual Care Foresight Research Project 1993

The following results summarise the research database of 367 Foresight couples using the information provided on the various Foresight Questionnaires.

2.1 Foresight Research Project Pregnancy Outcome Statistics

Table 2.1 shows that 89% of the Foresight couples involved in this research project had mono-birth children: 42% of which were male and 58% female. Only 11% of the Foresight couples (females) failed within the time period of the project to become pregnant. All Foresight children had an average birth weight (3265g) and average gestational age (38.5 weeks). Female babies were in general 60g less in birth weight than male babies. Figure 2.1 shows the relationship between birth weight and gestational age for the Foresight pregnancies.

Table 2.1 Foresight Research Project Outcome Statistics

Pregnancy/ Non-pregnancy		Birth weight (g)		Gestational age (wks)	
		Average	range	Average	range
Pregnancy	89%	3265	2368 – 4145	38.5	36–41
Males+	42%	3299	2484 – 4145	38.5	36–40
Females+	58%	3240	2368 – 4089	38.5	36–41
Non-pregnancy	11%				

* expressed as percentage of total Foresight Research number of cases
+ expressed as percentage of pregnancy cases

Whilst there is a slight spread in the data, a good correlation exists for both birth parameters.

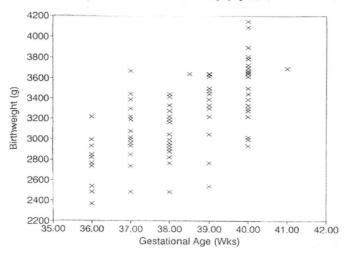

Figure 2.1 Birth Statistics for all Foresight pregnancies.

2.2 Influence of Previous Reproductive Problem History on Pregnancy Outcome

Table 2.2 shows the percentage of Foresight pregnant and non-pregnant cases as a function of their previous history of reproductive problems. Couples with no history of such problems subdivide into 96% who became pregnant and 4% non-pregnant. Couples who had reported histories of reproductive problems, such as infertility, miscarriage, therapeutic terminations or stillbirths in general had 73 to 83% success in having a Foresight baby, whilst 17 to 27% were non-pregnant. The very small number of SID's cases (n=3) were all non-pregnant. However, couples who were reporting histories of small-for-date (low birth weight) or malformations (spina bifida) had a 100% success rate for a Foresight pregnancy.

Table 2.2 Percentage of Foresight Pregnant and Non-Pregnancy Cases related to previous reproductive problems

Previous history	% Foresight Successfully Pregnant	% Non-pregnant
No history	96	4
Infertility	81	19
Miscarriage	83	17
Therapeutic Term	73	27
Stillbirths	80	20
SIDS		100
Small-for-dates (low birth weights)	100	0
Malformations	100	0

Hair Analysis Results, all done at the University of Surrey Laboratory

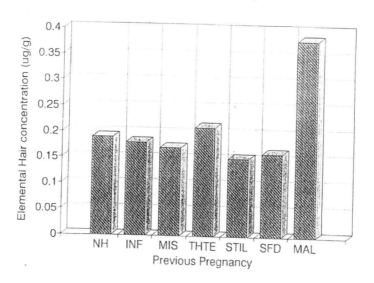

Hair Cd content and previous pregnancy history

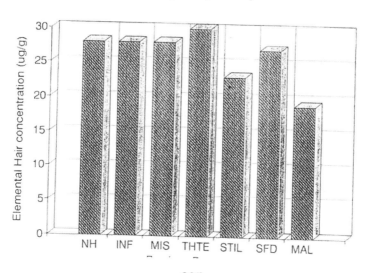

Hair Cu content and previous pregnancy history

Hair Fe content and previous pregnancy history

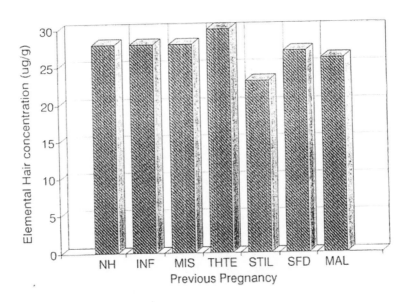

Hair Hg content and previous pregnancy history

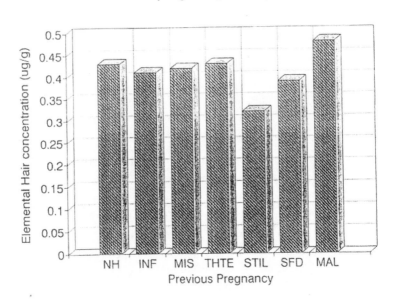

Hair Mn content and previous pregnancy history

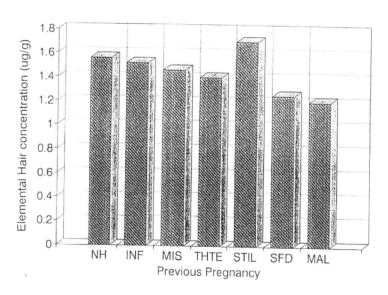

Hair Pb content and previous pregnancy history

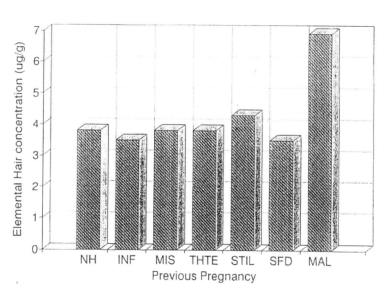

Hair Zn content and previous pregnancy history

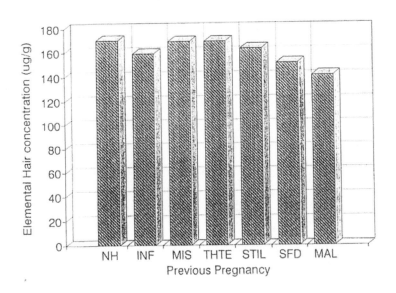

Male Fertility Status and Hair Element (Iron) Content (ug/g)

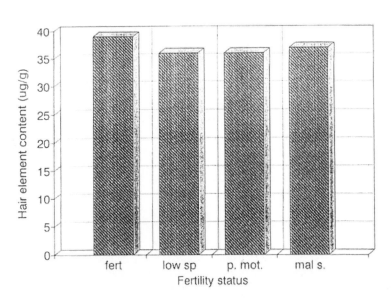

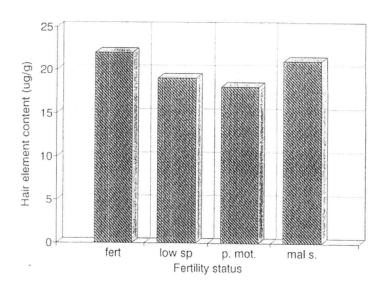

Male Fertility Status and Hair Element
(Copper) Content (ug/g)

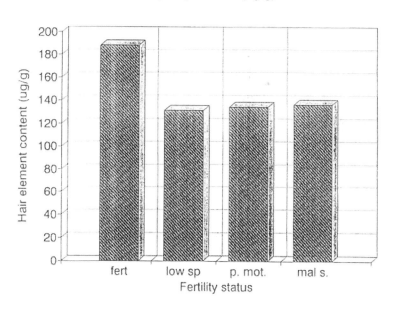

Male Fertility Status and Hair Element
(Zinc) Content (ug/g)

Male Fertility Status and Hair Element (Selenium) Content (ug/g)

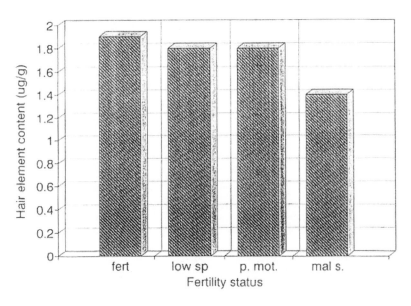

Male Fertility Status and Hair Element (Lead) Content (ug/g)

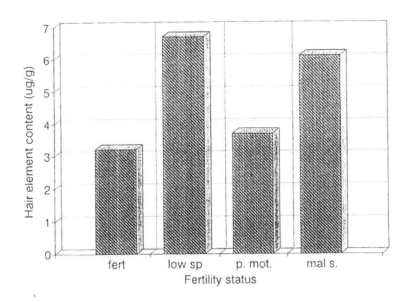

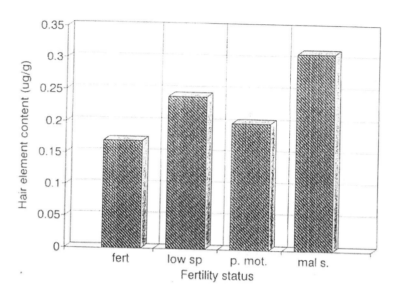

Male Fertility Status and Hair Element (Cadmium) Content (ug/g)

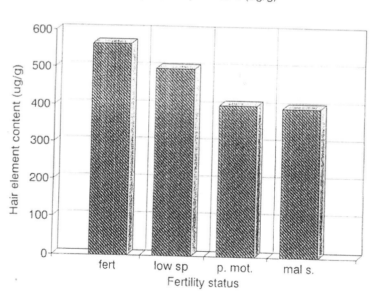

Male Fertility Status and Hair Element (Calcium) Content (ug/g)

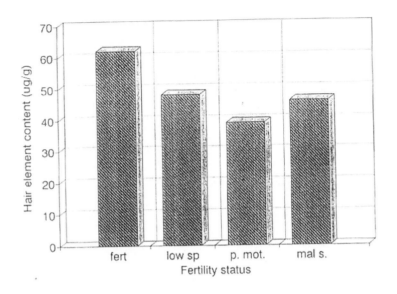

Male Fertility Status and Hair Element (Magnesium) Content (ug/g)

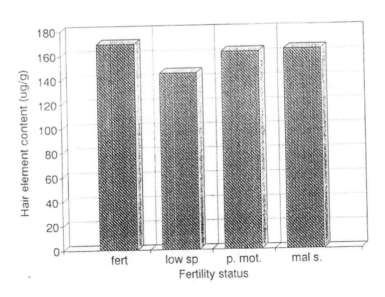

Male Fertility Status and Hair Element (Sodium) Content (ug/g)

Male Fertility Status and Hair Element (Potassium) Content (ug/g)

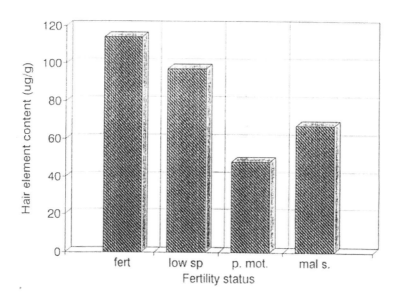

Hair Cd concentration and smoking activity

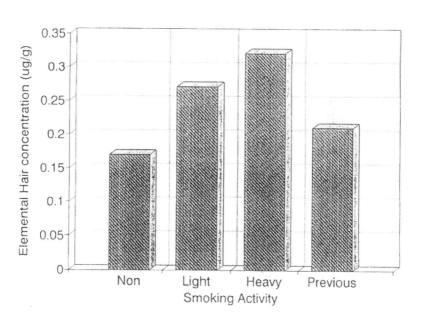

Hair Iron concentration and smoking activity

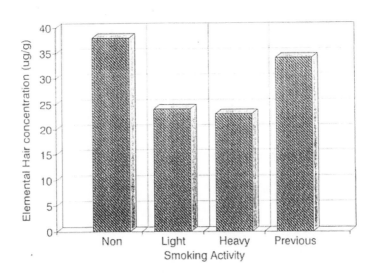

Hair Zinc concentration and smoking activity

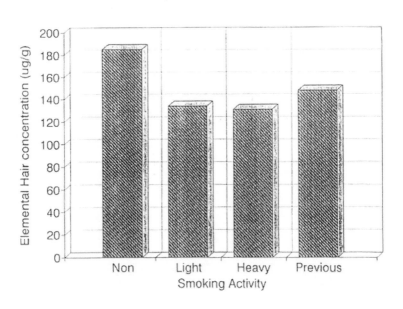

Male Hair Zn concentration and alcohol consumption

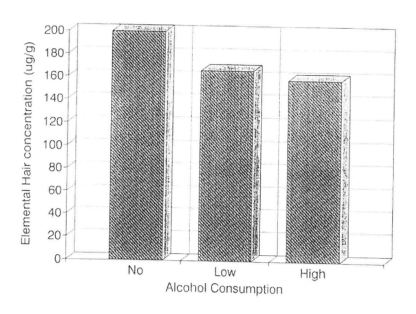

Hair Fe concentration and alcohol consumption

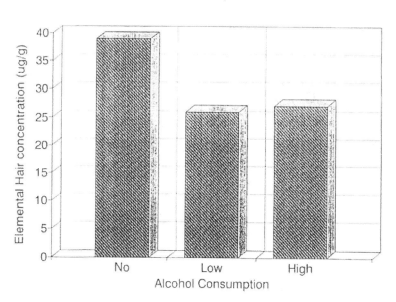